Extemporaneous Formulations: Filling the Gap in the Pharmaceutical Industry with Personalized Medicines

Extemporaneous Formulations: Filling the Gap in the Pharmaceutical Industry with Personalized Medicines

Guest Editors

Nunzio Denora
Antonio Lopalco

MDPI

Basel • Beijing • Wuhan • Barcelona • Belgrade • Novi Sad • Cluj • Manchester

Guest Editors

Nunzio Denora
Department of
Pharmacy-Pharmaceutical Sciences
University of Bari Aldo Moro
Bari
Italy

Antonio Lopalco
Department of
Pharmacy-Pharmaceutical Sciences
University of Bari "Aldo Moro"
Bari
Italy

Editorial Office
MDPI AG
Grosspeteranlage 5
4052 Basel, Switzerland

This is a reprint of the Special Issue, published open access by the journal *Pharmaceutics* (ISSN 1999-4923), freely accessible at: https://www.mdpi.com/journal/pharmaceutics/special_issues/6JPR840861.

For citation purposes, cite each article independently as indicated on the article page online and as indicated below:

Lastname, A.A.; Lastname, B.B. Article Title. *Journal Name* **Year**, *Volume Number*, Page Range.

ISBN 978-3-7258-6914-5 (Hbk)
ISBN 978-3-7258-6915-2 (PDF)
https://doi.org/10.3390/books978-3-7258-6915-2

Contents

About the Editors

Nunzio Denora

Nunzio Denora is a Full Professor of Pharmaceutical Technology at the Department of Pharmacy—Pharmaceutical Sciences, University of Bari Aldo Moro, Italy, where he heads a formulation research laboratory focused on advanced drug delivery systems. He obtained his degree in Pharmaceutical Chemistry and Technology at the University of Bari in 2001 and completed his PhD in Pharmaceutical Technology at the University of Palermo in 2004. After a postdoctoral position at the Department of Pharmaceutical Chemistry of the University of Kansas, USA (2005–2006), he joined the University of Bari as an academic staff member and research scientist in Pharmaceutical Technology. He has authored more than 220 peer-reviewed publications and is the inventor of 10 patents related to pharmaceutical formulations and diagnostic probes. He is a board member of the SITELF Italy Chapter, serves on advisory boards of international journals in pharmaceutics, and is a member of the scientific committee of the European Paediatric Translational Research Infrastructure (EPTRI). His research interests include the design and development of paediatric medicines using both conventional and innovative formulation technologies.

Antonio Lopalco

Antonio Lopalco is an Associate Professor at the Department of Pharmacy - Pharmaceutical Sciences, University of Bari Aldo Moro, Italy. He obtained his Master's degree in Chemistry and Pharmaceutical Technology from the University of Bari in 2008 and completed his PhD in Pharmaceutical Technology at the University of Palermo in 2012. Following postdoctoral research in Pharmaceutical Chemistry at the University of Kansas, USA, he was appointed as an Associate Researcher in the same department in 2015. He joined the University of Bari faculty in 2016 and progressed through the academic ranks, becoming Associate Professor in 2019. His research focuses on innovative drug delivery systems, age-related and patient-centric formulations, and extemporaneous pharmaceutical preparations. He is the author or co-author of more than 85 peer-reviewed publications and holds five patents. He serves as a reviewer for several international scientific journals and is a member of the Editorial Boards of the *Journal of Pharmaceutical Sciences* (Elsevier) and *Pharmaceutics* (MDPI).

Preface

Extemporaneous pharmaceutical formulations are customised medicines prepared on demand by pharmacists and healthcare professionals to meet specific patient requirements. By enabling tailored doses, appropriate excipient choices, and alternative routes of administration, compounding represents a practical expression of patient-centred and personalised medicine. Its relevance is particularly evident in paediatric and geriatric care, in rare diseases requiring orphan medicines, and whenever off-label use is unavoidable due to the lack of suitable authorised products.

This Reprint gathers contributions that reflect the current scientific and technological landscape of pharmaceutical compounding. It covers the design of dosage forms and the rational selection of excipients, with a strong emphasis on stability, compatibility, and fit-for-purpose quality control as essential elements to ensure safety, consistency, and reproducibility. It also highlights how modern compounding technologies, together with evolving regulatory and legislative frameworks, are shaping contemporary practice and supporting more robust preparation standards.

The motivation for this Reprint lies in the increasing need to address unmet medical needs, including scenarios where industrially manufactured medicines are unavailable or unsuitable, particularly in settings with limited access to healthcare resources. Innovation in compounding has the potential to bridge these gaps, improving access to essential therapies and supporting therapeutic continuity across diverse patient populations.

This Reprint is addressed to pharmacists, clinicians, researchers, regulators, and pharmaceutical stakeholders seeking an up-to-date overview of evidence-based approaches in extemporaneous formulation design and quality assurance and of their role in strengthening healthcare delivery.

Nunzio Denora and Antonio Lopalco
Guest Editors

pharmaceutics

Editorial

Extemporaneous Formulations: Filling the Gap in the Pharmaceutical Industry with Personalized Medicines

Antonio Lopalco * and Nunzio Denora *

Department of Pharmacy—Pharmaceutical Sciences, University of Bari Aldo Moro, 4, E. Orabona Street, 70126 Bari, Italy
* Correspondence: antonio.lopalco@uniba.it (A.L.); nunzio.denora@uniba.it (N.D.)

1. Introduction

The progressive shift of healthcare systems toward personalised and patient-centred therapeutic strategies has exposed the structural limitations of standardised pharmaceutical manufacturing. Although industrial drug development ensures high levels of quality, safety, and scalability, authorised medicinal products often fail to address the full spectrum of clinical needs encountered in practice. These gaps may result from the lack of appropriate dose strengths, rigid dosage forms, unsuitable excipient profiles, or the need for alternative routes of administration. In this context, extemporaneous pharmaceutical formulations remain an essential component of modern pharmacy practice, enabling the preparation of customised medicines tailored to individual patient requirements [1].

Across regulatory jurisdictions, pharmaceutical compounding is recognised as a legitimate professional activity performed by authorised healthcare professionals, primarily pharmacists, under a prescription or an established professional relationship. While legal contexts differ internationally, common principles are reflected in major pharmacopeial standards, including the European Pharmacopoeia and the United States Pharmacopeia–National Formulary (USP–NF), which define technical requirements and quality attributes for substances, excipients, and compounded preparations. Regulatory bodies such as the European Medicines Agency (EMA) and national competent authorities acknowledge compounding as necessary when industrially manufactured medicines are unavailable or unsuitable, provided it is conducted in accordance with professional standards and risk-based quality systems [2].

Extemporaneous formulations are relevant across all stages of life and in diverse clinical settings, including rare diseases, oncology, cardiology, dermatology, palliative care, and hospital therapies [3]. In this sense, compounding represents a practical implementation of personalised medicine at the point of care, allowing pharmacists and pharmaceutical scientists to translate formulation science into patient-specific therapeutic solutions [4].

Formulation development in extemporaneous compounding differs fundamentally from industrial pharmaceutical development. Compounded preparations are produced on demand, often within limited timeframes, and are not subject to centralised marketing authorisation. Consequently, their quality, safety, and suitability rely on professional competence, compliance with pharmacopeial standards, and adherence to beyond-use dating principles rather than pre-market regulatory approval [5]. Both the European Pharmacopoeia and USP–NF stress the control of critical quality attributes, including identity, purity, strength, stability, and microbiological quality, placing significant responsibility on the compounding pharmacist.

Within this context, pharmaceutical compounding strengthens the patient–physician–pharmacist triad and reinforces the integration of pharmaceutical sciences into clinical decision-making. Excipients play a crucial functional role by supporting solubilisation, stabilisation, preservation, and optimisation of drug delivery [6]. Their selection must be scientifically justified, pharmacopeia-compliant, and aligned with patient-specific needs to ensure safety and effectiveness.

This Special Issue, "Extemporaneous Formulations: Filling the Gap in the Pharmaceutical Industry with Personalized Medicines", provides a multidisciplinary overview of the scientific, technological, clinical, and regulatory aspects of pharmaceutical compounding. Contributions address formulation development, dosage forms and excipients, stability, compounding technologies, quality control, and legislative frameworks across healthcare systems. Particular attention is given to the interface between pharmacy practice and emerging drug delivery technologies, highlighting innovation within actual compounding environments.

2. Articles in This Special Issue

This Special Issue includes eleven contributions that collectively demonstrate how extemporaneous formulations can fill therapeutic gaps when authorised medicines are unavailable, unsuitable, or require individual adaptation. Across diverse clinical applications and compounding practices, the papers converge on a shared principle: modern pharmaceutical compounding increasingly relies on structured quality systems, analytical evidence, and patient-centric design to ensure reproducible preparation and safe use.

A broad and highly informative overview of pharmacy preparations within a national healthcare context is provided by Woerdenbag and co-workers, who describe the organisation, scope, and product care responsibilities associated with pharmacy preparations in the Netherlands. By highlighting specialist areas such as paediatric dosage forms, dysphagia-related administration, reconstitution of biologicals, and radiopharmaceutical practices, the article offers a valuable reference model illustrating how compounding can be integrated into healthcare pathways while maintaining a strong focus on governance, safety, and professional accountability [7].

Quality assurance and standardisation are further strengthened by the work of van den Born-Bondt and colleagues, who address a critical and often underestimated aspect of aseptic preparation: the qualification of personnel involved in the visual inspection of parenteral medicinal products manufactured under GMP conditions. By proposing an adaptable test set and a feasibility-oriented approach, the study supports harmonised training strategies and contributes to improving the reliability of visual inspection as a safeguard against defects and particulate contamination [8].

In a complementary quality-driven contribution, Aquino and co-workers propose a practical analytical methodology for managing residual compounded antiblastic drugs, encompassing small molecules and monoclonal antibodies. Their work is particularly relevant for high-cost oncology preparations, reinforcing the importance of stability evidence to support safe handling and rational decision making in hospital pharmacy services [9].

A central theme of this Special Issue is the role of extemporaneous preparation in paediatric care, where the lack of age-appropriate medicines often necessitates formulation adaptation. Pai and Nahata provide a comprehensive and timely review of global necessities, challenges, and opportunities for paediatric extemporaneous formulations. Their review article critically discusses excipient safety, acceptability, beyond-use dating, and regulatory variability, reinforcing the view that paediatric compounding should be guided by evidence-based approaches rather than empirical adaptation alone [10].

https://doi.org/10.3390/pharmaceutics18020209

Within paediatric neurology, Olivera and colleagues address a concrete therapeutic need by developing trihexyphenidyl orodispersible minitablets for the management of dystonia. This work illustrates how solid multiparticulate dosage forms can enable dose individualisation and improved acceptability, while offering robust performance and prolonged stability compared with less controlled liquid adaptations [11].

Beyond paediatrics, administration difficulties remain a major driver for extemporaneous formulation design, particularly in dysphagic patients. Logrippo and co-workers investigate gelled vehicles intended for oral drug administration in patients with swallowing impairment, demonstrating that the choice of carrier is a key determinant for swallowability, usability, and overall administration safety. This study reinforces that extemporaneous preparation often requires optimisation not only of the active ingredient but also of the administration vehicle [12].

A related patient-centred approach is presented by Trofimiuk and colleagues, who explore pharmacy-compounded oral gels as an alternative to conventional paediatric suspensions. By evaluating rheological and organoleptic properties alongside preservative-related considerations, the authors support the potential of semi-solid oral vehicles to improve acceptability and dosing reliability, particularly in home-care conditions where ease of administration and stability are essential [13].

Baratta and co-workers contribute a pragmatic example of "appropriate technology" compounding by developing a metronidazole suspension intended for paediatric use in developing countries. The study is framed within the A.P.P.A. project (Aid Progress Pharmacist Agreement), a collaborative initiative supporting the implementation of galenic laboratories and reproducible preparation protocols in contexts with limited healthcare resources. Using basic, low-cost excipients and a simple compounding approach, the work demonstrates how quality attributes such as content uniformity, dispersion behaviour, and pH stability can be systematically addressed even when advanced manufacturing infrastructure is unavailable. Beyond technical performance, the article effectively underscores the importance of palatability and acceptability in children, recalling the well-known message from the Walt Disney movie Mary Poppins that "a spoonful of sugar helps the medicine go down", thereby linking formulation design to patient adherence and practical feasibility [14].

Dermatological compounding is addressed by Lacassia and colleagues through a comparative evaluation of five ready-to-use bases for topical propranolol hydrochloride preparations. This contribution highlights the practical relevance of ready-to-use vehicles as enabling tools for extemporaneous dermatological formulations, facilitating the incorporation of active substances while supporting acceptable texture, spreadability, and chemical-physical stability. The selected active ingredient further strengthens the clinical significance of the work, as topical propranolol represents a paradigmatic case of off-label use and drug repurposing in dermatology, where compounding may offer accessible and adaptable options when authorised alternatives are limited. By providing evidence-based criteria for vehicle selection, the study supports more standardised topical compounding practices and improved reproducibility across preparation processes [15].

An alternative oral platform is described by Jovičić-Bata and co-workers, who investigate liquid- and semisolid-filled hard gelatin capsules containing alpha-lipoic acid. This work illustrates how capsule-based compounding may provide flexible administration strategies while addressing handling and stability considerations, representing a practical dosage form option when conventional preparations are unsuitable [16].

Finally, the Special Issue expands the compounding perspective to nuclear medicine, where extemporaneous preparation is often intrinsic to clinical practice and must comply with stringent quality requirements. Rizzello and co-workers review methodologies for

https://doi.org/10.3390/pharmaceutics18020209

gallium-68 extemporaneous preparations and provide an overview of the relevant regulatory context. The article clearly illustrates how galenic practice supports the preparation of medicinal products not only for conventional therapy but also for advanced diagnostic and therapeutic procedures in nuclear medicine, where short radionuclide half-lives impose strict time windows and demand robust, standardised processes. By linking feasibility, quality control, and compliance, the contribution reinforces the essential role of compounding in enabling patient access to modern radiopharmaceuticals within routine hospital workflows [17].

3. Conclusions

This Special Issue offers a contemporary perspective on the role and relevance of extemporaneous formulation in modern healthcare. Extemporaneous formulation represents a pragmatic and clinically driven approach to personalised medicine, enabling the adaptation of therapies when authorised products do not meet individual patient needs. Its value relies on the rational selection of dosage forms and excipients, supported by stability and compatibility assessment, microbiological control, and fit-for-purpose quality assurance. When performed within appropriate regulatory and professional standards, compounding can provide safe and reproducible preparations across a broad range of applications. In this perspective, extemporaneous formulation is not merely a substitute for industrial medicines but a complementary pharmaceutical strategy that supports therapeutic continuity and optimises patient care.

Author Contributions: Writing—original draft preparation, A.L. and N.D.; Writing—review and editing, A.L. and N.D. All authors have read and agreed to the published version of the manuscript.

Funding: This research received no external funding.

Acknowledgments: The Guest Editors would like to sincerely thank all authors for their valuable contributions to this Special Issue and for sharing their high-quality work, which has significantly enriched its scientific content and practical relevance. We also gratefully acknowledge the Editorial Office Team of *Pharmaceutics* for their professionalism, support, and assistance throughout the entire publication process.

Conflicts of Interest: The authors declare no conflicts of interest.

References

1. Allen, L.V., Jr. Contemporary pharmaceutical compounding. *Ann. Pharmacother.* **2003**, *37*, 1526–1528. [CrossRef]
2. Minghetti, P.; Pantano, D.; Gennari, C.G.; Casiraghi, A. Regulatory framework of pharmaceutical compounding and actual developments of legislation in Europe. *Health Policy* **2014**, *117*, 328–333. [CrossRef]
3. Ramtoola, Z.; Catibusic, A.; Ameen, H.; Cullen, S.; Barlow, J.W. Evaluation of the type and frequency of extemporaneous formulations dispensed in hospital and community pharmacies. *Explor. Res. Clin. Soc. Pharm.* **2023**, *12*, 100380. [CrossRef] [PubMed]
4. Carvalho, M.; Almeida, I.F. The Role of Pharmaceutical Compounding in Promoting Medication Adherence. *Pharmaceuticals* **2022**, *15*, 1091. [CrossRef] [PubMed]
5. Isles, M. Patient safety issues associated with the use of compounded medicines as alternatives to approved pharmaceutical products in Europe and how best practice can improve outcomes. *Int. J. Risk Saf. Med.* **2020**, *31*, 133–144. [CrossRef] [PubMed]
6. Van der Merwe, J.; Steenekamp, J.; Steyn, D.; Hamman, J. The Role of Functional Excipients in Solid Oral Dosage Forms to Overcome Poor Drug Dissolution and Bioavailability. *Pharmaceutics* **2020**, *12*, 393. [CrossRef] [PubMed]
7. Woerdenbag, H.J.; van Basten, B.; Oussoren, C.; Smeets, O.S.N.M.; Annaciri-Donkers, A.; Crul, M.; Maurer, J.M.; Schimmel, K.J.M.; Kemper, E.M.; Hooge, M.N.L.-d.; et al. Extemporaneous Compounding, Pharmacy Preparations and Related Product Care in the Netherlands. *Pharmaceutics* **2025**, *17*, 1005. [CrossRef] [PubMed]

https://doi.org/10.3390/pharmaceutics18020209

8. van den Born-Bondt, T.; Huizinga, H.P.S.; Kappert, K.R.; Westra, H.H.; van Zanten, J.; Woerdenbag, H.J.; Maurer, J.M.; Gareb, B. Development of an Adaptable Qualification Test Set for Personnel Involved in Visual Inspection Procedures of Parenteral Drug Products Manufactured Under Good Manufacturing Practice Conditions in Hospital Pharmacy Compounding Facilities. *Pharmaceutics* **2025**, *17*, 74. [CrossRef] [PubMed]
9. Aquino, R.P.; Falcone, G.; Russo, P.; Dal Piaz, F.; Auriemma, G.; de Francesco, F.M.; Cascone, S.; Nava, E.; Del Gaudio, P. Integrating Analytical Procedures in Routine Practices of Centralized Antiblastic Compounding Units for Valorization of Residual Compounded Drugs. *Pharmaceutics* **2025**, *17*, 101. [CrossRef] [PubMed]
10. Pai, V.B.; Nahata, M.C. Extemporaneous Formulations for Pediatric Patients: Global Necessities, Challenges and Opportunities. *Pharmaceutics* **2026**, *18*, 126. [CrossRef] [PubMed]
11. Olivera, C.; Boscolo, O.; Dobrecky, C.; Ortega, C.A.; Favier, L.S.; Cianchino, V.A.; Flor, S.; Lucangioli, S. Development and Characterization of Trihexyphenidyl Orodispersible Minitablets: A Challenge to Fill the Therapeutic Gap in Neuropediatrics. *Pharmaceutics* **2025**, *17*, 5. [CrossRef] [PubMed]
12. Logrippo, S.; Ganzetti, R.; Sestili, M.; Perinelli, D.R.; Cespi, M.; Bonacucina, G. Toward the Optimal Choice of Gelled Vehicles for Oral Drug Administration in Dysphagic Patients. *Pharmaceutics* **2025**, *17*, 251. [CrossRef] [PubMed]
13. Trofimiuk, M.; Sznitowska, M.; Winnicka, K. Oral Gels as an Alternative to Liquid Pediatric Suspensions Compounded from Commercial Tablets. *Pharmaceutics* **2024**, *16*, 1229. [CrossRef] [PubMed]
14. Baratta, F.; Zingarelli, C.; Fanton, F.; Lamy, E.; Di Lascio, G.; Brusa, P. Metronidazole Suspension for Paediatric Use in Developing Countries: Formulation, Quality, and Stability. *Pharmaceutics* **2025**, *17*, 787. [CrossRef] [PubMed]
15. Lacassia, C.; Cutrignelli, A.; la Forgia, F.M.; Fontana, S.; Lopalco, A.; Denora, N.; Lopedota, A.A. Evaluation of Five Ready-to-Use Bases for the Topical Administration of Propranolol Hydrochloride to Treat Infantile Hemangioma. *Pharmaceutics* **2025**, *17*, 83. [CrossRef] [PubMed]
16. Jovičić-Bata, J.; Todorović, N.; Krstonošić, V.; Ristić, I.; Kovačević, Z.; Vuković, M.; Lalić-Popović, M. Liquid- and Semisolid-Filled Hard Gelatin Capsules Containing Alpha-Lipoic Acid as a Suitable Dosage Form for Compounding Medicines and Dietary Supplements. *Pharmaceutics* **2024**, *16*, 892. [CrossRef] [PubMed]
17. Rizzello, M.; Pacelli, A.; De Bari, M.D.; Cutrignelli, A.; Iacobazzi, R.M.; Lopalco, A.; Denora, N. 68Ga Extemporaneous Preparations in Radiopharmacy. *Pharmaceutics* **2025**, *17*, 802. [CrossRef] [PubMed]

https://doi.org/10.3390/pharmaceutics18020209

pharmaceutics

MDPI

Review

Extemporaneous Formulations for Pediatric Patients: Global Necessities, Challenges and Opportunities

Vinita Balakrishna Pai [1,*] and Milap Chand Nahata [1,2,*]

1 Division of Pharmacy Practice and Science, College of Pharmacy, The Ohio State University, Columbus, OH 43210, USA
2 Institute of Therapeutic Innovations and Outcomes, Colleges of Pharmacy and Medicine, The Ohio State University, Columbus, OH 43210, USA
* Correspondence: pai.15@osu.edu (V.B.P.); nahata.1@osu.edu (M.C.N.)

Abstract

Many commercially available medications are often unapproved or unavailable in suitable dosage forms for specific patient populations, particularly infants and children. This necessitates the use of extemporaneously compounded formulations to deliver individualized doses based on body weight or body surface area, and when a medication is unavailable at an appropriate concentration or contains excipients potentially unsafe for certain patients. Extemporaneous compounding is required for oral liquids when patients are unable to swallow tablets or capsules. It is also needed for topical preparations and sterile dosage forms when commercial products are unavailable. Across regions, practices follow national pharmacopeial standards for both sterile and non-sterile compounding. Stability factors influencing the safety and efficacy of compounded formulations must be carefully considered when assigning appropriate beyond-use dates. While stability information is available for some medications in monographs, peer-reviewed literature, prescribing information, and investigator's brochures, such data is often lacking for many compounded preparations. Emerging extemporaneous formulations—such as orodispersible films, nanoparticle systems, and 3D-printed compounds—offer potential advantages over traditional compounded formulations but present unique challenges to widespread implementation. Despite the justified clinical need for extemporaneous compounding, significant barriers remain, including limited access to medications, insufficient compounding expertise or resources, gaps in pharmacokinetic and safety data, and regulatory constraints. This review critically appraises the current state of extemporaneous compounding—drawing primarily on the United States of America frameworks—and highlights its continued necessity, associated challenges, and pragmatic solutions for advancing personalized pharmacotherapy across pediatric age groups worldwide.

Keywords: extemporaneous formulations; pediatrics; compounding; personalized medicine

1. Introduction

The practice of compounding a dosage form to address the medical needs of an individual patient has existed since at least the early 1600s, when practitioners known as apothecaries, primarily chemists, mixed and sold medicines [1]. The demand for compounding declined as over 90% of medicinal products used in patient care began to be commercially manufactured [2,3]. Nevertheless, extemporaneous compounding remains essential where authorized products do not meet patient needs, anchoring the two themes of this work: the necessities driving patient-specific therapy and the challenges that constrain safe, high-quality practice. Extemporaneous compounding remains a key component of pediatric pharmacy practice, providing patient-specific, sometimes life-saving medications to patients whose health care needs cannot be met by commercially manufactured dosage forms. In the United States of America (US), the compounding of extemporaneous formulations is currently more commonly performed within hospital pharmacies or health systems. Community pharmacies often have limited resources and expertise for compounding, with approximately 7500 of 56,000 pharmacies in the US providing extemporaneous compounding as a specialized function [4]. Many such pharmacies operate with dedicated facilities and quality systems, providing both sterile preparations and non-sterile dosage forms such as oral liquids, oral solid dosage forms, and topical formulations.

The United States Pharmacopeia (USP) Chapter <795> Pharmaceutical Compounding—Nonsterile Preparations (USP <795>) describes compounding as "the preparation, mixing, assembling, altering, packaging, and labeling of a drug, drug-delivery device, or device in accordance with a licensed practitioner's prescription, medication order, or initiative based on the practitioner/patient/pharmacist/compounder relationship in the course of professional practice" [5].

According to the European Directive 2001/83/EC, compounding is classified as a magistral formula or an officinal formula. A magistral formula is any medicinal product prepared in a pharmacy according to a prescription for an individual patient. It is an extemporaneous preparation compounded for specific patients or patient groups and supplied immediately after preparation. The officinal formula is "any medicinal product which is prepared in a pharmacy in accordance with the prescriptions of a pharmacopoeia and is intended to be directly supplied to the patients served by the pharmacy" [6]. By contrast, stock preparations are compounded in advance and stored until a request for supply is received. On this basis, some European countries allow stock preparations alongside magistral or officinal formulas to ensure immediate availability at dispensing.

This article provides a comprehensive state-of-the art review of the role of extemporaneous compounding in current clinical practice involving pediatric patient care. It critically appraises the operational and regulatory challenges, including stability evidence and beyond-use dating, quality-system requirements, and regulatory heterogeneity, that influence safe implementation worldwide. We also highlight recent innovations, such as orodispersible films and tablets, nanoparticle formulations, and 3D-printed compounds. While these platforms can expand access to tailored therapies, they also introduce new validation, quality-control, and oversight requirements that must be addressed for routine clinical use. Finally, we outline pragmatic strategies and opportunities to improve quality, safety, and access, providing a concise framework for risk-based decision making by clinicians, pharmacists, and regulators. Relative to certain recent extensive review articles [7,8], the uniqueness of our critical review includes its broad scope, comprehensiveness, inclusion of the most recent studies and regulations, description of limitations of existing literature for application in patient care, and elaboration of opportunities as a roadmap for the future to advance the care of pediatric patients globally.

2. Literature Sources and Study Selection

For this narrative review, a literature search was conducted using the PubMed, Embase, Web of Science, and Scopus databases. Search terms included "extemporaneous", "compounding", "formulations", "stability," "pediatrics", 'prevalence", "novel", "3D-printing", "orodispersible films", "orodispersible tablets", and various combinations thereof. Articles published in non-English languages, not relevant to pediatric patient care, and only available as Abstracts were excluded. Priority was given to review articles and studies

https://doi.org/10.3390/pharmaceutics18010126

that focused on any aspect of extemporaneous compounding or extemporaneous formulations. Additionally, the bibliographies of selected articles were examined to identify further relevant publications. Both authors agreed on the inclusion and exclusion of articles for performing this review. Although PubMed includes citations dating back to the 1960s, this review was restricted to literature published between January 2000 and May 2025 to ensure a focus on contemporary practices and recent developments in the field.

3. Clinical Need for Extemporaneous Compounding

Compounding oral extemporaneous formulations is often a necessity for pediatric patient populations, particularly those who cannot swallow solid dosage forms or for whom commercially manufactured liquid formulations do not meet the individualized dosing requirements.

Drug doses for pediatric patients are typically calculated based on body weight (mg/kg) or body surface area (mg/m^2). This approach often results in specific doses that cannot be administered using commercially available formulations containing a fixed amount of the active pharmaceutical ingredient(s) (APIs) per tablet or capsule. In such cases, liquid dosage forms offer the advantage of enabling the administration of patient-specific doses. Many children under 6 years of age may be unable to swallow solid dosage forms, such as tablets or capsules, despite targeted training efforts [9]. Some infants may develop oral aversion and refuse to swallow food or medications, particularly if they have not utilized the oral route for an extended period. In such cases, the use of enteral feeding tubes—such as nasogastric (NG) or nasojejunal (NJ) tubes—may be required for both nutritional support and the administration of medications. It is essential that extemporaneously compounded formulations intended for these patients are appropriate for enteral tube delivery to ensure both the safety and efficacy of therapy. Oral aversion is not exclusive to the pediatric population; nearly 40% of adult patients may also experience oral aversion [10], particularly in relation to the administration of oral medications, thereby necessitating the use of NG or NJ tubes. In this context, compounded liquids should also consider viscosity/osmolality, material compatibility, and adsorption/occlusion risk to ensure reliable delivery via feeding tubes.

Certain drugs with a narrow therapeutic index, such as tacrolimus, require personalized therapy with careful dose titration to maintain serum concentrations within a defined therapeutic range, particularly in patients undergoing hematopoietic cell transplantation or solid organ transplantation. Achieving these individualized target concentrations may necessitate doses that are not commercially available, as tacrolimus is typically marketed only in capsule form. In such scenarios, the use of a liquid dosage formulation offers a practical solution, enabling precise dose adjustments to ensure effective and safe therapy. However, very low doses derived from concentrated stock solutions may increase measurement error; standardized dilutions and clear administration devices can mitigate this risk among pediatric patients.

In some cases, despite the availability of liquid dosage forms, compounding an extemporaneous formulation may be necessary because the dosage form contains excipients at concentrations that could be unsafe for the patient, especially premature newborns, neonates and infants. For example, dexamethasone intensol solution, 1 mg/mL for oral administration, contains a high concentration of alcohol (30% *v*/*v*), which may be harmful to premature newborns, term neonates, and infants. As a result, there is a need for extemporaneous compounding of a formulation that excludes alcohol to ensure safety and suitability for this vulnerable population. Extemporaneous compounding may be necessary if the concentration of the commercially available preparation is inappropriate for practical administration of a dose. Accurate dosing in pediatric patients can be dif-

https://doi.org/10.3390/pharmaceutics18010126

ficult when commercially available formulations contain high concentrations of API(s) intended for older populations, as the measurement of extremely small volumes for the doses required may lead to administration errors. For example, furosemide injection is commercially available in a 10 mg/mL concentration [11]. A 1 mg/kg dose of furosemide for a 750 g baby would be 0.75 mg or 0.075 mL of the undiluted medication, which would be difficult to prepare accurately without further dilution. Beyond excipient ethanol, other excipients (e.g., propylene glycol, sorbitol, benzoates) may warrant avoidance or tighter limits in neonates and young infants.

The treatment of rare diseases often relies on medications classified as orphan drugs, such as L-carnitine and L-arginine, which may not have commercially available formulations meeting the unique requirements of all patient populations [12]. Due to limited demand, pharmaceutical companies are often unwilling to invest in manufacturing appropriate dosage forms for these drugs, making extemporaneous compounding essential to meet individual patient needs. Sometimes specific combinations of APIs may be essential for effectively treating various dermatological conditions. However, these tailored formulations are frequently unavailable commercially, necessitating dermatologists to prescribe individualized combinations for compounding [13–15]. Extemporaneously compounded medications play a crucial role in the management of acute or chronic pain, as well as in the alleviation of symptoms during palliative and hospice care. In many cases, the specific therapeutic needs of patients may not be adequately addressed using commercially available products, making compounding an essential practice in these settings [16–18].

Shortages of commercially available dosage forms, particularly those used to address specific patient needs in acute care settings, have significantly contributed to a resurgence in extemporaneous compounding. Notable examples in the US include the shortages of ibuprofen suspension in 2023 and amoxicillin and oseltamivir suspensions in 2022 [19,20]. These shortages have been exacerbated by supply chain disruptions resulting from epidemics, pandemics, and natural disasters. As of March 2025, the American Society of Health-System Pharmacists (ASHP) reported 270 active drug shortages nationwide [21]. Collectively, these scenarios illustrate the clear clinical necessity for extemporaneous compounding but also highlight practical challenges—accurate low-dose measurement, tube-administration compatibility, excipient safety in vulnerable populations, and the need for justified beyond-use dates—that must be addressed to ensure safe, effective patient care.

3.1. Critical Review of Global Extemporaneous Compounding Practices in Pediatric Patient Care

Many drugs lack pediatric labeling and child-friendly formulations because research has traditionally focused on adults. To address this, the FDA's Best Pharmaceuticals for Children Act (BPCA) and Pediatric Research Equity Act (PREA), along with the European Medicines Agency (EMA), have established regulations to promote pediatric drug development [22–24]. Despite these efforts to increase pediatric labeling for newer drugs, many older, off-patent essential medicines—such as those on the WHO Model List of Essential Medicines for Children (EMLc) still lack appropriate pediatric dosage forms [25]. A review analyzing studies published between 2012 and 2022 across Europe, North America, Southeast Asia, Australia, and Africa found that off-label drug use remains prevalent in patients aged 0–18 years, with rates ranging from 3.3% of over 4 million prescriptions in Italy to 71.5% of nearly 2000 prescriptions in Indonesia [7].

Given the widespread global use of off-label medications in pediatric populations, we conducted a focused literature review (2000–2025) to assess the prevalence of extemporaneous compounding and identify the most commonly compounded formulations in children. Most of the 17 included studies used cross-sectional surveys and observational designs; a few employed prospective approaches, such as nested case–control or pilot stud-

https://doi.org/10.3390/pharmaceutics18010126

ies. These studies examined compounding practices, prevalence, and perceptions across healthcare settings in Europe, North America, Oceania, Asia, and Africa. Pharmacists, particularly those working in hospitals, communities, and independent settings, were the primary respondents. Some studies also surveyed physicians and nurses, especially in pediatric or hospital-based contexts. Five studies focused specifically on pediatric populations, targeting pediatric hospitals, formulations, or drug manipulation practices. Survey response rates ranged from 27.3% to 98%. Compounding was routinely performed across settings, with pharmacies averaging 12.5 compounded preparations per day and 3–12% of prescriptions requiring compounding. About 94% of pharmacists reported providing compounding services, and 20% of physicians prescribed medications requiring compounding. In pediatric inpatient settings, 28% of children received at least one extemporaneous liquid formulation. Frequent manipulation of oral dosage forms (e.g., splitting/crushing tablets) was consistently reported.

The findings indicated that non-sterile extemporaneous compounding is a routine practice in pediatric care worldwide. Oral liquid formulations and topical dermatologic preparations were the most frequently compounded dosage forms, followed by capsules, powder papers, and manipulated solid dosage forms such as tablets that were crushed or split. (Table 1). Commonly compounded drugs included spironolactone, furosemide, omeprazole, lansoprazole, captopril, sildenafil, hydrochlorothiazide, caffeine citrate, and prednisone/prednisolone. A 2024 global survey completed by 479 WHO regions found that oral liquids were the most frequently compounded preparations, with 90% of the participants doing so, and the diuretics, drugs for acid-related disorders, and beta-blockers were the top three compounded classes for the pediatric patients [26].

The reviewed studies offer valuable insights into extemporaneous compounding practices across diverse global settings. However, several methodological and contextual limitations impact the generalizability and comparability of the findings. Study designs were highly heterogeneous, ranging from surveys to observational assessments, with wide variation in the metrics and response rates used to evaluate compounding prevalence. Some studies reported the percentage of prescriptions compounded, while others quantified the volume, frequency, or number of manipulated dosage forms. The duration of data collection also varied from daily to monthly assessments. Conducted across multiple continents over an extended period, the studies reflect regional differences in regulatory frameworks, drug formularies, healthcare infrastructure, and access to commercially available pediatric formulations. Additionally, variation in study respondents, including pharmacists, physicians, and nurses, further contributes to the heterogeneity of the data. Taken together, these patterns underscore a clear clinical need for extemporaneous compounding but also pose persistent challenges for evidence synthesis—namely, heterogeneous metrics, variable time horizons, and region-specific regulatory contexts—that should be considered when interpreting comparative prevalence estimates.

https://doi.org/10.3390/pharmaceutics18010126

Table 1. Curated Overview of Prevalence of Non-sterile Extemporaneous Compounding Practices Across Countries.

Study Design/Reference	Geographic Locations	Compounded Prescriptions (Rx's) or Reported Use	Age Group	Most Compounded (c) or Manipulated (m) Dosage Form	Top 5 Drugs Frequently Compounded in Extemporaneous Formulations
Questionnaires answered by hospital pharmacists from 18 European countries to determine the most frequently extemporaneously compounded oral dosage forms, including the drug names, total volumes, and number of times the dosage forms were made in a 6-month period. Brion F et al. 2003 [27].	Belgium, Croatia, Denmark, England, Finland, France, Germany, Ireland, Italy, Norway, Scotland, Slovenia, Spain, Sweden, Switzerland	21/41 (51%) questionnaires returned. Over a six-month period: morphine was compounded 447 times, totaling 76,170 mL; isosorbide, totaling 4028 number of powder papers; hydrochlorothiazide, totaling 14,060 capsules	Pediatric (specific age distribution not provided)	Oral liquids >60% (c) in Denmark, England, Ireland, Norway, Sweden	Morphine, prednisolone, trimethoprim, captopril, midazolam
				Paper powders (c) in Finland, Italy, Scotland	Isosorbide, glycine, caffeine citrate, L-citrulline, vitamin E
				Capsules (c) in Belgium, Croatia, France	Hydrochlorothiazide, spironolactone, captopril, prednisolone, folic acid
Prospective, nested, case–control study of pharmacies (n = 79) dispensing Rx's for compounded medicines during one predetermined study day. Buurma H et al. 2003 [28].	The Netherlands	3.4% (991/28,711) Rx's/day were for compounded medicines 12.5 compounded medicines per pharmacy per day (mean)	Adults and pediatric patients (<12 years of age) more likely to receive Rx for compounding	Dermatological (62.1%) (c) Oral solutions (7.4%) (c) Ear, nose, throat products (7.1%) (c)	Specific drug names not provided Drugs affecting central nervous, cardiovascular, and gastrointestinal systems
Prospective, survey-based, observational study to determine the extent of Rx compounding in independent community pharmacies. McPherson et al. 2006 [29]; Martin KS et al. 2009 [30].	US (Illinois, Missouri, Kansas, Iowa)	22.92% (370/1610) response rate, 347 provided compounding; 333 analyzable 2.3% (7768/344,677) Rx's compounded/week ≥5% of the total Rx's compounded by 12.3% of the 347 compounders	Not specified	Dermatological (solutions, ointments, creams, gels) (90.7%) (c) Oral solutions (73.2%) (c) Oral suspensions (70.4%) (c) Dermatological and oral capsules are compounded at least once per week by 30% to 46% of the independent pharmacies	Not provided
Retrospective review of onsite logbooks to determine the extent and nature of extemporaneous compounding of liquid preparations in New Zealand. Kairuz T et al. 2007 [31].	New Zealand	2015 total products compounded over a 7-month period (in 2004); 252 per month (mean)	Pediatric patients (neonates, infants and children) included; inclusion of adult patients not specified	Oral dosage forms (152) (c) Topical dosage form (100) (c) Oral suspension is the most common oral dosage form compounded	Omeprazole, sotalol, labetalol, diazoxide, and clonidine

Table 1. *Cont.*

Study Design/Reference	Geographic Locations	Compounded Prescriptions (Rx's) or Reported Use	Age Group	Most Compounded (c) or Manipulated (m) Dosage Form	Top 5 Drugs Frequently Compounded in Extemporaneous Formulations
Prospective survey of children's hospitals ($n = 20$) to understand the scope, frequency, and use of extemporaneous liquid formulations. Lugo, R et al. 2009 [32].	US	28% of the median of 8400 inpatient admissions per hospital over a 12-month period received at least one extemporaneous liquid formulation	Pediatric (newborn to 18 years)	Liquid (c)	Lansoprazole, spironolactone, captopril, sildenafil, ursodiol
Cross-sectional descriptive survey of community pharmacists (stage 1) and physicians (stage 2) to determine the extent of prescription compounding by community pharmacists in the West Bank. Zaid, A et al. 2012 [33].	Cities and villages in the 11 districts of the West Bank	72.2% (153/212) of pharmacies provided compounding services. 1.55% (1973/126,840) of total Rx's were compounded 20.7% (37/179) of physicians prescribed a medication that required compounding and prescribed less than 20 Rx's per month	Not specified	Topical preparations (97.3%) (c) Oral solutions (78.4%) (c) Oral suspensions (43.2%) (c)	Not provided
Observational study (over 2 weeks) assessing the extent of drug manipulations conducted in clinical practice in inpatient settings. Questionnaire survey of experiences and views of pediatric nurses about these manipulations. Richey RH et al. 2013 [34].	Britain	Total 310 manipulations of drugs/dosage forms identified 258 potential drug manipulations reported in 27.3% (153/560) of questionnaires returned; 188 (73%) of these were valid manipulations	Pediatric (2 to 19 years of age)	Tablets (61.6%) (m) Intravenous injection (21%) (m) Sachet (9.7%) (m) Transdermal patch (3.2%) (m)	Analgesic, proton pump inhibitor, antimuscarinic agent, antiemetic, alginate preparation
Pilot study to determine the extent of compounding by reviewing batch records over a period of 24 months. Masupye IM et al. 2015 [35].	South Africa	27.6% preparations compounded per month (691 batch records assessed)	Not specified	Solutions 43.9% (c) Creams 33% (c) Ointments 13.6% (c)	Betamethasone, other corticosteroids

https://doi.org/10.3390/pharmaceutics18010126

Table 1. *Cont.*

Study Design/Reference	Geographic Locations	Compounded Prescriptions (Rx's) or Reported Use	Age Group	Most Compounded (c) or Manipulated (m) Dosage Form	Top 5 Drugs Frequently Compounded in Extemporaneous Formulations
Prospective cross-sectional study at three hospitals to assess the extent of manipulation of oral medicines, the type of and dosage form manipulated over a four-week period. Bjerknes K et al. 2016 [36].	Norway	17% (509/3070) of oral administrations were manipulated	Pediatric (newborn to 17 years of age) Number of manipulations by age: 28 days to 23 months—22.5% (175/777) 6–11 years—28.8% (276/957)	Tablets (87%) (m) Capsules (11%) (m)	Prednisolone, metronidazole, ketobemidone hydrochloride, nitrazepam, azathioprine
Observational study with cross-sectional descriptive survey conducted over 3 months to identify characteristics of extemporaneous compounding at Primary Health Care centers. Hapsari I et al. 2018 [37].	Indonesia	1229 formulations compounded for 1200 Rx's written	Pediatric and adult Preparations by age group 0 to 5 years—74% >5 years to <18 years—23% >18 years 2%	Paper powders 88.4% (c) Liquids (suspensions and syrups) 8% (c) Dermatological 3.6% (c)	Not provided
Cross-sectional survey of pharmacists in five districts of Yogyakarta province to assess the extent of prescription compounding in a typical month. Kristina et al. 2018 [38].	Indonesia	Survey response rate 72% (305/425) 94% (286/305) of pharmacists provided compounding services 11.55% (155/1342) Rx's per month requesting compounding	Not specified	Paper powders 32.1% (c) Capsules 25.3% (c) Syrup 21.9% (c)	Paracetamol, Chlorpheniramine, ambroxol
Cross-sectional survey of randomly selected community and hospital pharmacies (n = 431) in 12 governorates assessing the prevalence of extemporaneous compounding. Alkhatib H et al. 2019 [39].	Jordan	51.7% (223/431) provided compounding services A median of 1.5 of 20 daily prescriptions contained at least 1 compounding order	Not specified	Creams 99.6% (c) Ointments 91.5% (c) Solutions 23.3% (c) Suspensions 4.5% (c) Syrup 0.9% (c)	Not provided

https://doi.org/10.3390/pharmaceutics18010126

Table 1. *Cont.*

Study Design/Reference	Geographic Locations	Compounded Prescriptions (Rx's) or Reported Use	Age Group	Most Compounded (c) or Manipulated (m) Dosage Form	Top 5 Drugs Frequently Compounded in Extemporaneous Formulations
Cross-sectional examination of prescriptions sent to and the compounding logbook of the pharmacy department over a 4-month period in a 900-bed premier teaching hospital to determine the extent and prescribing pattern of, and labelling information provided for extemporaneous products. Yusuff KB et al. 2019 [40].	Nigeria	All (678) extemporaneous preparations were for liquid dosage form compounded for a total of 520 prescriptions involving 34 different API. 524/678 (77.2%) preparations were for pediatric patients in the Children's Emergency Ward, while 154/678 (22.7%) were ambulatory.	Pediatric (specific age distribution not provided)	Liquid 100% (c)	Zinc gluconate, spironolactone, hydrochlorothiazide, captopril, hydroxyurea
Cross-sectional survey of hospitals in Thailand ($n = 750$). Pitchayajittipong C et al. 2021 [41].	Thailand	52.7% (395/750) response rate; 59.75% (236/395) were involved in compounding formulations	Not specified	Solid (c) Liquid (c) Semisolid (c)	Oseltamivir, isoniazid, spironolactone, furosemide, special mouthwash
Cross-sectional survey of healthcare providers' (physicians, pharmacists, nurses) opinions on access to medicines in children collected over one month. Tiengkate P et al. 2022 [42].	Thailand	98% (218/223) response rate	Pediatric (specific age distribution not provided)	Not assessed	Omeprazole, prednisolone, sildenafil, spironolactone, aspirin
Evaluation of the type and frequency of extemporaneous compounding through an online survey administered to all community and hospital pharmacists registered with Pharmaceutical Society of Ireland. Ramtoola Z et al. 2023 [43].	Republic of Ireland	202/4361 (4.6%) pharmacists completed the survey. 170/202 prepared extemporaneous preparations 168 average number of Rx's per month received for compounding	Pediatric and adult	Dermatological 56% (c) community pharmacies Adult and under-12 years of age oral liquid formulations 11% (c) hospital pharmacies	Not provided

https://doi.org/10.3390/pharmaceutics18010126

Table 1. *Cont.*

Study Design/Reference	Geographic Locations	Compounded Prescriptions (Rx's) or Reported Use	Age Group	Most Compounded (c) or Manipulated (m) Dosage Form	Top 5 Drugs Frequently Compounded in Extemporaneous Formulations
Cross-sectional survey of 395 hospitals with on-site pharmaceutical production facilities to examine extemporaneous compounding practices over a 3-month period. Supapaan TS et al. 2023. [44].	Thailand	88/395 agreed to participate A total of 61 extemporaneous medicinal formulations were compounded		Oral liquids 57% (c) Semisolids 4.5% (c) Ophthalmic 38.4% (c)	Oseltamivir, isoniazid, spironolactone, furosemide, sodium bicarbonate
Survey of the International Pharmaceutical Federation (FIP) Pediatric Formulations Focus Group (PFFG). Fadda HM et al. 2024 [26].	WHO regions of the FIP PFFG Africa, Americas, Eastern Mediterranean, Europe, South-East Asia, Western Pacific	58% (736/1274) response rate 37.6% (479/1274) included in analysis	Pediatric	Oral liquids 90% (c) Capsules 44% (c) Powder papers 43% (c)	Omeprazole, captopril, spironolactone, propranolol, furosemide

c, compounded; m, manipulated; Rx's, prescriptions.

https://doi.org/10.3390/pharmaceutics18010126

3.2. Essential Components of Extemporaneous Compounding

3.2.1. Information Resources for Compounding

Extemporaneous compounding at the point of care is feasible only when the compounding facility possesses an established infrastructure that complies with applicable national regulations. For instance, in the US, USP Chapter <797> on Pharmaceutical Compounding—Nonsterile Preparations provides guidelines for the compounding of nonsterile products in accordance with established good practice standards.

Information on the formulation of an extemporaneous preparation—including ingredients, compounding methods, storage containers, optimal storage conditions, and reliable stability data may be obtained from various sources. The most accessible resource in a hospital setting is typically the country's pharmacopoeia and national formularies, provided they include official monographs for compounded preparations that encompass all relevant information. The USP-National Formulary (NF) currently has over 200 such monographs [45]. For drugs with approved pediatric labeling, relevant information may be found in the package inserts for brand-name products. Additionally, the investigator's brochure for drugs under study, particularly those focused on pediatric applications, may provide details on dose preparation or manipulation. However, obtaining this proprietary information can be challenging. Furthermore, the investigator's brochure content is trial-specific and not a substitute for validated compounding data; it should be used only if appropriate compatibility/stability and, where relevant, bioequivalence have been demonstrated. Tertiary references such as the Pediatric and Neonatal Dosage Handbook, Pediatric Drug Formulations, and Extemporaneous Formulations for Pediatric, Geriatric, and Special Needs Patients have compiled the necessary published information for compounding extemporaneous formulations and are periodically updated [46–48]. If these resources do not yield the required formulation information, a search of the primary literature should be conducted. Access to national pharmacopeias, formularies, and tertiary references may be limited due to cost. However, in such situations, freely available extemporaneous formulation recipes published by hospital pharmacies online may serve as alternatives (Table 2). Before use, it is essential to evaluate the accompanying stability data and ensure that the preparation meets national standards for non-sterile compounding.

If all attempts to acquire the necessary information fail, the drug can still be administered to the patient; however, this may necessitate manipulation and administration of the dose at the bedside for immediate administration. This process carries a significant risk of errors, particularly if the dose for an infant or young child represents a fraction of the commercially available dosage form. Additional complications may arise if the drug requiring bedside manipulation is hazardous, necessitating specific precautions while handling it.

Table 2. Information Resources Supporting Extemporaneous Compounding.

Country and Source	Source Type	Web Address
Children's Hospital of Eastern Ontario, Ontario, Canada	Online Free	Pharmacy compounding formulas—CHEO
The Hospital for Sick Children, Montreal, Canada	Online Free	Pharmacy Compounding Recipes | SickKids
Chu Sainte-Justine, Montreal, Canada	Online Free	Magistrales stadnardisées au Québec—Chu Sainte-Justine
The Montreal Children's Hospital		
Formulaire National, France	Online Free	https://ansm.sante.fr/pharmacopee/formulaire-national (accessed on 14 January 2026)

https://doi.org/10.3390/pharmaceutics18010126

Table 2. *Cont.*

Country and Source	Source Type	Web Address
Base de datos de formulas magistrales de la SEFH, Spain	Online Free	https://gruposdetrabajo.sefh.es/farmacotecnia/formulas-magistrales (accessed on 14 January 2026)
US Pharmacist Compounding	Online Free	https://www.uspharmacist.com/topic/compounding (accessed on 14 January 2026)
Fagron Formulary	Online—certain formulations available free; others need paid membership	https://www.fagron.com/formulary (accessed on 14 January 2026)
Nationwide Children's Hospital, US	Online Free	https://www.nationwidechildrens.org/specialties/pharmacy-services/compounding-formulas (accessed on 14 January 2026)
Deutscher Arzneimittel-Codex Neues Rezeptur-Formularium (DAC/NRF), Germany	Online registration necessary	https://dacnrf.pharmazeutische-zeitung.de/dac/nrf-wissen/rezepturenfinder/offen (accessed on 14 January 2026)

3.2.2. Non-Sterile Extemporaneous Formulations

1. Liquid Dosage Formulations for Personalized Patient Care

A comprehensive review of safe and effective extemporaneous formulation can be found in the most current USP or the technical bulletins published by ASHP [49,50]. These may also be available in the national pharmacopoeias of individual countries or published by their respective pharmacy organizations. Liquid formulations are the most frequently compounded for use in children [26]. Because many APIs in the commercially available solid dosage forms used in extemporaneous compounding of liquids are insoluble in water, suspensions are among the most commonly compounded formulations. The base vehicle for compounding suspensions typically consists of a suspending agent and a sweetening agent (e.g., syrup) in a 1:1 proportion. Numerous commercially made ready-to-use suspending agents, such as Ora-Plus®, and sweetening agents such as Ora-Sweet®, and others, including Ora-Blend Flavored®, SuspendRx®, and SyrSpend®, are available. Some of the sweetening agents are available in sugar-free form. However, these products may be cost-prohibitive or unavailable in some countries. A stable bedaquiline suspension was made using widely available cane sugar for preparing simple syrup and "Thick & Easy" food starch as a thickening agent for pediatric patients in Africa [51]. If a ready-to-use suspending agent is unavailable, an extemporaneous preparation may be made with regionally available ingredients—for example, a 1:1 mixture of 1% methylcellulose suspension and Simple Syrup USP. Other examples of extemporaneously compounded suspending agents may be found in each country's pharmacopoeia or national formulary. In the USP, examples include Vehicle for Oral Suspension, Suspension Structured Vehicle, and Sugar-Free Suspension Structured Vehicle USP [45].

The acceptance of extemporaneously compounded formulations is essential for ensuring patient adherence to medication regimens, particularly in pediatric patients. As noted, "a spoonful of sugar helps the medicine go down," which highlights the importance of palatability in treatment adherence. Organoleptic properties, including sweetness, taste, odor, texture, color, and flavor, play a critical role in the acceptance of these formulations. For patients with dietary carbohydrate restrictions, such as those with diabetes mellitus or following ketogenic diets, sugar-free sweetening agents provide suitable alternatives. A specific flavoring agent can be strategically added to mask undesirable tastes associated with certain APIs; for example, chocolate can effectively disguise bitterness [52]. Chocolate Syrup USP may be used both as a sweetening and flavoring agent [45]. Other examples of extemporaneously compounded flavoring agents that can also serve as sweetening

https://doi.org/10.3390/pharmaceutics18010126

agents may be found in each country's pharmacopoeia or national formulary. In the USP, examples include Cherry Syrup, Orange Syrup, Peppermint spirit, and Vanilla tincture [45]. Additionally, flavors can be paired with coloring agents to enhance aesthetics. However, their addition should be approached with caution, especially if they were not included in the original formulation with stability data, as it may compromise the formulation's stability and safety. Changes in temperature, pH, light exposure, and the presence of oxidizing or reducing substances can adversely affect added colors. In cases where stability data for flavoring or coloring agents are lacking, these agents may be added to individual doses as needed immediately before administration. Availability and affordability vary by country; where products are not available, in-house vehicles must be prepared and documented according to local standards.

To stabilize and preserve, certain formulations may require the addition of acids, bases, pH buffering agents, or solubilizing agents such as propylene glycol, ethanol, and glycerol, as well as preservatives like parabens and benzyl alcohol. However, caution is necessary when using these additives, as the original dosage form intended for extemporaneous compounding may already contain one or more of them, increasing the total exposure and risk of toxicity—particularly in premature newborns, neonates, and infants, thereby raising the potential for adverse effects (Table 3) [53,54]. Under such circumstances, additives should be used in minimal amounts or not at all, while still meeting the stability, palatability, and safety criteria for the dosage form.

Using extemporaneously compounded liquid dosage forms for pediatric patients may not always be feasible, particularly when the beyond-use-date (BUD) is very short, necessitating frequent visits to the pharmacy for prescription refills. This can prove impractical due to work obligations, distance from the pharmacy, or lack of transportation. In such cases, manufactured tablets may be cut or split, and capsules may be opened with their contents mixed with food items such as applesauce, pudding, or ice cream, or liquids like water, juice, or formula. However, these methods may compromise the physical and chemical stability of the medication, particularly if the original formulation is extended-release, delayed-release, or enteric-coated, which could lead to dosing errors from inaccurate splitting, spillage, or loss of specific release technology during reconstitution. Additionally, mixing with large quantities of food should be avoided, as patients may not consume the entire portion, resulting in inadequate dosing. For water-soluble APIs, crushed tablets or capsule contents can be mixed with a desired volume of water to achieve a precise dose based on mg/mL; however, this process carries the risk of preparation and calculation errors. Any manipulation should be supported by clear instructions, appropriate measuring devices, and, where feasible, compatibility/stability information to minimize pharmacokinetic and pharmacodynamic variability.

Table 3. Excipients with Potential Harmful Effects on Pediatric Patients [53,54].

Excipients	Harmful Effects and Recommendations	Admissible Amount for Intake
	Artificial Sweeteners	
Aspartame	Headaches, seizures, neurotoxicity, hallucinations Use contraindicated in patients with phenylketonuria	40 mg/kg/day
Saccharine	Nausea, diarrhea, hives, itching, increased sensitivity to light. Limit use in pregnant women and children.	2.5 mg/kg/day

https://doi.org/10.3390/pharmaceutics18010126

Table 3. *Cont.*

Excipients	Harmful Effects and Recommendations	Admissible Amount for Intake
Sorbitol	Gastrointestinal disorders such as diarrhea, flatulence, abdominal pain. Hepatotoxicity. Do not use in patients with fructose intolerance. Use not recommended in hypoglycemic patients	0 to 2 years of age 5 mg/kg/day >2 years of age 140 mg/kg/day
Sucralose	Composition of gut microbiome, blood glucose, insulin and glucagon-like peptide levels altered	15 mg/kg/day
Sucrose	Dental carries. Use not recommended in children with type 1 diabetes	Not available
	Preservatives	
Benzalkonium Chloride	Bronchoconstriction—use with caution in patients with asthma. Ototoxicity, hypersensitivity	Not available
Benzyl alcohol	Metabolic acidosis and respiratory depression—contraindicated in newborns and children under 3 years of age due to immature metabolism. Cerebral palsy and developmental delay. Hypersensitivity	5 mg/kg/day
Parabens (methyl, ethyl, propyl)	Cross reactions in patients allergic to acetylsalicylic acid. Avoid use in newborns and neonates to avoid hyperbilirubinemia	10 mg/kg/day
	Solvents and Solubilizing Agents	
Ethyl alcohol	Hypoglycemia, acidosis, electrolyte abnormalities. CNS effects such as stupor, coma Can also be used as a preservative	6 mg/kg/dose Acceptable ethanol content in a formulation: >12 years of age = <10% *v*/*v* 6–12 years of age = <5% *v*/*v* <6 years of age = <0.5% *v*/*v*
Polyethylene Glycol	Gastrointestinal: diarrhea, flatulence, abdominal pain Nephrotoxicity Use with caution in newborns and infants	10 mg/kg/day
Propylene Glycol	CNS depression; diarrhea on oral administration due to high osmolality. Avoid in children < 4 years of age due to immature metabolism	Neonates: 1 mg/kg/day <5 years of age: 50 mg/kg/day Adults: 500 mg/kg/day
	Coloring Agents	
Tartrazines, quinolines, triphenylmethane, xanthines	Hypersensitivity reactions in patients sensitive to tartrazines Azo colorants share cross-sensitivity with acetylsalicylic acid. Use in pediatric formulations not recommended	Not available

https://doi.org/10.3390/pharmaceutics18010126

2. Novel Extemporaneous Solid Dosage Formulations for Personalized Patient Care

Assuming the patient's ability to swallow is unimpaired, commonly compounded solid oral dosage forms include powder papers (sachets), capsules, and tablets, all of which are resource- and labor-intensive to prepare, even with access to capsule-filling and tablet-compression equipment.

Novel dosage forms—such as orally disintegrating tablets, fast-dissolving tablets, orodispersible films, lozenges, hard candy, and troches are classified as oral transmucosal drug delivery systems [55–57]. They facilitate systemic administration of the API, particularly in patients who are unable to swallow traditional solid or liquid dosage forms or who require rapid drug release and a prompt clinical response. Drug release from these dosage forms occurs primarily through dissolution in saliva, followed by absorption across the oral mucosa, which can bypass first-pass hepatic metabolism and enhance bioavailability. The selected excipients must facilitate the disintegration and release of the API within 10–15 min or less, to ensure timely mucosal absorption and therapeutic effects. Given their prolonged contact with the oral mucosa, these dosage forms must also possess acceptable taste, flavor, and texture. Their formulation and use should be supported by documented stability data.

Orally dissolving films and orally disintegrating tablets may offer the advantages of ease of medicine administration, rapid onset of action, increased bioavailability, and improved adherence [56]. Buprenorphine, ondansetron, levocetirizine, rizatriptan, clobazam, diazepam, nicotine, sildenafil, tadalafil, dextromethorphan and diphenhydramine are among the commercially available medicines approved by the FDA as films. Loratadine, cetirizine, ondansetron, and tramadol are examples of orally disintegrating tablets approved by the FDA. These technologies are rarely used for preparing extemporaneous formulations for many reasons stated above.

The use of three-dimensional (3D) printing technology in extemporaneous compounding is an emerging and promising approach that significantly advances the practice of personalized medicine [58,59]. This flexible platform enables the digital design and fabrication of solid dosage forms using specialized software and computer-aided design (CAD) tools, which define the geometry and dimensions of the final product. In this process, a 3D-printer is loaded with a mixture of APIs and excipients and constructs the dosage form layer by layer. The printing parameters—such as resolution, temperature, and speed—are programmed based on the physicochemical properties of the drug, the type of printer used, and the desired characteristics of the final product. Among the various 3D-printing technologies, stereolithography (SLA) is particularly notable for its high resolution and precision, with the ability to achieve fine structural details. 3D-printing has demonstrated the potential to individualize drug delivery systems by tailoring the release profile to the patient's specific pharmacokinetic data. The 3D approach enables the development of complex dosage forms such as polypills, which incorporate multiple APIs into a single unit, thereby improving patient convenience and adherence. Furthermore, 3D-printing facilitates the production of tablets in various shapes, sizes, colors, and flavors, which can enhance patient acceptability, especially in pediatric populations. Unlike traditional pharmaceutical manufacturing, 3D-printing supports on-demand, point-of-care production of personalized medications, representing a transformative advance in extemporaneous compounding and precision pharmacotherapy. Current advancements in 3D-printing of pharmaceuticals are focused on the development of specialized printers, printing software, and suitable pharmaceutical excipients that enable the formulation of dosage forms with predictable drug release profiles and acceptable stability with assurance of quality and reproducibility. In parallel, evidence of economic feasibility (cost-effectiveness/scalability), regulatory frameworks, assurance of drug excipient compatibility in the printing process, potential

https://doi.org/10.3390/pharmaceutics18010126

occupational exposure risks for pharmacy staff, and potential impact of this technology on patient care and safety must be established before this technology can be widely adopted in the pharmaceutical industry and clinical practice. It is not surprising that levetiracetam is the only commercially available 3D-printed medicine approved by the FDA, and this technology has not been used much for preparing extemporaneous formulations among patients in the US, largely due to regulatory, technical, and cost barriers.

Medicines in nanoparticles can be delivered to targeted areas (e.g., pathogens or cancer cells) while minimizing harm to healthy cells, improving bioavailability and releasing API(s) gradually for sustained therapeutic effectiveness [60]. Examples of commercially available medicines in the US are liposomal amphotericin B, doxorubicin, daunorubicin, cytarabine and vincristine, PEGylated nanoparticles in pegfilgrastim, and crystalline nanoparticles in Elixophyllin®. However, this technology is largely used in industrial manufacturing and rarely employed in preparing extemporaneous formulations due to many limitations similar to 3D-printed medicines.

3.3. Factors Influencing Utilization of Extemporaneous Formulations in Clinical Practice

The efficacy and safety of compounded formulations depend on their ability to remain stable throughout clinical use. Therapeutic stability ensures that the drug's therapeutic effect remains unchanged until the BUD, the date beyond which the physical, chemical, microbiological, therapeutic, and toxicological stability of the compounded formulation cannot be guaranteed [5]. This date is determined from the time the formulation is compounded and cannot be directly extrapolated from the expiration date of the commercial dosage form used in the compounding process. As a general expectation, formulations with storage parameters and BUDs that maintain the potency of active ingredients within 90 to 110% of the initial concentration, along with assurance of physical, chemical, and microbiological stability, are recommended. Bioavailability, pharmacokinetic, efficacy, safety and outcomes studies are rarely available for extemporaneously prepared formulations.

When a BUD for a formulation that meets physical, chemical, microbiological, and therapeutic stability is unavailable, the BUD recommendations provided in the pharmacopoeia applicable to the respective country or USP <795> for non-sterile preparations should be utilized. These BUDs are applicable in the absence of stability information for specific preparations through a USP-NF monograph or published stability literature specific to the formulation. The BUD must not exceed the expiration date of any components used in the compounding process. In the revised USP <795>, the determination of BUDs for non-sterile oral liquid formulations is based on "water activity" ("a_w") (Table 4), which is critical in determining the susceptibility of a non-sterile preparation to microbial growth [40]. Additionally, it also informs the potential for degradation of the active ingredient due to chemical reactions that may be induced by the presence of water. The update places greater emphasis on microbial risk (as reflected by "a_w") and, where applicable, on the performance of the preservative system; default BUDs may be extended only when supported by appropriate, stability-indicating data.

These BUDs should be applied with caution in certain cases. For example, captopril (0.75 mg/mL) in Cherry Syrup remains stable for only 2 days at room temperature or when refrigerated. It is stable for $\leq$10 days in a 1:1 mixture of Ora-Sweet® and Ora-Plus® or Ora-Sweet® SF and Ora-Plus®, depending on the storage temperature [61]. Therefore, without specific stability data, labeling these captopril formulations with a BUD of 14 days in accordance with USP guidelines would be inappropriate. The 2023 revised USP addresses this concern by recommending a shorter BUD if the physical and chemical stability of the compounded formulation is less than the USP-recommended BUD (Table 4). In practice, compounders should default to the shorter of: (i) the USP default BUD based on

https://doi.org/10.3390/pharmaceutics18010126

dosage form and "a_w", or (ii) the BUD supported by formulation-specific stability data. Further, it is crucial to ensure that the BUDs were determined from well-designed studies utilizing validated methodologies, analyses and interpretations of the data for application in patient care.

Table 4. United States Pharmacopeia BUDs [1] for Compounded Nonsterile Preparations.

Formulation Category	USP <795> (2014)	USP <795> (2023)
Aqueous—Oral	Water-containing oral formulations: 14 days (refrigerated)	Non-preserved aqueous ("a_w" ≥ 0.60): 14 days (refrigerated) [49]
Aqueous—Preserved (Oral)		Preserved aqueous ("a_w" ≥ 0.60): 35 days (controlled room temperature or refrigerated) [49]
Aqueous—Topical/Dermal/Mucosal	Water-containing topical/dermal/mucosal/oral formulations: 30 days	Managed as "aqueous" based on "a_w" and presence/absence of preservative (apply the 14- or 35-day defaults as appropriate) [49]
Nonaqueous—Oral Liquids		Nonaqueous oral liquids ("a_w" < 0.60): 90 days (controlled room temperature or refrigerated) [49]
Nonaqueous—Other Dosage Forms	Nonaqueous formulations: 6 months (180 days)	Other nonaqueous dosage forms (e.g., capsules, tablets, granules, powders) ("a_w" < 0.60): 180 days (controlled room temperature or refrigerated) [49]

[1] BUD by type of preparation only in the absence of a USP–NF Compounded Preparation Monograph or formulation-specific stability information.

3.4. Challenges and Safety Concerns with Extemporaneous Compounding

3.4.1. Clinical Challenges in Assigning BUDs for Compounded Non-Sterile Preparations

With revised BUDs per USP <795>, any extemporaneously compounded oral liquid dosage form with an "a_w" of ≥0.6, devoid of a preservative, is assigned a BUD of 14 days in the absence of a USP-NF monograph or specific stability data for compounded non-sterile preparations [49]. This raises the question of whether the BUDs recommended in published stability studies for non-preserved aqueous oral dosage forms remain valid if such formulations contain no preservatives. Adding a preservative to an existing formulation with established stability data to extend the BUD beyond 14 days could potentially compromise its stability. Consequently, these updates necessitate repeating or supplementing published stability studies with the inclusion of preservatives to ensure that the API concentration remains within 90–110% of its original level for the recommended BUDs. However, preserved aqueous formulations are generally limited to a BUD of 35 days when stored under controlled conditions or refrigerated, regardless of how long the API remains within 90–110% of its original concentration. The BUD may be extended—up to the time point at which the API remains within 90–110% of its initial concentration or 180 days, whichever is shorter—only if the formulation passes antimicrobial effectiveness testing in accordance with USP <51> [62]. The revised USP <795> permits the use of bracketing in stability studies, employing validated analytical methods and antimicrobial effectiveness testing at both the lowest and highest concentrations of the API. If both concentrations meet the required criteria, the resulting stability data may be extrapolated to support BUDs for all intermediate strengths within that range. Adhering to the revised BUDs for oral liquid formulations may necessitate substantial workflow adjustments for pharmacists and pharmacy technicians in healthcare system pharmacies. Shorter default BUDs and

https://doi.org/10.3390/pharmaceutics18010126

preservative requirements will require more frequent compounding, increasing demands on time and resources. Additionally, significant investment will be needed to reformulate many existing extemporaneous preparations with the addition of preservatives, despite previously demonstrated API stability under recommended storage conditions. Physical, chemical, therapeutic, and microbiological stability testing will also need to be repeated to comply with the updated requirements.

3.4.2. Regulatory Oversight and Safety of Compounded vs. Commercially Manufactured Drug Products

Drug regulatory agencies require preclinical and clinical studies to demonstrate the safety and efficacy of dosage forms prior to approval. Commercial manufacturing of approved formulations is regulated by national laws enforcing current good manufacturing practices (cGMP). In the US, cGMP regulations under the Federal Food, Drug, and Cosmetic Act (FD&C Act) set minimum standards for manufacturing, packaging, and marketing [63]. The WHO also issues cGMP guidelines, adopted into national laws by many countries [64]. In contrast, compounding pharmacies in most countries, including the US, are not subject to centralized regulatory oversight by agencies that govern pharmaceutical manufacturing, nor are they required to comply with cGMP. In the US, pharmacy practice, including compounding, is regulated by state boards of pharmacy. Most states require adherence to USP Chapter <795> for non-sterile compounding and Chapter <797> for sterile compounding. Compounded drugs are not held to the same safety, potency, or efficacy standards as those enforced by cGMP for commercially available products. Commercial drugs must include national FDA-approved labeling, whereas compounded drugs are subject only to state-level labeling rules. Adverse event reporting and FDA advertising regulations also do not apply to compounding pharmacies.

Extemporaneously compounded formulations have been associated with significant safety concerns. A 2001 FDA survey found that one-third of compounded products failed potency testing, compared to just 2% of the commercial drugs [65]. A 2006 follow-up revealed no improvement, with potencies ranging from 68% to 268%. Inconsistent procedures were implicated as likely contributors to safety issues. From 2001 to 2019, 1562 adverse events linked to compounding errors were reported in the US, including 116 deaths [66]. Common causes included contamination of sterile products, excipients of unknown grade, incorrect potencies, and mislabeling of ingredients. The lack of cGMP compliance and limited oversight were identified as key factors contributing to these incidents.

Sterile product compounding presents specific safety concerns. It remains uncertain whether USP <797> standards ensure sterility to the same degree as terminally sterilized, cGMP-manufactured products. Multiple outbreaks linked to bacteremia, blindness, and fungal meningitis have been traced to contaminated sterile preparations [67,68]. The 2012 fungal meningitis outbreak from preservative-free methylprednisolone resulted in 793 infections and 76 deaths, highlighting the dangers of large-scale compounding under lax oversight [69]. The growth of home infusion services and the outsourcing of parenteral products has expanded extemporaneous compounding beyond hospital pharmacies, leading to the creation of large-scale compounding facilities. These facilities resemble drug manufacturers but operate under pharmacy regulations. This regulatory gap contributed to the 2012 fungal meningitis outbreak [69].

In response, the 2013 Drug Quality and Security Act created Sections 503A and 503B of the FD&C Act [70]. Section 503A governs patient-specific compounding, regulated by state boards and USP standards. These pharmacies are not required to comply with cGMP but must conduct environmental monitoring and may establish expiration dates using internal or published stability data. Section 503B covers FDA-registered outsourcing facilities engaged in bulk compounding, which must comply with cGMP, register with the

https://doi.org/10.3390/pharmaceutics18010126

FDA and Drug Enforcement Agency, and undergo risk-based inspections. The US FDA maintains an active website that provides compounding risk alerts to inform health care professionals and compounders about risks associated with compounded drugs, including adverse events, outbreaks, and drug quality concerns. These alerts are intended to help practitioners more effectively protect patients from unsafe, ineffective, or poor-quality compounded medications [71]. Canada adopted a similar approach in 2009, with the Health Products and Food Branch Inspectorate distinguishing between compounding and manufacturing [72]. These adverse events have increased the legal liability of prescribers and compounding pharmacists. The FDA discourages compounding when approved alternatives exist, and professional societies now recommend informed consent when using compounded drugs as alternatives to commercially available dosage forms.

3.4.3. US and EU Regulatory Responses to Gaps in Pediatric Labeling and Formulations

The US legislative initiatives, the BPCA and PREA, encouraged pediatric drug development and labeling. Between 2002 and 2019, 768 products received pediatric labeling changes, 63% under PREA, 21% under BPCA, and 16% under both, demonstrating the stronger influence of PREA's mandatory approach compared to BPCA's voluntary incentive [73]. The EU's 2007 Paediatric Regulation led to significant advances in pediatric drug development, with over 260 child-specific authorizations by 2016 and more than 1000 pediatric investigation plans (PIPs) initiated [74]. Although 60% of PIPs were completed by 2019, only 55% qualified for extended market protection. These extensions delay competition and increase industry revenue, often at added cost to consumers and insurers.

Despite regulatory progress, only one-third of the drugs on the WHO EMLc have age-appropriate formulations, particularly for children aged 1–5 years. This gap persists largely because the EMLc primarily includes older or off-patent medications, which are not subject to the mandates or incentives provided under BPCA, PREA, or the EU Paediatric Regulation.

3.4.4. Standardizing Extemporaneous Formulation Concentrations to Improve Efficiency and Reduce Errors

Medication errors causing grievous harm can occur with extemporaneously compounded formulations even when stability data are available. The lack of standardized concentrations for extemporaneously compounded formulations poses a significant risk of medication errors, particularly for those formulations that have varying stability and BUDs for different concentrations. Patients and caregivers typically report drug doses in milliliters when the dosage form is a suspension or solution. However, when a drug has multiple extemporaneous formulations with different concentrations, failing to confirm the concentration being used by the patient can lead to dosing errors. Documenting the dose in milliliters without inquiring about the specific concentration may result in incorrect dosing. A medication error involving extemporaneous formulations is likely to occur when prescriptions are transferred between different settings (e.g., from inpatient to outpatient or from one healthcare institution to another) if the concentration of the compounded formulation varies at any step in the transition and the dose is not adjusted accordingly based on the concentration.

Standardization of these formulations could substantially reduce the incidence of medication errors during compounding, dispensing, or administration. The American Society of Health-System Pharmacists (ASHP) has recommended standardized concentrations for intravenous and oral liquid dosage forms for use across all healthcare settings [75]. This ASHP "Standardize 4 Safety Initiative" provides a list of standardized concentrations for intravenous medications and compounded oral liquids for both adult and pediatric

https://doi.org/10.3390/pharmaceutics18010126

patients. Healthcare systems are encouraged to adopt these standard concentrations to minimize medication errors in patient care.

3.4.5. Affordability of Extemporaneously Compounded Preparations

The costs of compounding, testing, and storing extemporaneous formulations pose significant challenges. Health systems operating 503A pharmacies, especially those with high compounding volume, may benefit from investing in in-house stability testing facilities. Reimbursement could help offset these expenses, but in the US, obtaining reimbursement can be difficult. Insurers may require time-consuming prior authorizations, and payment may not fully cover costs, particularly when using high-cost injectable ingredients. Many compounding pharmacies bill patients directly, increasing their financial burden.

In contrast, countries with nationally funded healthcare systems (e.g., much of Europe) are less affected by reimbursement limitations, while in nations without insurance coverage, such as parts of Africa and Asia, costs are typically paid out of pocket. Where demand is high, outsourcing to 503B facilities may offer a practical solution not only for patient-specific needs but also for supplying health systems more broadly. Further, economic modeling has been rarely done to establish the cost–benefit or cost-effectiveness of extemporaneous formulations.

4. Future Roadmap of Opportunities and Conclusions

The practice of extemporaneous compounding is essential in addressing the critical gap in medication availability for vulnerable pediatric populations, such as infants and children, who often require tailored or off-label dosage forms. Each country should identify the highest priorities based on its unique needs and resources to meet the needs of pediatric populations. Emerging extemporaneous solid dosage forms such as orodispersible films and 3D-printed compounds hold great promise for advancing personalized pharmacotherapy. However, their widespread use remains limited by technical, regulatory, quality control and cost constraints. While the necessity for individualized formulations cannot be overstated, the challenges associated with compounding practices, ranging from resource and expertise limitations to regulatory and reimbursement hurdles, pose significant barriers to effective implementation. In addition, default BUD frameworks and heterogeneous evidence for stability, preservative efficacy, and bioavailability introduce operational complexity that must be actively managed. Where feasible, standardizing concentration and documenting compatibility for enteral administration can further reduce error and variability. It is imperative for all stakeholders, including healthcare professionals, payors, and regulatory bodies, to collaborate on developing harmonized, risk-based guidelines and providing resources that enhance the safety, effectiveness, and accessibility of compounded medications in diverse health-system contexts. Global priorities include the needs for: (i) well-deigned and validated stability-indicating studies aligned with "a_w" and, where applicable, antimicrobial effectiveness testing; (ii) strengthened quality systems and control, training, and capacity-building (especially in low- and middle-income settings); (iii) documentation of outcomes studies of effectiveness, safety and patient- and caregiver acceptance and adherence of the formulations among patients when feasible; (iv) shared, open access formularies or repositories of validated formulations and standard concentrations adopted by hospital networks/consortia; (v) regulatory harmonization among countries; (vi) increased funding of research to improve the access and use of effective and safe extemporaneous formulations for infants and children; and (vii) reimbursement and procurement models that recognize the true cost of safe compounding in both publicly funded and out-of-pocket payment systems. By doing so, we can optimize

https://doi.org/10.3390/pharmaceutics18010126

therapeutic outcomes and ensure that all pediatric patients—regardless of region—receive the individualized care they deserve.

Author Contributions: Conceptualization, V.B.P. and M.C.N.; methodology, V.B.P. and M.C.N.; data curation V.B.P. and M.C.N.; writing—original draft preparation, V.B.P.; writing—review and editing, V.B.P. and M.C.N. All authors have read and agreed to the published version of the manuscript.

Funding: This research received no external funding.

Institutional Review Board Statement: Not applicable.

Informed Consent Statement: Not applicable.

Data Availability Statement: No new data were created or analyzed in this study.

Conflicts of Interest: The authors declare no conflicts of interest.

Abbreviations

The following abbreviations are used in this manuscript:

APIs	Active Pharmaceutical Ingredients
ASHP	American Society of Health-System Pharmacists
BPCA	Best Pharmaceuticals for Children Act
BUDs	Beyond-Use Dates
C	Compounded
CSPs	Compounded Sterile Preparations
cGMP	current Good Manufacturing Practices
EMA	European Medicines Agency
EU	European Union
FD&C Act	Federal Food, Drug, and Cosmetic Act
FDA	Food and Drug Administration
ISO	International Standards Organization
M	Manipulated
EMLc	Model List of Essential Medicines for Children
NG	Nasogastric
NJ	Nasojejunal
NF	National Formulary
PIPs	Pediatric Investigation plans
PREA	Pediatric Research Equity Act
Rx's	Prescriptions
3-D	Three-dimensional
US	United States of America
USP	United States Pharmacopeia
WHO	World Health Organization

References

1. Higby, G.J. Lewis & Clark Bought Imported Drugs!! Apothecary's Cabinet 2004, No. 8 (Fall). Available online: https://aihp.org/wp-content/uploads/2017/07/AC8.pdf (accessed on 9 January 2026).
2. Minghetti, P.; Pantano, D.; Gennari, C.G.M.; Casiraghi, A. Regulatory framework of pharmaceutical compounding and actual developments of legislation in Europe. *Health Policy* **2014**, *117*, 328–333. [CrossRef]
3. Daemmrich, A. Pharmaceutical Manufacturing in America: A Brief History. *Pharm. Hist.* **2017**, *59*, 63–72. [CrossRef]
4. American Pharmacists Association. Frequently Asked Questions About Pharmaceutical Compounding. Available online: https://www.pharmacist.com/Practice/Patient-Care-Services/Compounding/Compounding-FAQs (accessed on 15 May 2025).
5. U.S. Pharmacopeial Convention; United States Pharmacopeial Compounding Compendium. *General Chapter <795> Pharmaceutical Compounding—Nonsterile Preparations*; USP-NF 2022, Issue 3; U.S. Pharmacopeial Convention: Rockville, MD, USA, 2022.

https://doi.org/10.3390/pharmaceutics18010126

6. European Union. Directive 2001/83/EC of the European Parliament and of the Council of 6 November 2001 on the Community Code Relating to Medicinal Products for Human Use. Available online: https://eur-lex.europa.eu/eli/dir/2001/83/oj (accessed on 15 May 2025).
7. Petkova, V.; Georgieva, D.; Dimitrov, M.; Nikolova, I. Off-Label Prescribing in Pediatric Population—Literature Review for 2012–2022. *Pharmaceutics* **2023**, *15*, 2652. [CrossRef]
8. Yuliani, S.H.; Putri, D.C.A.; Virginia, D.M.; Gani, M.R.; Riswanto, F.D.O. Prevalence, Risk, and Challenges of Extemporaneous Preparation for Pediatric Patients in Developing Nations: A Review. *Pharmaceutics* **2023**, *15*, 840. [CrossRef] [PubMed]
9. Harman, J.L.; Scott, A.; Jurbergs, N. Pill-Swallowing Training in Very Young Children with Cancer: A Case Series and Developmental Considerations. *J. Pediatr. Oncol. Nurs.* **2020**, *38*, 61–63. [CrossRef] [PubMed]
10. McCloskey, A.P.; Penson, P.E.; Tse, Y.; Abdelhafiz, M.A.; Ahmed, S.N.; Lim, E.J. Identifying and addressing pill aversion in adults without physiological-related dysphagia: A narrative review. *Br. J. Clin. Pharmacol.* **2022**, *88*, 5128–5148. [CrossRef]
11. U.S. Food and Drug Administration. Drugs@FDA: FDA-Approved Drugs. Available online: https://www.accessdata.fda.gov/scripts/cder/daf/index.cfm?event=overview.process&ApplNo=018667 (accessed on 9 January 2026).
12. Dooms, M.; Carvalho, M. Compounded medication for patients with rare diseases. *Orphanet J. Rare Dis.* **2018**, *13*, 1. [CrossRef] [PubMed]
13. Staubach, P.; Salzmann, S.; Peveling-Oberhag, A.; Weyer, V.; Zimmer, S.; Gradl, G.; Lang, B.M. Extemporaneous formulations in Germany—Relevance for everyday clinical practice. *JDDG J. Der Dtsch. Dermatol. Ges.* **2018**, *16*, 566–574. [CrossRef]
14. Chang, R.-K.; Raw, A.; Lionberger, R.; Yu, L. Generic Development of Topical Dermatologic Products: Formulation Development, Process Development, and Testing of Topical Dermatologic Products. *AAPS J.* **2012**, *15*, 41–52. [CrossRef]
15. Selam, M.N.; Ababu, A. Extemporaneous Compounding Practice for Dermatologic Preparations in Ethiopian Public Hospitals: Regulatory Requirements and Quality Concerns. *Risk Manag. Healthc. Policy* **2021**, *ume 14*, 1933–1938. [CrossRef]
16. Latta, K.S. Extemporaneous Compounding of Pain and Symptom Control Medications. *J. Pain Palliat. Care Pharmacother.* **2002**, *16*, 51–60. [CrossRef]
17. Sylvester, R.K.; Schauer, C.; Thomas, J.; Steen, P.; Weisenberger, A. Evaluation of Methadone Absorption After Topical Administration to Hospice Patients. *J. Pain Symptom Manag.* **2011**, *41*, 828–835. [CrossRef]
18. Ancedy, D.; Sebti, M.; Postaire, M.; Vidal, F.; Cisternino, S.; Schlatter, J. Stability of 10-mg/mL and 50-mg/mL ketamine oral solutions. *Am. J. Health-Syst. Pharm.* **2021**, *78*, 825–831. [CrossRef] [PubMed]
19. American Society of Health-System Pharmacists. Drug Shortages List. Available online: https://www.ashp.org/drug-shortages/current-shortages/drug-shortages-list?loginreturnUrl=SSOCheckOnly (accessed on 9 January 2026).
20. American Society of Health System Pharmacists. Amoxicillin Oral Presentations. Available online: https://www.ashp.org/drug-shortages/current-shortages/drug-shortage-detail.aspx?id=875&loginreturnUrl=SSOCheckOnly (accessed on 9 January 2026).
21. American Society of Health-System Pharmacists. Drug Shortage Statistics: National Drug Shortages January 2001 to March 2025. Available online: https://www.ashp.org/drug-shortages/shortage-resources/drug-shortages-statistics (accessed on 15 May 2025).
22. National Institutes of Health. Best Pharmaceuticals for Children Act (BPCA). Available online: https://www.nichd.nih.gov/research/supported/bpca/about (accessed on 22 April 2025).
23. U.S. Food and Drug Administration. Pediatric Research Equity Act (PREA). Available online: https://www.fda.gov/drugs/development-resources/pediatric-research-equity-act-prea (accessed on 15 May 2025).
24. European Union. Regulation (EC) No 1901/2006 of the European Parliament and of the Council of 12 December 2006 on Medicinal Products for Paediatric Use and Amending Regulation (EEC) No 1768/92, Directive 2001/20/EC, Directive 2001/83/EC and Regulation (EC) No 726/2004 (Text with EEA Relevance). Available online: https://eur-lex.europa.eu/eli/reg/2006/1901/oj (accessed on 15 May 2025).
25. World Health Organization. Web Annex B: WHO Model List of Essential Medicines for Children—9th List, 2023. In *The Selection and Use of Essential Medicines 2023: Executive Summary of the Report of the 24th WHO Expert Committee on the Selection and Use of Essential Medicines, 24–28 April 2023*; WHO/MHP/HPS/EML/2023.03; World Health Organization: Geneva, Switzerland, 2023.
26. Fadda, H.M.; Weiler, H.; Carvalho, M.; Lee, Y.Z.; Dassouki, H.; AbuBlan, R.; Iurian, S.; Hamid, A.; Şeremet, G.; Li, Z.; et al. Pediatric oral extemporaneous preparations and practices: International Pharmaceutical Federation (FIP) global study. *Eur. J. Pharm. Biopharm.* **2024**, *204*, 114483. [CrossRef] [PubMed]
27. Brion, F.; Nunn, A.; Rieutord, A. Extemporaneous (magistral) preparation of oral medicines for children in European hospitals. *Acta Paediatr.* **2003**, *92*, 486–490. [CrossRef]
28. Buurma, H.; de Smet, P.A.G.M.; van den Hoff, O.P.; Sysling, H.; Storimans, M.; Egberts, A.C.G. Frequency, nature and determinants of pharmacy compounded medicines in Dutch community pharmacies. *Pharm. World Sci.* **2003**, *25*, 280–287. [CrossRef] [PubMed]
29. McPherson, T.B.; Fontane, P.E.; Jackson, K.D.; Berry, T.; Chereson, R.; Bilger, R.; Martin, K.S. Prevalence of Compounding in Independent Community Pharmacy Practice. *J. Am. Pharm. Assoc.* **2006**, *46*, 568–573. [CrossRef]
30. Martin, K.S.; McPherson, T.B.; Fontane, P.E.; Berry, T.; Chereson, R.; Bilger, R. Independent Community Pharmacists' Perspectives on Compounding in Contemporary Pharmacy Education. *Am. J. Pharm. Educ.* **2009**, *73*, 54. [CrossRef]

31. Kairuz, T.; Chhim, S.; Hasan, F.; Kumar, K.; Lal, A.; Patel, R.; Singh, R.; Dogra, M.; Garg, S. Extemporaneous compounding in a sample of New Zealand hospitals: A retrospective survey. *N. Z. Med. J.* **2007**, *120*, U2466.
32. Lugo, R.; Cash, J.; Trimby, R.; Ward, R.; Spielberg, S. A Survey of Children's Hospitals on the Use of Extemporaneous Liquid Formulations in the Inpatient Setting. *J. Pediatr. Pharmacol. Ther.* **2009**, *14*, 154–192. [CrossRef]
33. Zaid, A.N.; Al-Ramahi, R.; Shahed, Q.; Saleh, B.; Elaraj, J. Determinants and Frequency of Pharmaceutical Compounding in Pharmacy Practice in Palestine. *Int. J. Pharm. Pract.* **2012**, *20*, 9–14. [CrossRef] [PubMed]
34. Richey, R.H.; Shah, U.U.; Peak, M.; Craig, J.V.; Ford, J.L.; Barker, C.E.; Nunn, A.J.; Turner, M.A. Manipulation of drugs to achieve the required dose is intrinsic to paediatric practice but is not supported by guidelines or evidence. *BMC Pediatr.* **2013**, *13*, 81. [CrossRef]
35. Masupye, E.M.; Suleman, F.; Govender, T. Investigating extemporaneous compounding practices in the Polokwane tertiary hospital pharmacies in South Africa—A pilot study. *Afr. J. Pharm. Pharmacol.* **2015**, *9*, 1099–1105. [CrossRef]
36. Bjerknes, K.; Bøyum, S.; Kristensen, S.; Brustugun, J.; Wang, S. Manipulating tablets and capsules given to hospitalised children in Norway is common practice. *Acta Paediatr.* **2017**, *106*, 503–508. [CrossRef] [PubMed]
37. Hapsari, I.; Marchaban, M.; Wiedyaningsih, C.; Kristina, S.A. The Extemporaneous Compounding at Primary Health Care Centers: Characteristic and Personnel. *Glob. J. Health Sci.* **2018**, *10*, 112. [CrossRef]
38. Kristina, S.A.; Wiedyaningsih, C.; Widyakusuma, N.N.; Aditama, H. Profile and Determinants of Com-pounding Services among Pharmacists in Indonesia. *Asian J. Pharm.* **2018**, *12*, S966–S972.
39. AlKhatib, H.S.; Jalouqa, S.; Maraqa, N.; Ratka, A.; Elayeh, E.; Al Muhaissen, S. Prevalence, determinants, and characteristics of extemporaneous compounding in Jordanian pharmacies. *BMC Health Serv. Res.* **2019**, *19*, 816. [CrossRef]
40. Yusuff, K.B. Extent of extemporaneous compounding and pattern of prescribing and use of extemporaneous medicines in a developing setting. *J. Pharm. Health Serv. Res.* **2019**, *10*, 255–260. [CrossRef]
41. Pitchayajittipong, C.; Sriboon, S.; Kulmee, S.; Prachuabaree, L.; Srisawai, K.; Wattanawong, W.; Sripa, S.; Anderson, C.; Supapaan, T. An Overview of Pharmaceutical Production in Thai Hospitals. *Hosp. Pharm.* **2019**, *56*, 265–275. [CrossRef]
42. Tiengkate, P.; Lallemant, M.; Charoenkwan, P.; Angkurawaranon, C.; Kanjanarat, P.; Suwannaprom, P.; Borriharn, P. Gaps in Accessibility of Pediatric Formulations: A Cross-Sectional Observational Study of a Teaching Hospital in Northern Thailand. *Children* **2022**, *9*, 301. [CrossRef]
43. Ramtoola, Z.; Catibusic, A.; Ameen, H.; Cullen, S.; Barlow, J.W. Evaluation of the type and frequency of extemporaneous formulations dispensed in hospital and community pharmacies. *Explor. Res. Clin. Soc. Pharm.* **2023**, *12*, 100380. [CrossRef] [PubMed]
44. Supapaan, T.S.; Jamlongpeng, C.; Yangyuen, N.; Srisawai, K.; Prachuabaree, L.; Wattanawong, W.; Anansushatgul, J.; Songmuang, T.; Sripa, S.; Pitchayajittipong, C. Enhancing extemporaneous preparations in Thai Hospitals: Exploring variation, common formulations, and challenges and needs related to extemporaneous preparations. *Pharm. Pr. (Internet)* **2024**, *21*, 01–12. [CrossRef]
45. U.S. Pharmacopeial Convention; USP Compounding Compendium. *Section 4—Compounded Preparation Monographs*, June ed.; U.S. Pharmacopeial Convention: Rockville, MD, USA, 2022.
46. Taketomo, C.K. *Lexicomp Pediatric and Neonatal Dosage Handbook*, 30th ed.; Wolters Kluwer: Riverwoods, IL, USA, 2023.
47. Nahata, M.C.; Pai, V.B. *Pediatric Drug Formulations*, 7th ed.; Harvey Whitney Books Company: Cincinnati, OH, USA, 2018.
48. Jew, R.K.; Soo-Hoo, W.; Amiri, E.; Gomes, J.M. *Extemporaneous Formulations for Pediatric, Geriatric, and Special Needs Patients*, 4th ed.; eBook; American Society of Health-System Pharmacists: Bethesda, MD, USA, 2021.
49. U.S. Pharmacopeial Convention; United States Pharmacopeial Compounding Compendium. *General Chapter <795> Pharmaceutical Compounding—Nonsterile Preparations*; USP-NF 2023, Issue 1; U.S. Pharmacopeial Convention: Rockville, MD, USA, 2023.
50. American Society of Health-System Pharmacists. ASHP Technical Assistance Bulletin on Compounding Nonsterile Products in Pharmacies. Technical Bulletins Published by ASHP. Available online: http://12.53.28.72/pharmacy-practice/policy-positions-and-guidelines/browse-by-document-type/technical-assistance-bulletins?loginreturnUrl=SSOCheckOnly (accessed on 17 May 2025).
51. Taneja, R.; Nahata, M.C.; Scarim, J.; Pande, P.G.; Scarim, A.; Hoddinott, G.; Fourie, C.L.; Jew, R.K.; Schaaf, H.S.; Garcia-Prats, A.J.; et al. Stable, compounded bedaquiline suspensions to support practical implementation of pediatric dosing in the field. *Int. J. Tuberc. Lung Dis.* **2023**, *27*, 189–194. [CrossRef]
52. Tekade, R.K. *Basic Fundamentals of Drug Delivery*; Elsevier: Amsterdam, The Netherlands, 2019.
53. Belayneh, A.; Tadese, E.; Molla, F. Safety and Biopharmaceutical Challenges of Excipients in Off-Label Pediatric Formulations. *Int. J. Gen. Med.* **2020**, *ume 13*, 1051–1066. [CrossRef]
54. Rouaz, K.; Chiclana-Rodríguez, B.; Nardi-Ricart, A.; Suñé-Pou, M.; Mercadé-Frutos, D.; Suñé-Negre, J.M.; Pérez-Lozano, P.; García-Montoya, E. Excipients in the Paediatric Population: A Review. *Pharmaceutics* **2021**, *13*, 387. [CrossRef]
55. Lam, J.K.; Xu, Y.; Worsley, A.; Wong, I.C. Oral transmucosal drug delivery for pediatric use. *Adv. Drug Deliv. Rev.* **2014**, *73*, 50–62. [CrossRef]
56. Khan, Q.-U.; Siddique, M.I.; Sarfraz, M.; Rehman, K.; Sohail, M.F.; Katas, H. Oral Dispersible Films from Product Development to End-User Acceptability: A Review. *Crit. Rev. Ther. Drug Carr. Syst.* **2022**, *39*, 33–64. [CrossRef]

https://doi.org/10.3390/pharmaceutics18010126

57. Khadivi, Y.; Monajjemzadeh, F. Advancement in the Formulation and development of orally disintegrating tablets: Innovation, challenges, and future perspective. *J. Drug Deliv. Sci. Technol.* **2025**, *108*. [CrossRef]
58. Beer, N.; Kaae, S.; Genina, N.; Sporrong, S.K.; Alves, T.L.; Hoebert, J.; De Bruin, M.L.; Hegger, I. Magistral Compounding with 3D Printing: A Promising Way to Achieve Personalized Medicine. *Ther. Innov. Regul. Sci.* **2022**, *57*, 26–36. [CrossRef] [PubMed]
59. Gayakwad, S.; Patel, A.; Shah, N. A Review of 3D Printing Techniques for Dosage Form Development. *Int. J. Pharm. Sci.* **2025**, *3*, 3032–3048. [CrossRef]
60. Cheng, H.; Ta, Y.N.; Hsia, T.; Chen, Y. A quantitative review of nanotechnology-based therapeutics for kidney diseases. *WIREs Nanomed. Nanobiotechnol.* **2024**, *16*, e1953. [CrossRef]
61. Lv, L.V.A.; Erickson, M.A. Stability of baclofen, captopril, diltiazem hydrochloride, dipyridamole, and flecainide acetate in extemporaneously compounded oral liquids. *Am. J. Health-Syst. Pharm.* **1996**, *53*, 2179–2184. [CrossRef]
62. U.S. Pharmacopeial Convention; United States Pharmacopeial Compounding Compendium. *General Chapter <51> Antimicrobial Effectiveness Testing*; USP-NF 2022, Issue 3; U.S. Pharmacopeial Convention: Rockville, MD, USA, 2022.
63. Center for Drug Evaluation and Research. Current Good Manufacturing Practice (CGMP) Regulations. FDA. Available online: https://www.fda.gov/drugs/pharmaceutical-quality-resources/current-good-manufacturing-practice-cgmp-regulations (accessed on 30 December 2021).
64. World Health Organization. Good Manufacturing Practices. Available online: https://www.who.int/teams/health-product-policy-and-standards/standards-and-specifications/norms-and-standards/gmp (accessed on 22 April 2025).
65. Gudeman, J.; Jozwiakowski, M.; Chollet, J.; Randell, M. Potential Risks of Pharmacy Compounding. *Drugs R&D* **2013**, *13*, 1–8. [CrossRef]
66. The Pew Charitable Trusts. U.S. Illnesses and Deaths Tied to Compounded or Repackaged Medications, 2001–2019. Available online: https://www.pewtrusts.org/en/research-and-analysis/data-visualizations/2020/us-illnesses-and-deaths-associated-with-compounded-or-repackaged-medications-2001-19 (accessed on 22 April 2025).
67. Staes, C.; Jacobs, J.; Mayer, J.; Allen, J. Description of outbreaks of health-care-associated infections related to compounding pharmacies, 2000–2012. *Am. J. Health-Syst. Pharm.* **2013**, *70*, 1301–1312. [CrossRef] [PubMed]
68. Gonzalez, S.; Rosenfeld, P.J.; Stewart, M.W.; Brown, J.; Murphy, S.P. Avastin Doesn't Blind People, People Blind People. *Arch. Ophthalmol.* **2012**, *153*, 196–203.e1. [CrossRef] [PubMed]
69. Arnold, C. Fungal meningitis outbreak affects over 700. *Lancet Neurol.* **2013**, *12*, 429–430. [CrossRef] [PubMed]
70. United States Food and Drug Administration. Food, Drug, and Cosmetic Act: Provisions that Apply to Human Drug Compounding. Available online: https://www.fda.gov/drugs/human-drug-compounding/compounding-laws-and-policies (accessed on 22 April 2025).
71. U.S. Food and Drug Administration. Compounding Risk Alerts. Available online: https://www.fda.gov/drugs/human-drug-compounding/compounding-risk-alerts (accessed on 19 November 2025).
72. Health Products and Food Branch Inspectorate. Policy on Manufacturing and Compounding Drug Products in Canada (POL-0051). Available online: https://www.canada.ca/en/health-canada/services/drugs-health-products/compliance-enforcement/good-manufacturing-practices/guidance-documents/policy-manufacturing-compounding-drug-products.html (accessed on 22 April 2025).
73. United States Department of Health and Human Services; Food and Drug Administration; Center for Drug Evaluation and Research (CDER); Center for Biologics Evaluation and Research. Pediatric Drug Development: Regulatory Considerations—Complying with the Pediatric Research Equity Act and Qualifying for Pediatric Exclusivity Under the Best Pharmaceuticals for Children Act. Available online: https://www.fda.gov/regulatory-information/search-fda-guidance-documents/pediatric-drug-development-regulatory-considerations-complying-pediatric-research-equity-act-and (accessed on 22 April 2025).
74. European Union. State of Paediatric Medicines in the EU. 10 Years of the EU Paediatric Regulation. Report from the Commission to the European Parliament and the Council. Available online: https://health.ec.europa.eu/system/files/2017-11/2017_childrensmedicines_report_en_0.pdf (accessed on 22 April 2025).
75. American Society of Health-System Pharmacists. Standardize 4 Safety Initiative. Available online: https://www.ashp.org/pharmacy-practice/standardize-4-safety-initiative (accessed on 22 April 2025).

pharmaceutics

MDPI

Review

Extemporaneous Compounding, Pharmacy Preparations and Related Product Care in the Netherlands

Herman J. Woerdenbag [1,*], Boy van Basten [2], Christien Oussoren [3], Oscar S. N. M. Smeets [3], Astrid Annaciri-Donkers [3], Mirjam Crul [4], J. Marina Maurer [5], Kirsten J. M. Schimmel [6], E. Marleen Kemper [7], Marjolijn N. Lub-de Hooge [5], Nanno Schreuder [8], Melissa Eikmann [9], Arwin S. Ramcharan [9], Richard B. Lantink [10], Julian Quodbach [11], Hendrikus H. Boersma [5], Oscar Kelder [12], Karin H. M. Larmené-Beld [13], Paul P. H. Le Brun [6], Robbert Jan Kok [11], Reinout C. A. Schellekens [14], Oscar Breukels [15], Henderik W. Frijlink [1] and Bahez Gareb [5]

[1] Department of Pharmaceutical Technology and Biopharmacy, Groningen Research Institute of Pharmacy (GRIP), University of Groningen, Antonius Deusinglaan 1, 9713 AV Groningen, The Netherlands; h.w.frijlink@rug.nl

[2] Department of Pharmaceutical Technology and Biopharmacy, School of Science and Engineering (SSE), University of Groningen, Antonius Deusinglaan 1, 9713 AV Groningen, The Netherlands; b.van.basten@rug.nl

[3] Royal Dutch Pharmacists Association (KNMP), Alexanderstraat 11, 2514 JL Den Haag, The Netherlands; c.oussoren@knmp.nl (C.O.); o.s.n.m.smeets@knmp.nl (O.S.N.M.S.); a.annaciri-donkers@knmp.nl (A.A.-D.)

[4] Department of Clinical Pharmacology and Pharmacy, Amsterdam University Medical Center, Location Vrije Universiteit, De Boelelaan 1117, 1081 HV Amsterdam, The Netherlands; m.crul@amsterdamumc.nl

[5] Department of Clinical Pharmacy and Pharmacology, University Medical Center Groningen (UMCG), Hanzeplein 1, 9713 GZ Groningen, The Netherlands; m.maurer@umcg.nl (J.M.M.); m.n.de.hooge@umcg.nl (M.N.L.-d.H.); h.h.boersma@umcg.nl (H.H.B.); b.gareb01@umcg.nl (B.G.)

[6] Department of Clinical Pharmacy and Toxicology, Leiden University Medical Center (LUMC), Albinusdreef 2, 2333 ZA Leiden, The Netherlands; k.j.m.schimmel@lumc.nl (K.J.M.S.); pphlebrun@icloud.com (P.P.H.L.B.)

[7] Apotheek A15, Buys Ballotstraat 2, 4207 HT Gorinchem, The Netherlands; m.kemper@apotheeka15.nl

[8] GE HealthCare Radiopharmacy Zwolle, Dokter Spanjaardweg 1A, 8025 AC Zwolle, The Netherlands; nanno.schreuder@gehealthcare.com

[9] Transvaal Apotheek, Kempstraat 113, 2572 GC Den Haag, The Netherlands; m.eikmann@transvaalapotheek.nl (M.E.); a.ramcharan@transvaalapotheek.nl (A.S.R.)

[10] Laboratorium Ofichem, Heembadweg 5, 9561 CZ Ter Apel, The Netherlands; lantink@ofichem.com

[11] Division of Pharmaceutics, Utrecht Institute for Pharmaceutical Sciences (UIPS), Utrecht University, Universiteitsweg 99, 3584 GC Utrecht, The Netherlands; j.h.j.quodbach@uu.nl (J.Q.); r.j.kok@uu.nl (R.J.K.)

[12] Ziekenhuis Groep Twente (ZGT) Apotheek, Boerhaavelaan 63, 7555 BB Hengelo, The Netherlands; okelder@home.nl

[13] Department of Clinical Pharmacy, Isala Hospital, Dokter van Heesweg 2, 8025 AB Zwolle, The Netherlands; k.h.m.beld@isala.nl

[14] Fagron Sterile Services Nederland, Dieselstraat 3, 7903 AR Hoogeveen, The Netherlands; reinout.schellekens@fagron.nl

[15] Department of Hospital Pharmacy, Meander Medisch Centrum Amersfoort, Maatweg 3, 3813 TZ Amersfoort, The Netherlands; o.breukels@meandermc.nl

* Correspondence: h.j.woerdenbag@rug.nl

Abstract

Background/Objectives: In many parts of the world, pharmacists hold the primary responsibility for providing safe and effective pharmacotherapy. A key aspect is the availability of appropriate medicines for each individual patient. When industrially manufactured medicines are unsuitable or unavailable, pharmacists can prepare tailor-made medicines. While this principle applies globally, practices vary between countries. In the Netherlands, the preparation of medicines in pharmacies is well-established and integrated into routine healthcare. This narrative review explores the role and significance of extemporaneous compounding, pharmacy preparations and related product care in the Netherlands. **Methods**: Pharmacists involved in pharmacy preparations across various professional sectors, including community and hospital pharmacies, central compounding facilities, academia, and the professional pharmacists' organisation, provided detailed and expert insights based on the literature and policy documents while also sharing their critical perspectives. **Results**: We present arguments supporting the need for pharmacy preparations and examine their position and role in community and hospital pharmacies in the Netherlands. Additional topics are discussed, including the regulatory and legal framework, outsourcing, quality assurance, standardisation, education, and international context. Specific pharmacy preparation topics, often with a research component and a strong focus on product care, are highlighted, including paediatric dosage forms, swallowing difficulties and feeding tubes, hospital-at-home care, reconstitution of oncolytic drugs and biologicals, total parenteral nutrition (TPN), advanced therapy medicinal products (ATMPs), radiopharmaceuticals and optical tracers, clinical trial medication, robotisation in reconstitution, and patient-centric solid oral dosage forms. **Conclusions**: The widespread acceptance of pharmacy preparations in the Netherlands is the result of a unique combination of strict adherence to tailored regulations that ensure quality and safety, and patient-oriented flexibility in design, formulation, and production. This approach is further reinforced by the standardisation of a broad range of formulations and procedures across primary, secondary and tertiary care, as well as by continuous research-driven innovation to develop new medicines, formulations, and production methods.

Keywords: advanced therapy medicinal products (ATMPs); biologicals; community pharmacy; extemporaneous compounding; hospital pharmacy; legislation and regulations; oncolytic medicinal products; personalised medicine; pharmaceutical product care; pharmacy education; pharmacy preparations; radiopharmaceuticals; total parenteral nutrition (TPN)

1. Introduction and Aim

Pharmacists are an indispensable link in the healthcare chain, providing reliable pharmaceutical care to patients globally. Yet, while this core task is universal, specifics will differ from country to country, guided by national laws, regulations, customs and history. In the Netherlands, both community and hospital pharmacists legally share responsibility with other healthcare professionals for the pharmacotherapeutic treatment of patients. Dutch pharmacists are heavily involved in patient-centred tasks, such as counselling, instructing correct medication use, informing about possible adverse reactions, and supplying patients with the most appropriate medicine, either licensed or unlicensed [1].

Most prescribed and dispensed medicines are industrially manufactured and often mass-produced. These medicines are licensed, meaning that marketing authorisation has been granted following a registration procedure via a competent authority such as the European Medicines Agency (EMA) [2], or a national equivalent such as the Medicines Evaluation Board (MEB) (Dutch: College ter Beoordeling van Geneesmiddelen; CBG) in the Netherlands [3]. This procedure and the subsequent authorisation ensure the quality, effectiveness and safety of a pharmaceutical product. Although the vast majority of prescriptions in the Netherlands involve registered medicines nowadays [4,5], the market cannot always (sufficiently) provide the optimal medication for each specific patient or patient group. In such cases, pharmacists are allowed to either prepare (customised) medicines or outsource the preparation thereof to specialised central compounding facilities before dispensing them to the patient. This practice is known as extemporaneous compounding, yielding so-called pharmacy preparations [6].

Worldwide, extemporaneous compounding is acknowledged and defined as the practice in which a licensed pharmacist, or a person under the supervision of a licensed pharmacist, mixes or alters ingredients based on a prescription to create a pharmacy preparation tailored to the medical needs of an individual patient or patient group, in cases where treatment with a commercially available medicinal product is not possible [7–10]. In Europe, pharmacy preparations are considered indispensable for meeting the specific demands of individual patients [7,10]. They are an integral part of daily pharmacy practice in the Netherlands, though the extent varies depending on the pharmacy setting, and they fall under the umbrella of pharmaceutical product care.

In the Netherlands, the concept of pharmaceutical product care refers to ensuring that patients receive the most appropriate medicine upon prescription, in an optimal dosage form, and of the highest possible quality. It encompasses the procurement, storage, preparation (or outsourcing thereof, where applicable), and dispensing of medicines, along with providing patients with instructions on their use. Pharmaceutical product care is intrinsically linked to effective pharmacotherapeutic treatment and pharmaceutical patient care [11].

Non-industrially prepared medicines are unlicensed; they lack the rigorous governmental control of licensed products. Extemporaneous compounding, however, is closely regulated in the Netherlands. To ensure quality and safety, pharmacists must adhere to specific guidelines and rules that have been developed based on those for industrially manufactured products, such as Good Manufacturing Practice (GMP) [12–14], International Conference on Harmonisation (ICH) [15], and Pharmaceutical Inspection Convention/Pharmaceutical Inspection Co-operation Scheme (PIC/s) [16]. Furthermore, as a member state of the European Union (EU), all medicinal products should comply with the European Pharmacopoeia (Ph. Eur.) monograph 'Pharmaceutical Preparations' [6].

Knowledge of a product's composition, structure, and functionality, as well as the production process and the implications of its properties for efficacy and safety, primarily falls within the domain of pharmacists. They are the only healthcare professionals who combine pharmaceutical–technological insight with pharmacotherapeutic knowledge to cater to specific patient needs. Product knowledge is essential for responding to clinical enquiries. It is also essential for making informed purchasing decisions and for ensuring safe working conditions in a pharmacy environment, particularly in managing health risks for staff handling or preparing medicines [1].

A comprehensive six-year university programme, integrating scientific, practical, and clinical training, equips future pharmacists in the Netherlands with the knowledge and competencies required to meet professional standards [1,17]. The Royal Dutch Pharmacists Association (Dutch: Koninklijke Nederlandse Maatschappij ter bevordering der Pharmacie; KNMP) supports the professional field through standards, guidelines, knowledge bases, and helpdesks. Information and guidance are aligned with the latest scientific and practice-oriented developments [18,19]. Specific professional support for hospital pharmacists is provided by the Dutch Association of Hospital Pharmacists (Dutch: Nederlandse Vereniging voor Ziekenhuisapothekers; NVZA) [20].

This article aims to provide a comprehensive overview of the current state of extemporaneous compounding, pharmacy preparations and related product care within the pharmaceutical profession and healthcare system in the Netherlands. Topics presented and discussed include the types of pharmacy preparations and clinical needs, the organisation around pharmacy preparations in community and hospital pharmacies, the regulatory and legal framework, outsourcing, quality assurance, education, and international benchmarking. Specific topics linked to pharmacy preparations, often with a research component and a strong focus on product care, are highlighted: optimising individual treatment, specialist product groups, and technological innovations. Paediatric dosage forms, swallowing difficulties and feeding tubes, hospital-at-home care, reconstitution of oncolytic drugs and biologicals, total parenteral nutrition (TPN), advanced therapy medicinal products (ATMPs), radiopharmaceuticals and optical tracers, clinical trial medication, robotisation in reconstitution, and patient-centric solid oral dosage forms are addressed. Good practices are highlighted and examples from practice are given.

2. Rationale of Pharmacy Preparations

2.1. What to Dispense

Upon receiving a prescription from a healthcare provider, the pharmacist is responsible for verifying the pharmacotherapeutic rationale, a prerequisite for dispensing any medicinal product to a patient. In most cases (>95% of all prescriptions), the first choice is a licensed commercially available product [5]. If such a product is not available, or unable to provide the best solution for the patient, a standardised pharmacy preparation is preferred. If that is also not available, a non-standardised pharmacy preparation may be considered. A non-standardised pharmacy preparation can be an unvalidated modification of a standardised preparation while adhering to general and established procedures for preparing specific dosage forms (see Section 5.2). It can also be a product formulation that is designed from scratch; however, this carries the highest risk of quality loss. Only a minimal set of quality requirements is available, and the composition, stability, and biopharmaceutical performance may not be scientifically validated. Figure 1 shows the decision tree to be followed.

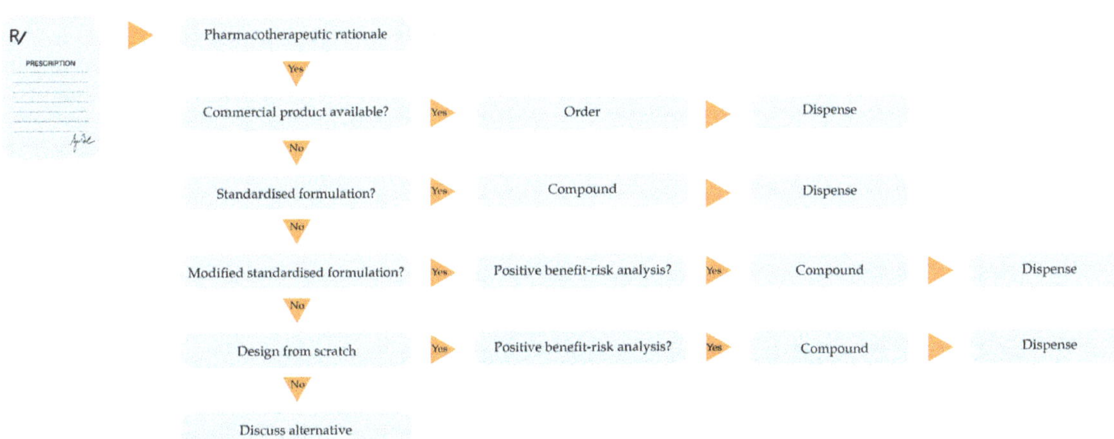
R/
PRESCRIPTION
Pharmacotherapeutic rationale
Yes
Commercial product available?
Yes
Order
Dispense
No
Standardised formulation?
Yes
Compound
Dispense
No
Modified standardised formulation?
Yes
Positive benefit-risk analysis?
Yes
Compound
Dispense
No
Design from scratch
Yes
Positive benefit-risk analysis?
Yes
Compound
Dispense
No
Discuss alternative

Figure 1. Decision tree for the medicinal product to be dispensed to a patient upon receipt of a prescription from a healthcare provider; based on [21].

In all cases, a benefit–risk assessment should be conducted on the pharmacotherapeutic benefit against any potential loss of product quality. In this context, it is important to consider that, in most instances, a non-standardised or self-designed product will be made for a single patient. If the pharmacy preparation does not meet the highest possible quality level but can provide the best therapy to the patient, the benefit–risk assessment may favour it. An alternative, especially in community pharmacy, may be to consider together with the prescriber a different commercially available or a different standardised product as a substitute, provided that the desired pharmacotherapeutic outcome will be similar [21]. In hospital pharmacy, however, it more frequently occurs that the only treatment option for a patient is a substantiated and well-considered ad hoc preparation.

2.2. Types of Pharmacy Preparations

Three types of pharmacy preparations are distinguished and covered by Dutch guidelines: (1) products entirely prepared from raw materials, (2) the modification of commercially available products, and (3) the reconstitution of purpose-designed products [22–24]. Always, product care is essential to obtain a high-quality and safe product.

Modifying a licensed product beyond its Summary of Product Characteristics (SmPC) yields an unlicensed product, shifting the responsibility for quality from the industrial manufacturer to the compounding pharmacist. Since this practice is associated with pharmaceutical–technological and biopharmaceutical challenges, in-depth product knowledge is required. Examples are pulverising tablets and mixing the powder with excipients to make capsules, and the conversion of an oral solid dosage form into an oral liquid dosage form such as a suspension.

In the case of reconstitution, a licensed product is designed to undergo final handling as specified in the SmPC before it is administered to a patient. A reconstituted product remains licensed [25]. Reconstitution of a product is classified as a manipulation rather than compounding in regulatory frameworks [12–16,22]. However, similar handlings are carried out while maintaining comparable product care measures. Reconstitution is common in both community and hospital pharmacies. Examples include reconstitution of an injection fluid, diluting a concentrate into an infusion bag (admixing), and dissolving a freeze-dried antibiotic in water to obtain an oral liquid dosage form. Reconstitution in excess of an SmPC legally yields an unlicensed preparation [25]. Examples are the use of a reconstitution solution not mentioned in the SmPC, or a differently assigned shelf life.

2.3. Justification of Pharmacy Preparations

Choosing a pharmacy preparation is justified when no commercial product is available to meet the patient's specific needs. Optimal pharmacotherapy can then be achieved with a tailored approach, often improving patient compliance and providing greater flexibility. Dose adjustment, dosage form adjustment, or modification of a formulation are common in this context, especially for children and the elderly. A patient with an allergy or hypersensitivity to a certain excipient can be served with an adapted, compounded formulation. Products with a short shelf life can only be made on demand by extemporaneous compounding. Furthermore, for the production of early-stage investigational medicinal products (IMPs), extemporaneous compounding is needed. Medicine shortage, a current major problem in the Netherlands, may be alleviated with pharmacy preparations. Finally, recent developments such as individualised therapies based on a patient's genetic profile are expected to increase the demand for patient-tailored medicines that are not commercially available [26–30].

3. The Dutch Healthcare System and Pharmacy Preparations

3.1. Demographic Data

At the start of 2025, the Netherlands had more than 18 million inhabitants, with a nearly equal share of males and females. The country is facing an ageing population. On 1 January 2025, 54% of the population was older than 40 years and 21% older than 65 years. For comparison, this was 45% and 13%, respectively, on 1 January 2000. The median age in 2020 was 41.5 years; in 2000, it was 36.2 years [31,32]. An ageing population places an increased demand on the healthcare system and necessitates a more personalised approach, including tailor-made pharmacy preparations.

3.2. Professional Organisations and Support

The KNMP offers extensive support to daily practice of the pharmaceutical profession in the Netherlands [33]. A key service is the KNMP Knowledge Bank (Dutch: Kennisbank), a digital information resource available via paid subscription for pharmacists and pharmacy teams [21]. It includes services aimed at pharmaceutical product care and compounding provided by the Laboratory of Dutch Pharmacists (Dutch: Laboratorium der Nederlandse Apothekers; LNA). The LNA serves as the knowledge centre for pharmaceutical product care within the KNMP, focusing on ensuring the quality and availability of pharmaceutical products for patients. The LNA conducts research on pharmaceutical raw materials, semi-finished and finished products, dosage forms, and packaging materials for both human and veterinary use, as well as for clinical research [33].

LNA's services include the Formulary of Dutch Pharmacists (Dutch: Formularium der Nederlandse Apothekers; FNA), LNA Messages, LNA Procedures, Oralia VTGM, Parenteralia VTGM, and RiFaS, the Risk Instrument for Pharmaceutical Substances. Further support is offered by the Special Interest Group (SIG) 'Product Care and Preparation' (Dutch: Productzorg en Bereiden), consisting of pharmacists who share commitment to pharmaceutical product care.

The FNA is a collection of nationally standardised formulations for medicinal products for community and hospital pharmacies that produce pharmacy preparations (see Section 5.2).

LNA Messages (Dutch: LNA Mededelingen) are irregularly appearing newsletters from the LNA, to ensure pharmacists stay informed about FNA formulations, LNA procedures, and other LNA resources. These newsletters cover topics such as medicine availability, counterfeit drugs, and pharmacy working conditions, along with background information on new and existing pharmacy preparations. As part of quality assurance, the newsletters support pharmacists in ensuring consistency, safety and efficacy in individual and small-scale preparations.

LNA procedures are instructional documents that outline actions, processes and methods related to pharmaceutical product care. Oralia VTGM provides guidance on the preparation of oral medicines for patients with swallowing difficulties or those requiring administration with a feeding tube. Parenteralia VTGM offers information on the preparation, stability, admixture compatibility, and storage of parenteral medicines (see Section 5.4). RiFaS delivers tailored advice on the safe handling of pharmaceutical substances, taking the available equipment in the pharmacy and the duration of exposure into account [34].

The KNMP has established the Directive Pharmacy Preparations (Dutch: Richtlijn Bereiden) to provide community pharmacists with GMP-based guidelines for high-quality small-scale preparations [35]. This directive outlines protocols covering key aspects including quality control, risk assessment, documentation, and correct labelling of pharmacy preparations.

For hospital pharmacies, support is also provided by the NVZA, in addition to the KNMP [19]. A key NVZA document is the GMP-Z (Good Manufacturing Practice for hospital pharmacies) [21], which serves as the foundational standard for the preparation of medicinal products in hospitals. The NVZA has dedicated working groups focused on pharmaceutical product care within the hospital settings and is internationally affiliated with the European Association of Hospital Pharmacists (EAHP) [36]. GMP-Z is aligned with the requirements of the Health and Youth Care Inspectorate (Dutch: Inspectie Gezondheidszorg en Jeugd; IGJ) [22,37].

3.3. *Community Pharmacy*

Primary care in the Netherlands, which is primarily focused on outpatient services, included 1953 community pharmacies as of 1 January 2024 [38]. In 2023, 2.8% of all medications dispensed by these pharmacies were compounded preparations, with topical and oral products accounting for the majority, at 53% and 33%, respectively [38,39]. Over the past decades, compounding in community pharmacies has declined significantly. Today, only around 125 pharmacies regularly perform in-house extemporaneous compounding activities [40], while the remainder fully outsource these tasks to specialised compounding pharmacies. This shift is largely driven by the high costs, as well as the need for specialised resources, trained personnel, and infrastructure required to meet strict regulatory and quality standards. However, despite the decline in extemporaneous compounding, reconstitution remains a routine practice in all community pharmacies.

A compounding community pharmacy should have a dedicated compounding area that meets defined standards for cleanliness, organisation, and safety. This includes space for the appropriate storage of raw materials and compounded medications, where applicable in validated refrigerators. A separate, designated area must be available for the cleaning and sanitisation of equipment to prevent cross-contamination, especially when preparing multiple formulations or handling hazardous substances. Basic compounding equipment includes balances, mortars and pestles, mixing spatulas, a capsule filling and closing apparatus, a dust extraction cabinet, hot plates or other heating devices, homogenisers and mixers, a laminar flow cabinet, and an autoclave. Pharmacy technicians involved in compounding must possess specialised qualifications (see also Section 3.5).

Compounding pharmacy software is used to manage and streamline various operational processed, including inventory control, formulation management, and the weighing of active pharmaceutical ingredients (APIs) and excipients. It improves efficiency, supports compliance with regulatory standards, ensures accuracy, and ultimately enhances patient safety.

Table 1 presents the most common types of pharmacy preparations produced in compounding community pharmacies in the Netherlands.

Table 1. Common types of pharmacy preparations produced in compounding community pharmacies in the Netherlands.

Product Type	Specification and Examples
Topical preparations	Creams, ointments, and gels are compounded for patients who require specific formulations for skin disorders (e.g., eczema, psoriasis, or fungal infections). Lotions are used for conditions like dandruff, seborrheic dermatitis, and acne.
Oral preparations	Liquid formulations can be prepared as alternatives to medication typically available as tablet or capsule for patients who have difficulty swallowing solid medication, such as children and the elderly. Capsules can be either compounded from raw materials or from ground commercially available tablets, for example, to allow dose adaptation.
Paediatric formulations	Medicines may be compounded with flavours to make them more palatable for children. Dosages can be adjusted to suit the child's weight or age.
Suppositories	Rectal or vaginal suppositories are compounded for medications that need to be administered via these routes, often for treating conditions such as haemorrhoids and vaginal infections.
Sterile solutions	Intravenously administered medications include antibiotic solutions dispensed in disposable infusion pumps or infusion bags for home treatment. Subcutaneous medications, such as morphine or lidocaine, are prepared for pain management when precise dosing is required or when commercial formulations are unavailable.

After compounding and dispensing a pharmacy preparation, the pharmacy submits a reimbursement claim to the patient's health insurance company. All Dutch citizens are required to have health insurance. The reimbursement procedure typically involves three steps. First, the medical necessity is verified based on the prescription and the patient's medical condition. Second, a cost assessment is conducted, which includes evaluating the price of raw materials, labour costs for compounding, and any additional pharmacy overhead. Insurance companies may negotiate reimbursement rates or set maximum limits for compounded products. Third, a claim is either approved or denied. If the compounded medication does not meet the insurer's criteria, the reimbursement claim is denied, and the patient must cover the full cost. Decisions on reimbursement claims can be postponed for up to two years after dispensing, which exposes compounding pharmacies to significant financial risks [41].

3.4. Hospital Pharmacy

Hospital pharmacists primarily manage specialised pharmaceutical patient care for patients in general hospitals (secondary care) and specialised, often academic, hospitals (tertiary care). In 2025, the Netherlands had 69 hospital organisations, including 8 academic medical centres, 113 hospital locations (academic, general and children's hospitals), and 137 outpatient clinics. While the number of hospital organisations is decreasing due to mergers, the total number of locations providing hospital care has remained relatively stable owing to a growing number of outpatient clinics [42].

In all Dutch hospital pharmacies, the reconstitution of parenteral products is routine daily practice. Many, but not all hospitals also prepare medications for individual patients. These preparations can, in principle, encompass the full range of dosage forms. However, stock preparations are prepared in only a limited number of hospital pharmacies, primarily focusing on sterile and aseptic products (syringes, infusions, ampoules) as well as a selection of non-sterile products (oral liquids, oral drops, cutaneous preparations) that are not commercially available. In cases where pulmonary drug administration is requested, the compounding of pressurised metered dose inhalers or dry powder inhalers is not feasible, because of technical requirements related to their production and quality control. However, aqueous solutions suitable for nebulisation can be prepared by hospital pharmacies or specialised compounding pharmacies. When compounding such solutions, it is essential that quality attributes such as the particle size of the aerosol and output rate are determined, requiring specialised equipment which is not generally available in most pharmacies [43].

The NVZA issues the professional guideline GMP-Z, which hospital pharmacies are required to follow. Introduced in 1996, GMP-Z is regularly revised and updated to reflect advancements in hospital pharmacy practice [20,22].

Like community pharmacies, hospital pharmacies also outsource pharmacy preparations, either to centralised compounding facilities or to other hospital pharmacies. These facilities must fully comply with GMP manufacturing requirements and are required to obtain a 'toleration declaration' (Dutch: gedoogverklaring) from the IGJ [44]. Some of these facilities hold a GMP manufacturing license (Manufacturing and Importation Authorisation (MIA); Dutch: fabrikantenvergunning) for producing pharmacy preparations for third parties [45].

An alternative to outsourcing patient-specific preparations is the 'carry-over' regulation, whereby the prescription is transferred from the dispensing to the compounding pharmacy. The compounding pharmacy takes responsibility for preparing the medication, while tasks such as dosage verification and interaction checks may remain with the dispensing pharmacy, depending on the terms of the contract. This regulation, which does not require a toleration declaration, is particularly useful for cytostatic drugs, radiopharmaceuticals, and medications for metabolic diseases [46].

In hospital pharmacies, both parenteral individual and stock preparations are produced in cleanrooms that comply with GMP [12,47] and GMP-Z [22] requirements. Due to the wide range of products handled, different items are often manufactured on the same production line and/or within the same working area. This imposes stringent demands on the cleanroom type, cleaning and disinfection procedures, cross-contamination prevention strategies, and personnel qualifications. Particular emphasis is placed on personnel training, especially in aseptic procedures and quality assurance. Staff are required to constantly develop and maintain their skills through periodic requalification to demonstrate ongoing competence [22]. In larger hospital pharmacies, both sterile and non-sterile compounding from raw materials to produce individual and intermediate-scale stock preparations is common practice.

Hospital pharmacies play a crucial role in the reconstitution of complex medications, particularly sterile products such as chemotherapy, immunotherapy, TPN, ready-to-use (RTU) and ready-to-administer (RTA) syringes. They are also involved in preparing personalised medicines for specific patient groups, such as paediatric patients and those with swallowing difficulties (see also Sections 7.1.1 and 7.1.2).

To further enhance patient safety, there is a growing demand for RTA and RTU products prepared by hospital pharmacies. This approach has been shown to reduce medication errors and prevent microbial contamination [48,49]. One way to ensure the availability of RTA products on hospital wards is to have pharmacy assistants prepare them in dedicated rooms located on or near the ward. Alternatively, preparation can be centralised in the hospital pharmacy, where the syringes are aseptically filled. However, these syringes have a limited shelf life of weeks and must be stored refrigerated, which poses challenges for storage capacity in larger-scale production. Consequently, hospital pharmacies have increasingly developed and implemented the production of prefilled sterilised syringes (PFSSs) in recent years. PFSSs offer the advantage of a long shelf life (up to three years) at room temperature, along with high quality and an efficient, automated production process that saves time. Approximately one-third of parenterally administered medications in a hospital are suitable for delivery in RTA formulations. This can significantly improve medication safety and saves time for nursing staff [48–50].

Inpatient medication costs, including those for pharmacy preparations, are covered by the hospital's central budget. As a result, hospital pharmacies calculate internal cost prices and develop business cases for reconstitution activities, with quality improvement being a key factor in the decision to undertake these services.

3.5. *Pharmacy Technicians and Pharmacy Assistants*

Pharmacy technicians and assistants play a vital role in Dutch pharmacies. To become a certified pharmacy technician, individuals must complete a three-year vocational programme covering topics such as diseases, medication effects, patient communication, pharmaceutical calculations, and quality assurance [51]. Graduates earn the title of pharmacy technician and are eligible for registration in the public register for healthcare professionals (see also Section 4.1) [52,53]. In addition to technicians, most pharmacies also employ pharmacy assistants who do not undergo the same formal education. Instead, they are trained either on the job or through shorter, less comprehensive training programmes, including final examinations, as offered by several commercial course providers [54,55]. The average of pharmacist-to-technician/assistant ratio in Dutch community pharmacies is estimated at approximately 1:7, though this varies between pharmacies [40].

Pharmacy technicians handle prescription verification, medication dispensing, patient counselling, and the preparation and reconstitution of medicines. Pharmacy assistants perform logistic tasks, support pharmacy technicians, and help at the pharmacy's production site.

Pharmacy technician training has increasingly focused on communication, clinical pharmacy services, and patient counselling, leaving graduates with limited preparation and reconstitution skills. As a result, employers must provide additional training, including a supervised onboarding programme and commercial e-learning modules [55,56].

Training follows a three-stage process: observation, hands-on practice under direct supervision, and independent execution under indirect supervision. Upon completion, a pharmacy assistant is qualified to perform one or more specific tasks. For aseptic handling, a KNMP guideline [57] outlines the initial person-specific qualification, which involves completing 30 individual handling steps using a culture media fill protocol. This qualification must be renewed at least annually. While not mandatory, it is considered good practice to implement an additional requalification protocol for both pharmacy technicians and assistants. This may include the periodic production of worst-case preparations and the requirement for a minimum number of hours or days per month or year which staff should perform preparation tasks [58].

Excluding preparation and production-related content from pharmacy technician training limits their fundamental understanding of pharmaceutical compounding. While on-the-job training can teach individuals to perform tasks correctly and follow established protocols, a lack of insight into the underlying scientific principles and rationale increases the risk of errors. Furthermore, reliance on an educational model that emphasises simply 'repeating what others already do' may restrict the capacity for innovation and hinder the ability to adapt to new developments. In the long term, this could pose a threat to the sustainability of the current system.

In addition to pharmacy technicians, there is a growing trend towards employing pharmaceutical managers (Dutch: farmakundigen) in pharmacies. These professionals act as intermediaries between pharmacy technicians and (hospital) pharmacists. Their training enables them to support pharmacists in specialised tasks such as organising production workflows, planning work schedules, and assisting with product development and financial management. They may also become involved in overseeing compounding-related processes and their quality assurance [59].

The pharmacist retains ultimate responsibility for the quality of the preparations produced in the pharmacy. The pharmacist is also responsible for providing adequate training programmes to ensure that pharmacy staff are properly qualified, as well as for ensuring the availability of appropriate infrastructure, compounding equipment, standard operating procedures, and production protocols.

4. The Dutch Regulatory and Legal Framework for Pharmacy Preparations

4.1. The Position and Qualification of the Dutch Pharmacist

Two specific activities are exclusively reserved for pharmacists registered in the Netherlands: dispensing and preparing medicines [60]. The legal and regulatory framework surrounding pharmacy preparations is defined by various national laws and guidelines, which are currently being aligned with updated EU pharmaceutical legislation [61]. According to the Medicines Act (Dutch: Geneesmiddelenwet; GW) [62], which governs the manufacture, distribution and sale of medicines, pharmacists are legally permitted to prepare medication for patients in their own pharmacy upon receiving a health practitioner's prescription. A prerequisite is that the pharmacist must be competent to perform this task through appropriate education, training, and practical experience. In addition, all preparation activities must adhere to strict standards of safety, quality, and hygiene. The Medical Treatment Contracts Act (Dutch: Wet op de Geneeskundige Behandelingsovereenkomst; WGBO) [63] establishes that pharmacists are co-responsible for a patient's treatment, together with physicians. This shared responsibility may result in deciding that the preparation of an extemporaneous, non-commercially available medication is the most appropriate therapeutic option for a specific patient.

Pharmacists who are actively working in healthcare in the Netherlands must be registered in a public register for healthcare professionals (the so-called BIG register), according to the Professions in Individual Health Care Act (Dutch: Wet op de Beroepen in de Individuele Gezondheidszorg; Wet BIG) [53,60].

4.2. *Extemporaneous Pharmacy Preparations*

One of the primary objectives of the general EU pharmaceutical legislation is to ensure the safety, efficacy and quality of medicines available on the EU market [64,65]. As such, the manufacturing, distributing and marketing of medicines require appropriate licenses. However, extemporaneous pharmacy preparations are exempt from these licensing requirements, as they are considered unlicensed products.

In the Netherlands, two situations regarding pharmacy preparations are distinguished. The first involves medicines prepared within a pharmacy for direct supply to patients of that same pharmacy (see Section 4.2.1). The second concerns the supply of compounded medicines from one pharmacy to other, commonly referred to as pharmacy-to-pharmacy delivery or outsourcing (see Section 4.2.2).

4.2.1. Medicines Prepared in a Pharmacy for Own Patients

The general rule in the Netherlands is that manufacturing and supplying medicines without the appropriate manufacturing licenses is prohibited. However, this requirement does not apply to medicines compounded by a pharmacist (or by a qualified pharmacy assistant or technician under the responsibility of a pharmacist) within a pharmacy, provided the medicine is intended for direct supply to a patient of that specific pharmacy. This exception is derived from Article 3 of Directive 2001/83/EC [64].

In a letter to the Dutch Parliament on 8 April 2019 [66], the Minister of Healthcare outlined the conditions under which a pharmacy preparation is allowed. Based on the Medicines Act [62], these conditions are as follows:

- The preparation takes place in the pharmacy, based on a medical prescription for an individual patient or as stock for patients yet to be determined by that pharmacy;
- The preparation complies with the Ph. Eur.;
- The preparation is intended for dispensing on a small scale.

The third condition, dispensing on a small scale, is subject to a numerical criterion, intended to provide clarity to stakeholders. As defined by the Minister of Healthcare, small-scale dispensing means:

- Dispensing to up to approximately 50 unique patients per month for long-term use of the medication;
- Dispensing to approximately 150 patients per month for short-term use.

Short-term use is one week or less, while long-term use is more than one week.

If all of the above-mentioned conditions are met, pharmacists are permitted to compound on a small scale for their own patients, even when a medicinal product with marketing authorisation is available on the market. However, it should be noted that the numerical criteria have not yet been included in a generally binding regulation.

The European GMP guidelines [12] are primarily designed for the industrial manufacture of medicines. However, their principles are also relevant to all pharmaceutical preparation processes carried out in community and hospital pharmacies. Since these guidelines do not provide sufficient detail for the preparation of medicines in pharmacies, the KNMP and the NVZA have developed supplementary GMP-based guidelines specially tailored to pharmacy settings to ensure the quality of pharmacy preparations. These include the following:

- KNMP: Directive Pharmacy Preparations, for community pharmacies [35];
- NVZA: GMP-Z, for hospital pharmacies [22].

The IGJ is the supervisory authority responsible for enforcing of these guidelines, thereby safeguarding the quality and safety of medicines prepared in pharmacies throughout the Netherlands [37].

4.2.2. Pharmacy-to-Pharmacy Delivery and Outsourcing

As outlined in Section 4.2.1, pharmacies in the Netherlands are generally only permitted to compound for their own patients, and in small quantities. However, societal and professional developments have made it increasingly difficult to maintain operational compounding facilities, expertise, and proficiency in every community and hospital pharmacy. In addition, focus clinics and other care institutions without an in-house pharmacy also need compounded products. At the beginning of the 21st century, this insight led to a consensus among the government, the IGJ and pharmacists that a different model was necessary. The goal was twofold: to ensure continued patient access to necessary compounded medicines, and to enable compounding at a larger scale, thereby justifying the considerable investments in facilities, quality systems, training and expertise.

The supply of compounded preparations from one pharmacy to another and the outsourcing compounding to specialised pharmacies, also known as 'collegial supply', has been fully regulated since 2017 [67]. This was outlined in the IGJ document 'Circulaire handhavend optreden bij collegiaal doorleveren van eigen bereidingen door apothekers' (translation: Circular on enforcement action in the event of collegial forwarding of own preparations by pharmacists; hereafter referred to as the 'IGJ circular'). The IGJ formulated six restrictive conditions under which pharmacy-to-pharmacy delivery is permitted [68] (see Table 2). If all conditions are met, no enforcement action is taken (so-called 'tolerance policy').

The quantitative restrictions for small-scale compounding by pharmacies for their own patients do not apply to pharmacy-to-pharmacy delivery and outsourcing arrangements.

As of 1 February 2025, the IGJ circular [68] was replaced by a policy rule with a legal base in Dutch administrative law [71–73]. The policy rule maintains the approach that pharmacy-to-pharmacy delivery of compounded products is permitted without marketing authorisation, provided that the specified conditions are met (Table 2). The policy rule may contribute to the ongoing revision of the EU directive and regulation on medicinal products for human use [74].

In 2025, the outsourcing landscape in the Netherlands has evolved to include approximately 20 specialised compounding pharmacies operating under various legal structures. Unlike in some other countries, there are no legal restrictions on ownership. Both pharmacies and private companies are active in supplying compounded products to community pharmacies, hospital pharmacies, focus clinics, and outpatient services.

Table 2. The conditions, formulated by the IGJ, under which pharmacy-to-pharmacy delivery and outsourcing in the Netherlands are allowed [68].

Condition	Explanation
Unmet need	The compounded product may only be outsourced, compounded, and delivered if the patient's condition cannot be adequately treated with a product that is licensed (registered) in the Netherlands. Both the dispensing and compounding pharmacies are responsible for verifying this requirement.
Notification	The compounding pharmacy is obligated to register its product in the national medicinal products database used by all healthcare stakeholders (the G-Standard, maintained and updated by Z-Index [69]). This ensures transparency regarding the products available and the pharmacy involved in pharmacy-to-pharmacy delivery.
Product file	For each product, the compounding pharmacy must maintain a file that justifies the product and its design. This file should include the medical application (pharmacotherapy), as well as the chemical and pharmaceutical aspects, such as composition, preparation method, quality controls, stability studies and expiration date, microbiological controls, and other relevant data.
GMP	The compounding pharmacy is required to comply with the EU-GMP standards, which necessitates the implementation of a fully functioning pharmaceutical quality system. Compliance is monitored by the IGJ through its on-site inspection programme. Typically, regulatory inspections are conducted every three years.
Pharmacovigilance	Compounding pharmacies must implement a pharmacovigilance system to document and assess (potential) adverse reactions on severity and causality, which should be reported to the national pharmacovigilance centre Lareb [70].
Promotion	The promotion, advertisement and/or offering of incentives for compounded products is prohibited. It is permitted to send a price list to interested dispensing pharmacies and to respond to information requests.

These pharmacies generally follow established FNA formulations and procedures or adopt a quality-driven approach in the development of new formulations. When supported by appropriate quality measures, outsourcing ensures that compounded products are prepared in accordance with GMP standards and meet the required quality criteria.

The product portfolios of central compounding pharmacies primarily consist of non-sterile products, although there is a growing trend towards ophthalmic preparations and patient-specific sterile products for homecare. Additionally, the available expertise and infrastructure of these facilities are often leveraged to manufacture orphan drugs.

Hospital-based compounding facilities primarily serve hospital pharmacies. Their portfolios typically include parenteral products, supplied in RTA or RTU formats, which help reduce medication errors and ease the burden on nursing staff by eliminating the need for bedside preparation of infusions and injectables. Furthermore, the available expertise and facilities are often used to manufacture IMPs for investigator-initiated clinical trials (see Section 7.2.5).

Both public institutions and private companies use their infrastructure to mitigate drug shortages. Examples are ipratropium bromide inhalation fluid, pethidine hydrochloride ampoules, and suxamethonium chloride ampoules. Recently, in response to global supply chain disruptions following the destruction of a major production site in the USA caused by hurricane Helene in October 2024, Dutch hospital pharmacies produced sodium chloride and glucose infusion bags to address the resulting shortages [75,76].

4.3. Enforcement

The IGJ monitors compliance with pharmaceutical standards and regulations [37,62,68,72]. Pharmacy inspections or audits are conducted to assess adherence to the required standards related to cleanliness, equipment, procedures, and personnel qualifications involved in pharmacy preparations. These inspections also ensure compliance with the European GMP standards or applicable derived guidelines. The IGJ recognises the GMP-Z guidelines as the standard for pharmaceutical compounding in Dutch hospital pharmacies. The GMP-Z was developed and is maintained in collaboration with the IGJ, and any update to the guideline only takes effect following IGJ approval [22,37].

4.4. International Context

In most European countries, extemporaneous compounding is an integral part of routine pharmacy practice, particularly when commercial products are unavailable or inadequate to meet specific patient needs [7,10,24]. Compounding practices in Dutch pharmacies share many features with general European approaches while also reflecting distinctive national characteristics. Europe does not have a unified regulatory framework for pharmacy compounding, but the legal framework governing medicinal products excludes pharmacy preparations from its scope, meaning that marketing authorisation and manufacturing authorisation are not required. Additionally, in cases of specific medical needs, individual EU member states are allowed to establish their own regulations regarding the use of unlicensed products [64].

In general, EU countries recognise that extemporaneous compounding is a competence reserved to pharmacies that dispense medicines directly to patients. The percentage of pharmacies that actually perform in-house compounding activities varies across European countries and is influenced by whether outsourcing is permitted [77–79]. However, reliable benchmarking data on this matter are not readily available.

There is always great emphasis on the quality and safety of compounded medication, but there are differences in the extent of standardisation of formulations (see Section 5.2). The Netherlands and Germany (Deutscher Arzneimittel-Codex/Neues Rezeptur-Formularium (DAC/NRF; translated: German Drug Codex/New German Formulary) [80]) have a well-developed regulatory framework in this respect, while in other European countries and in the USA, compounding practices are less streamlined.

The EAHP plays a key role in promoting and guiding pharmaceutical compounding practices within European hospitals by setting standards, developing policy and guidelines, providing training programmes, and supporting research and innovation [7,36].

In most European countries, outsourcing is typically not permitted. However, in some northern European countries, including the Netherlands, Belgium, Germany, Sweden, Ireland, and the United Kingdom, pharmacies are allowed to outsource the preparation of compounded or unlicensed products within defined national legal frameworks. These frameworks usually stipulate that outsourcing is only permitted when no licensed product can adequately meet a patient's therapeutic needs [7,10,24]. Outsourcing facilities generally operate on a larger scale, and GMP requirements for such operations vary by country.

The USA employs a more commercialised system compared to Europe, with larger outsourcing facilities, alongside traditional compounding pharmacies [81]. The U.S. Food and Drug Administration (FDA) regulates pharmaceutical compounding to ensure patient safety and product quality [8]. Compounding pharmacies are categorised into two distinct types under Sections 503A and 503B of the Federal Food, Drug, and Cosmetic Act. [81].

Pharmacies operating under Section 503A focus on preparing customised medications for individual patients based on specific prescriptions. These are typically traditional compounding pharmacies, often located in community or hospital settings. Section 503B, introduced in 2013 in response to safety concerns, created the category of 'outsourcing facilities', which are permitted to produce compounded medications at a larger scale and must comply with stricter GMP standards [81]. This dual regulatory structure enables the

U.S. healthcare system to meet a broad range of patient and clinical needs while ensuring the quality and safety of compounded medicines [82].

5. Quality Assurance of Pharmacy Preparations

5.1. Quality by Design (QbD)

Licensed and unlicensed medicinal products are prepared under different conditions, which has implications for their quality and quality assurance. Industrially manufactured products are required to meet the highest possible quality standards along with evidence of product safety and efficacy, as this is required for registration.

Pharmaceutical companies commonly adopt the QbD approach in product development to ensure the quality of medicines. QbD is a systematic, proactive methodology that focuses on understanding and controlling variability in materials, processes, and formulations to maintain consistent product quality, safety, and efficacy. By managing all variables from the outset, QbD ensures that each batch consistently meets the required quality standards. Regulatory agencies such as the EMA and the FDA strongly support the use of QbD, making it a standard practice in the pharmaceutical industry [83,84].

While the QbD approach enhances product quality, it can also lead to longer development timelines and higher production costs. The scale of production generally determines the extent of substantiation required for the pharmacotherapeutic and technical design. In the context of small-scale preparations, QbD is generally not feasible. Nevertheless, although small-scale production is more customised and less standardised than large-scale manufacturing, pharmacotherapeutic and technical design can still be applied using standardised formulations.

5.2. Standardisation of Formulations

The KNMP supports the professional field by providing standardised formulations that are not commercially available but needed in daily practice. The LNA, a division of the KNMP, developed and maintains the FNA, a comprehensive formulary containing standardised formulations and guidelines for compounded preparations, accessible through the KNMP Knowledge Bank [21,33].

On 1 May 2025, the FNA included 226 nationally standardised formulations for pharmacy preparations [85], which can be produced in community, hospital, and specialised compounding pharmacies. Each formulation includes detailed information on the qualitative and quantitative composition, preparation method, recommended packaging, storage conditions, shelf life, and quality requirements. Extensive background information, including reference to scientific literature, underpins the formulation design and preparation method, along with a pharmacotherapeutic assessment of each preparation. Shelf life and usage periods are generally based on real-life stability testing. For most FNA preparations, analytical protocols have been established, including methods for qualitative and quantitative analysis of active substances and excipients. Where relevant and feasible, information on the degradation of active substances is included. The LNA develops its analytical protocols based on pharmacopeial standards or through in-house development of non-standardised methods [21,33].

Because both the design of the composition and the preparation methods are carefully developed and validated, the formulations are robust. When prepared by a trained professional (pharmacist or pharmacy assistant), the quality of the final product will be assured and consistent, resulting in reproducible outcomes. Consequently, the responsible pharmacist can guarantee the quality of such compounded preparations.

Regular updates and ongoing maintenance of the FNA are essential to ensure that pharmacists have access to the most current and reliable information on individual and small-scale formulations. New formulations are added to the FNA for various reasons, for instance, when licensed medications are unavailable in the appropriate dose for paediatric patients (e.g., Fluoxetine capsules 5 mg, Hydrochlorothiazide 0.5 mg/mL oral solution). The FNA also provides formulations for medicinal products that are no longer commercially available (e.g., Metoclopramide hydrochloride suppositories 10 mg) or to improve and standardise commonly used preparations (e.g., Clobetasol propionate mouthwash 0.25 mg/mL) [21].

For preparations not described in the FNA, the LNA has developed standardised procedures that provide comprehensive guidelines and validated methods for various dosage forms. The procedures include specifications for formulation design, preparation methods and equipment, raw material selection, and quality control measures.

5.3. Product File and Production Batch Record

For each product prepared in a (compounding) pharmacy or hospital pharmacy, a product file is compiled in advance to support and substantiate the pharmacy preparation. The product file contains the pharmacotherapeutic rationale and all information pertaining to the preparation and the manufacturing process. It covers specifications for the API and excipients, batch size, composition, preparation method, materials and equipment used, in-process controls and final quality controls, test results of trial preparations, storage conditions, shelf life, packaging, labelling, and patient information [86].

For each product to be made, a production batch record (protocol) should be available. This is derived from a master file, which is supported by the corresponding product file. A master file serves as a template for the production batch record for each individual batch or product. The release of the preparation by an authorised pharmacist is based on a completed production batch record containing all the data recorded during and after preparation. This document is archived for traceability and accountability. The entire procedure follows the principles of GMP.

5.4. Preparation for Administration and Reconstitution

In addition to supporting the preparation of compounded medicines, the LNA provides guidance on the preparation of licensed medicines for administration. Two dedicated databases are accessible via the KNMP Knowledge Bank: Oralia VTGM and Parenteralia VTGM [21]. VTGM is a practice meaning 'voor toediening gereedmaken' in Dutch, which can be translated as 'preparation handlings needed for administration'. A prepared VTGM product is considered an RTA product, requiring no further handling prior to administration to a patient.

Oralia VTGM contains more than 600 individual monographs that offer practical guidance for the safe administration of medicines to patients with swallowing difficulties and those who require a feeding tube. Designed for pharmacists and pharmacy staff, the database consolidates all available information into a single resource. Each monograph is primarily based on product information, data provided by pharmaceutical companies, the scientific literature, and practical research. The monographs provide guidance on the safe handling of specific medicines and formulations. Where possible, a licensed formulation is recommended, but the monographs also suggest alternative administration routes and substitute medicines to consider. If no alternatives are available, the monographs provide recommendations for safe handling of the medicinal product, including instructional videos. Table 3 illustrates the typical content of a monograph in Oralia VTGM.

Table 3. Typical content of a monograph in Oralia VTGM [21].

- Information about handling or manipulation of the medicinal product
- Pharmaceutical alternatives
- Therapeutic alternatives
- Enteral tube administration
- Enteral nutrition and food interactions
- Interaction with tubing material
- Route of administration
- Background information on the active substance for (hospital) pharmacists
- Health and safety

In addition to the Oralia VTGM database, another dedicated website, Oralia.nl [87], has been developed for healthcare professionals other than pharmacy staff, such as nurses. It presents the same essential information as Oralia VTGM, but in a simplified format, omitting technical details that are not relevant to nursing practice, such as the explanation of why a medicine can or cannot be processed.

Parenteralia VTGM provides fundamental information on processing licensed medicines intended for parenteral administration. It includes data on stability, raw materials, and compatibility, as well as specific product-related details such as preparation instructions and the final concentrations. Serving as a reference source, it enables pharmacists to answer daily queries regarding parenteral medicines. Nurses require direct instructions on how to prepare, administer, and store specific medicines but have no direct access to the information on the KNMP Knowledge Bank [21]. Therefore, (hospital) pharmacists can use Parenteralia VTGM to develop monographs and instructions tailored to the needs of nursing staff.

Parenteralia VTGM covers all commercially available parenteral medicines, as well as those for which an FNA formulation exists. However, due to their specific nature, no VTGM monographs are available for cytostatic drugs, (X-ray) contrast agents, radiopharmaceuticals, dialysis fluids, and additives for TPN. Additionally, the database includes VTGM products for 50 medicines intended for paediatric patients from one month of age. For consistency, the format is aligned as closely as possible with that of adult VTGM monographs. However, paediatric preparations often require dilution due to the higher concentrations present in the available commercial products. The database also provides calculation examples for pump setting and/or starting doses. The information in Parenteralia VTGM is organised by active substance and presented in the form of monographs (see Table 4).

Table 4. Typical content of a monograph in Parenteralia VTGM [21].

- Methods of administration
- Shelf life
- Influence on stability
- Compatibilities
- Duration/rate of administration

Table 4. *Cont.*

• Maximum concentration • Other administration information • Literature

5.5. Raw Materials

Pharmacy preparations should only be manufactured with pharmaceutical-grade raw materials, with sufficient knowledge of their origin and quality, meeting pre-set requirements.

Active substances and excipients used in pharmacy preparations must be manufactured in accordance with EU GMP part II and must comply with the Ph. Eur. monograph 'Substances for pharmaceutical use' [6,12]. Where specific monographs exist for individual raw materials, their quality must also meet the requirements outlined in those monographs. If the Ph. Eur. provides no or insufficient information, the British Pharmacopoeia (BP), the United States Pharmacopeia (USP), the Japanese Pharmacopoeia (JP) or another reputable pharmacopoeia should be consulted. In the absence of any applicable monograph, the required quality of the raw materials must be defined and documented based on a risk assessment tailored to their intended use and associated risks [88]. If insufficient knowledge is available, the pharmacist should refrain from using such raw materials for production.

For licensed medicinal products, the quality requirements of the active substance are evaluated by a regulatory authority such as the EMA, as part of the Marketing Authorisation Application (MAA) procedure. The active substance manufacturer provides all pivotal information to the Marketing Authorisation Holder (MAH), while the full dossier, including confidential details, is submitted directly to the regulatory authority. This process protects the manufacturer's intellectual property while ensuring that the MAH retains full responsibility for the quality of the active substance [89].

In contrast, for pharmacy preparations, the licensed pharmacist is responsible for assessing the quality and suitability of the raw materials used, supported by a documented risk assessment. While most information can be obtained from the active substance manufacturer, confidential details typically reviewed by regulatory authorities are often unavailable to the pharmacist.

It is strongly recommended that active substances used in pharmacy preparations be accompanied by a Certificate of Suitability to the Monographs of the European Pharmacopoeia (CEP) or a certificate of analysis referring to the Ph. Eur. [90]. A CEP certifies that the quality of a substance can be adequately controlled using a relevant Ph. Eur. monograph. As part of the CEP procedure, all information about the active substance is submitted independently from an MAH to the European Directorate for the Quality of Medicines and HealthCare (EDQM). The EDQM evaluates whether the substance complies with the applicable Ph. Eur. monograph, along with any additional applicable requirements. Once approved, a CEP is issued for the substance. If a raw material cannot be procured with a CEP, it is recommended that the compounding pharmacist performs a due diligence investigation on the quality and purity of the substance and on GMP standards at the manufacturing site.

Using active substances with a CEP allows pharmacists to rely on the certificate as a proof of quality, thereby reducing the need to evaluate detailed manufacturing and quality control data themselves. While CEP-certified substances help ensure quality, pharmacies must still maintain a comprehensive pharmaceutical quality system (PQS) to effectively manage their raw material suppliers. It is important to note that CEP certificates are not available for all substances listed in the Ph. Eur. As a result, the suitability of the raw material often still needs be assessed by the pharmacist.

In contrast with industrial-scale pharmaceutical companies, hospitals and compounding pharmacies may lack the resources to implement extensive supplier management and qualification systems. Nevertheless, a certain level of vendor management is also required for small-scale pharmaceutical production. In the Netherlands, the KNMP, in close collaboration with the NVZA, has established a vendor management programme aimed at conducting audits at all major supplier sites for APIs, excipients, and packaging materials. The outcomes of these audits are available to members of both organisations and can serve as a valuable tool for evaluating vendors [91].

It is also important to note that many hospital pharmacies are included in vendor management processes conducted by the pharmaceutical industry itself. Participation in clinical trials often results in quality assurance (QA) involvement from the pharmaceutical industry, particularly concerning GMP and Good Clinical Practice (GCP) regulations. The capacity to carry out these tasks must be established and should be included in the costs charged to the sponsor of the clinical trial. Ideally, revenue generated from GMP-related tasks in sponsored clinical trials should be reinvested into the organisation to support its own QA and GMP infrastructure and personnel [22].

Sourcing raw materials can also be challenging, particularly for low-volume orders. Specialised companies can assist with sourcing, qualification, and analysis of raw materials. They provide high-quality raw materials, along with the necessary qualification documentation, supply chain transparency, and supplier qualifications.

6. Pharmacy Education in the Netherlands

6.1. Universities and Pharmacy (-Related) Programmes

After secondary school, students who pass their state exams in mathematics, physics and chemistry are eligible to study pharmacy or pharmaceutical sciences. Four universities in the Netherlands offer such degree programmes (Table 5): Leiden University (LU), the University of Groningen (UG), Utrecht University (UU) and the Vrije Universiteit Amsterdam (VU). All Bachelor of Science (BSc) programmes are three-year programmes (180 ECTS (European Credit Transfer System)), whereas the connecting Master of Science (MSc) programmes are either two years (120 ECTS) for pharmaceutical sciences, or three years (180 ECTS) for pharmacy.

Table 5. Overview of all pharmacy and pharmaceutical sciences degree programmes in the Netherlands.

University	Level	Programme	Duration (ECTS) (1)	Access to MSc Pharmacy? (2)	Qualifies as Pharmacist?
Leiden University	Bachelor	Bio-Pharmaceutical Sciences	180	No (3)	-
	Master	Bio-Pharmaceutical Sciences	120	-	No
	Master	Pharmacy	180	-	Yes
University of Groningen	Bachelor	Pharmacy	180	Yes (4)	-
	Master	Medical Pharmaceutical Sciences	120	-	No

Table 5. *Cont.*

University	Level	Programme	Duration (ECTS) [(1)]	Access to MSc Pharmacy? [(2)]	Qualifies as Pharmacist?
	Master	Molecular Medicine and Innovative Treatment	120	-	No
	Master	Pharmacy	180	-	Yes
Utrecht University	Bachelor	College of Pharmaceutical Sciences	180	Yes [(5)]	-
	Bachelor	Pharmacy	180	Yes	-
	Master	Drug Innovation	120	-	No
	Master	Pharmacy	180	-	Yes
Vrije Universiteit Amsterdam	Bachelor	Pharmaceutical Sciences	180	No	-
	Master	Drug Discovery Sciences	120	-	No

[(1)] In the Netherlands, 1 ECTS equals 28 h of workload. [(2)] Direct access, excluding additional programmes such as a pre-Master's. [(3)] With the Pharmacy specialisation, this programme grants access to the MSc Pharmacy at Leiden University. [(4)] With the Pharmacy major. [(5)] With elective courses that address compounding and pharmacotherapy.

Approximately 200 to 250 students qualify as pharmacists each year [92], for which they must obtain the MSc Pharmacy degree. The BSc Pharmacy programmes give automatic access to this Master's programme; BSc programmes in pharmaceutical sciences either only provide indirect access (usually with additional requirements) or no access at all. Ordinarily, students who have completed such a BSc programme will instead continue in one of the MSc programmes in pharmaceutical sciences, which are generally more research-oriented.

6.2. Alignment with the Professional Field

The content of the Dutch MSc Pharmacy programmes is initially dictated by the Besluit opleidingseisen apotheker (Decree on training requirements for pharmacists) [93]. This educational decree details the core knowledge and skills a newly qualified pharmacist should have, as well as the subjects the programme should cover and additional stipulations, such as mandatory pharmacy internships.

In 2016, the LU, UG and UU, together with the KNMP, composed the Pharmacist Competency Framework & Domain-specific Frame of Reference for the Netherlands [1]. These documents not only expand on the basic educational decree, but also take the wishes and demands of the professional field into account, thereby closely aligning the education of Pharmacy students with professional practice.

The Frame of Reference outlines the pharmacist's areas of responsibility and identifies important developments in the field of pharmacy, whereas the Competency Framework defines the learning outcomes for the Bachelor's and Master's Pharmacy programme within the context of the Frame of Reference. These learning outcomes are described in terms of competencies based on the CanMEDS model [94]. This competency profile consists of seven complementary areas of competence, with pharmaceutical expertise at its core. The remaining six areas are communication, collaboration, leadership and organisation, health advocacy and social responsibility, knowledge and science, and professionalism (see Figure 2). Within the confines of the Competency Framework, each university can design their Pharmacy education, resulting in programmes with distinctive profiles, yet all providing the necessary training required for a newly qualified pharmacist [17].

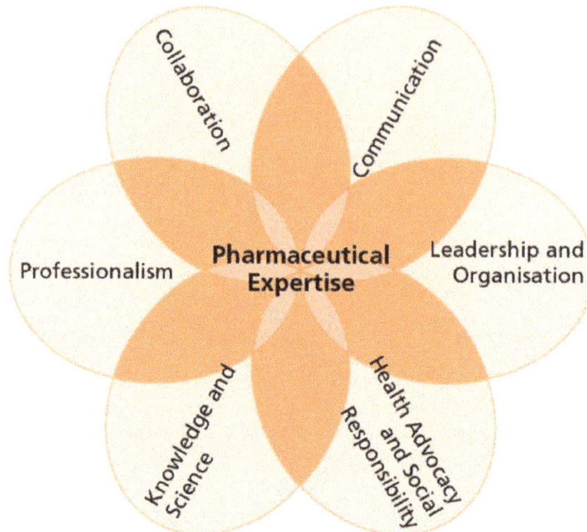

Figure 2. CanMEDS model for the competencies of a Dutch pharmacist. Taken from [1] with permission.

The Competency Framework is currently under revision, and a new version of the Frame of Reference is expected to be published later in 2025. The revised documents will be expanded to explicitly include pharmaceutical sciences and the corresponding university programmes in order to cover the full scope of the pharmaceutical field more thoroughly. The new developments identified in the Frame of Reference are now described in 'knowledge domains' for the students: drug development, manufacturing and product expertise; education; pharmaceutical care on a population level; and pharmaceutical care on an individual (patient) level. The programmes in pharmaceutical sciences will mainly focus on the first two knowledge domains, while the MSc Pharmacy programmes will include all four domains.

6.3. Bachelor's Pharmacy Programme

Pharmacy and pharmaceutical sciences as academic disciplines are positioned in the centre of life sciences. It connects the natural sciences, mainly chemistry, biology and physics, to medical sciences. The current Competency Framework reflects this multidisciplinary nature in over 40 learning outcomes for the Pharmacy Bachelor's programmes, categorised into three core domains: knowledge and understanding, skills and professional behaviour. These learning outcomes lay the foundation for the development of the competencies defined for the Pharmacy Master's programmes and should be considered entry requirements.

The Pharmacy programmes cover pharmaceutical preparations and compounding in the broader context of pharmaceutical product care, motivated by the notion that students should become experts on pharmaceutical products to the fullest extent. In the current Competency Framework, six learning outcomes of the Bachelor's programme deal implicitly or explicitly with pharmaceutical product care (Table 6A) [1]. In short, during the Bachelor's programme, students will obtain knowledge and understanding of the (physico)chemical properties of pharmaceutical ingredients and excipients, the properties of different dosage forms and basic pharmaceutical compounding.

Table 6. Product care-related learning outcomes for the Dutch Bachelor's (**A**) and Master's (**B**) Pharmacy programmes [1].

(A)
Bachelor's Pharmacy Programme
Students who complete a Bachelor of Pharmacy degree programme possess knowledge and understanding of:
• The processes and factors that a play role in the route of administration and biological action of medicines and the pharmacon released in the body. • The chemical and physicochemical properties and analysis of low- and high-molecular-weight active pharmaceutical ingredient and auxiliary pharmaceutical substances. • The compounding of medicines in appropriate pharmaceutical dosage forms and the associated quality criteria. • How the physicochemical properties of chemical compounds affect their potential use as medicine. • The main patient characteristics and product properties that may influence the effects of medicines and the diagnostic measurement methods used to assess them. • The processes involved in the development of medicines.
(B)
Master's Pharmacy Programme
Pharmaceutical Expertise
Pharmacists are able to:
• Apply a wide range of knowledge and skills to pharmaceutical matters across the full spectrum of pharmaceutical practice. ○ Apply scientific reasoning in approaching and analysing pharmaceutical matters where possible. In the area of product care this involves the application of basic principles of chemistry, physics and biology. ○ Approach and analyse pharmaceutical issues from the user's perspective. In the case of product care, this applies primarily to the pharmaceutical dosage form and its application. • Apply knowledge and skills appropriately, responsibly and ethically to relevant matters in the areas of responsibility of Product Care, Patient Care and Medication Policy in pharmaceutical practice. ○ Design high quality pharmaceutically rational and active products that are safe. ○ Assess whether a medicine meets all of the criteria to achieve the desired pharmacotherapeutic effect. ○ Select the right pharmaceutical dosage form and route of administration to achieve optimal therapeutic effect. ○ Make valid statements regarding the bioequivalence of different preparations that contain the same active substance, in the same concentration, in the same pharmaceutical dosage form. ○ Assess the rationale and feasibility of a compounding request. ○ Describe a pharmaceutical product in technical pharmaceutical and biopharmaceutical terms. ○ Develop and implement a protocol or procedure for small-batch compounding of pharmaceutical ingredients or preparation of medicines for administration. ○ Evaluate and assess the design, composition, production method and packaging of medicines. ○ Compile inspection requirements and carry out inspections. ○ Interpret the results of product inspections and make statements regarding the deliverability of products based on the interpretation of the results. ○ Determine and document optimal conditions for the transport and storage of medicines.
Communication
Pharmacists are able to:
• Provide pharmaceutical supervision for the patient and those involved with the patient. ○ Motivate the patient and provide practical solutions in response to questions regarding, and problems with, the use of medicines or medical devices, such as difficulty with compliance.

Table 6. *Cont.*

Pharmacists are able to:
• Provide verbal and written information, and report findings, regarding outcomes of (consultation on) product care, patient care, medication policy, quality assurance and their own research. ○ Keep records of relevant aspects of product care in a product file. ○ Document product care and quality assurance processes in protocols.
Knowledge and Science
Pharmacists are able to:
• Critically assess and interpret (sources of) pharmaceutical and related medical information. ○ Develop (or contribute to the development of) protocols for patient care, medication policy, product care and quality assurance. ○ Assess the overall quality of guidelines and protocols.
Health Advocacy and Social Responsibility
Pharmacists are able to:
• Take appropriate action in response to incidents and risks associated with product and patient care at the level of the individual patient and society. • Help control pharmacotherapy costs by, among other things, monitoring and minimising spillage, dispensing in appropriate quantities, and promoting responsible recycling of unused medicines. • Help protect the environment from medicine waste. ○ Show understanding of the potential environmental impact of medicines. ○ Actively promote safe disposal of unused medicines through designated facilities.

6.4. Master's Pharmacy Programme

The Pharmacy Master's programme is designed to provide students with competencies required for professional roles in both community and hospital pharmacy in five areas of responsibility of a pharmacist: product care, patient care, medication policy, quality assurance, and research, education and innovation. Students may further specialise in the professional and clinical fields after graduation.

The learning objectives of the Pharmacy Master's programme are described in the form of competencies belonging to the seven competency areas and in relation to these five areas of responsibilities of the pharmacist. Together, they form a matrix with 140 learning outcomes [1]. Product care is covered by multiple competency areas: while most learning outcomes can be found in the Pharmaceutical Expertise core competency, product care related learning outcomes are also part of the Communication, Knowledge and Science, and Health Advocacy and Social Responsibility competencies (Table 6B), illustrating how closely interwoven product care and patient care are in the Dutch Pharmacy programme (and in pharmacy daily practice).

6.5. Post-Master's Specialisation Programmes and Post-Academic Education

After obtaining the MSc Pharmacy degree, a newly qualified pharmacist can choose to further specialise as either a community or a hospital pharmacist. The KNMP has set up the Specialists Registration Committee, which oversees the quality of these specialisations and the (re-)registration of pharmacy specialists [95].

6.5.1. Community Pharmacy Specialist

The community pharmacist specialisation is a two-year programme offered by the Charlotte Jacobs Institute (CJI), the KNMP's training institute for community pharmacy.

During this post-master's programme, the pharmacist in training is employed by a certified training pharmacy and works and learns under the supervision of an experienced community pharmacist. Following on-the-job learning, the pharmacist in training partakes in CJI-organised educational activities. Product care is an explicit part of the first year of this training programme [96].

6.5.2. Hospital Pharmacy Specialist

The hospital pharmacist specialisation is a four-year programme overseen by the NVZA. Similar to the community pharmacist specialisation, the hospital pharmacist in training will learn on the job in a hospital pharmacy. The first half of the specialisation has a standard programme, which includes individual medicine preparations and reconstitution as one of the areas of expertise. In the second half, the pharmacist in training can further specialise in a specific hospital pharmacy topic by choosing a so-called differentiation (Dutch: differentiatie). Regardless of the chosen differentiation, both product care and patient care ought to be part of it [97]. Hospital pharmacists in training can further specialise by choosing the differentiation Preparations and Pharmaceutical Analysis (Dutch: Bereidingen en Farmaceutische Analyse). During this differentiation, all aspects of pharmacy preparations are prominently covered, which equips the pharmacist with broad theoretical and practical skills required for pharmacy preparations prepared in a hospital pharmacy.

6.5.3. Post-Academic Education

To maintain the registration as a specialist, a pharmacist must regularly update the knowledge and skills by attending a predetermined amount of post-academic educational activities. To this end, different providers have developed courses, often in collaboration with the universities offering the Pharmacy programmes. Accreditation for these courses is regulated by the KNMP for community pharmacists and by the NVZA for hospital pharmacists [98]. Life-long learning is a must for community and hospital pharmacists.

6.6. Textbook

In 1992, the first edition of the textbook Recepteerkunde was published, consolidating decades of knowledge and practical experience in pharmaceutical compounding into a formalised reference. In the years that followed, Recepteerkunde served as both a guide for practicing pharmacists and a textbook for pharmacy students at Dutch universities. Five editions of Recepteerkunde were published (supported by the KNMP), gradually shifting its focus from small-scale compounding specifically to pharmaceutical product care in general.

Other European countries recognised the need for a formalised collection of knowledge and experience. At the 'EDQM symposium on European Co-operation & Synergy and the BEAM compounding course' in 2010, the idea for a European-wide textbook on pharmaceutical compounding was proposed. The fifth edition of Recepteerkunde would serve as the basis for this book, leading to the publication of Practical Pharmaceutics in 2015 (supported by the KNMP, NVZA and EAHP). Practical Pharmaceutics is a collaborative effort between European experts on pharmaceutical compounding and product care. It covers a wide range of topics, from basic principles (e.g., biopharmaceutics, physical chemistry and microbiology) to preconditions for compounding (such as raw materials, containers, premises and equipment) and the various specific dosage forms [99]. A second edition of Practical Pharmaceutics was published in 2023, supported by the KNMP and NVZA. This updated edition incorporates new developments and insights, such as ATMPs and 3D printing [100]. Practical Pharmaceutics has become an internationally recognised source of pharmaceutical–technological knowledge in relation to pharmacy preparations.

It is used as a reference book in pharmacy practice and during the Pharmacy curriculum of universities in the Netherlands and several other countries.

7. Special Topics Linked to Pharmacy Preparations

This section discusses specific pharmacy preparations and related product care, primarily within hospital settings in the Netherlands. These preparations include, amongst others, customised medications tailored to individual patients and require specialised handling and care characteristics of compounding practices. Often, they are linked to research focused on product development and/or optimising pharmacotherapy with dedicated pharmaceutical formulations. The emphasis is placed on specific patient groups, product categories, and techniques employed in their preparation.

7.1. Optimising Individual Treatment

7.1.1. Paediatric Dosage Forms

Pharmacists play a crucial role in the preparation of paediatric medications, ensuring that treatments are tailored to meet the specific needs of young patients. Major challenges include dosage adjustments, swallowability and palatability. Alternative dosage forms, such as flavoured oral solutions, suspensions, or chewable tablets, can improve adherence to treatment regimens. Age-appropriate dosage forms, such as liquid suspensions or small capsules, are prepared based on a child's weight and age. This is particularly important for medicines that are not available in paediatric-friendly strengths [101–104].

Common excipients in medicines for adults, such as alcohol, certain preservatives, or artificial colouring agents, are less or even unsuitable for children. It is the pharmacist's responsibility to replace these ingredients with safer alternatives or to find a way to omit them, minimising the risk of adverse effects and improving overall safety [105]. An example is the preparation of medication for paediatric patients with epilepsy who follow a ketogenic diet. The pharmacist can formulate sugar-free liquid oral solutions or capsules, ensuring that the medication is both effective and compatible with the child's dietary restrictions.

Another important aspect of paediatric pharmacy is the tailor-made preparation of injection and infusion fluids. Although not fundamentally different from preparations for adults, this specialised type of preparation for children is often carried out by pharmacy technicians due to the increased risk of preparation errors—frequently caused by calculation mistakes—resulting from the broader dosing range required for paediatric patients. In addition, these preparations may involve more dilution steps. For example, lower doses of peptides such as insulin often require the addition of albumin as an extra formulation step to prevent the insulin from adsorption to surfaces of parts of the syringe.

Many of these preparations take place in a cleanroom located near the paediatric ward, following specialised reconstitution procedures in accordance with GMP-Z regulations.

The Netherlands maintains a national paediatric formulary (www.kinderformularium.nl (accessed on 25 May 2025)) that provides dosing guidance and lists dosage forms to achieve the calculated dose, including compounded formulations described in the FNA (Section 5.2). The formulary is well coordinated, ensuring alignment between dosing recommendations and available formulations [106]. Additionally, several FNA formulations have been explicitly designed to meet the needs of paediatric patients.

With their expertise in formulation design, drug stability, compatibility issues and paediatric pharmacology, pharmacists play an essential role in optimising paediatric care by creating safe, effective, and tailored medicines for this specific patient population.

7.1.2. Swallowing Difficulties and Feeding Tubes

The correct administration of oral solid medicinal products to patients with swallowing difficulties (mostly children and the elderly) and patients with an enteral feeding tube remains a challenge. Information on the necessary adaptations is limited and associated with reduced efficacy, increased toxicity, and in the case of feeding tubes, a risk of tube obstruction.

The Oralia VTGM database (see Section 5.3) [21] provides guidance on the safe handling and transformation of solid formulations into liquid forms that can be easily swallowed or administered via a feeding tube. Instructional videos are provided as well. Whenever possible, a licensed administration route should be used as outlined in the SmPC of a product. The monographs in Oralia VTGM also suggest alternative administration routes and products to consider. In general, immediate-release tablets and unsealed (uncoated) hard capsules may undergo such handling, while sustained-release oral dosage forms may not. Unfortunately, not all immediate-release tablets can be pulverised and suspended into a viscous vehicle (suspension base, also commercially available). For these specific products, alternative approaches are provided (Table 7).

Table 7. Approaches in Oralia VTGM to convert an oral solid dosage form into an oral liquid dosage form. The preferred method depends on the product [21].

- Disintegrate the tablet in (warm) water in a spoon, glass or cup.
- Disintegrate the tablet in (warm) water in a syringe.
- Crush the tablet with a tablet crusher and mix the powder with water or semi-solid food.
- Open the capsule and mix the content with water or semi-solid food.

Similar information, but without technical background information, is available to healthcare providers other than pharmacy staff (e.g., nurses) through the website www.oralia.nl (accessed on 26 March 2025) [89].

For tablet crushing, commercially available manual crushers can be used, while both manual and electric grinders are available for tablet grinding. The performance of these devices varies: manual crushers generally produce a coarse powder, whereas manual or electric grinders result in a fine powder. When sufficient size reduction is required for administration via a feeding tube, as is common in hospitals and nursing homes, a grinder is preferred. To ease swallowing, oral swallowing gels are available as a substitute for water or semi-solid food for taking crushed or pulverised medication [107].

7.1.3. Hospital-at-Home Care

Outpatient parenteral therapy is increasingly used in clinical practice due to its associated cost savings, reduction in inpatient hospital days, and decreased risk of hospital-acquired infections [108–110]. Antimicrobials were among the first types of drugs to be administered parenterally at home, a practice known as OPAT (outpatient parenteral antimicrobial therapy) [111]. To date, a wider range of parenteral drugs is administered at home, including diuretics, analgesics, immunomodulators, oncolytic agents, and TPN.

Various types of containers are used for the preparation of these medicines, such as infusion bags, cassettes, and elastomeric infusion pumps. For administration, infusion bags and cassettes require electronic infusion devices, whereas elastomeric infusion pumps are independent of a power source [112].

In the Netherlands, parenteral medication for home administration is aseptically prepared in community pharmacies, hospital pharmacies, or compounding pharmacies under GMP-Z conditions. To support the development of hospital-at-home care, several initiatives have been launched, some of which have received government funding, such as the 'OPAT praktijkgids' (practical guide for OPAT) [113].

7.2. Specialist Product Groups

7.2.1. Reconstitution of Oncolytic Medicinal Products and Biologicals

Since the 1990s, it has been standard practice in the Netherlands for oncolytic medicinal products to be reconstituted in dedicated cleanrooms in hospital pharmacies rather than on the wards [114,115]. Oncolytic medicinal products include 'classical' chemotherapeutic agents (commonly referred to as cytotoxic medicinal products or cytotoxic drugs), oral targeted medicinal products, and biologicals.

Several factors necessitate the reconstitution of cytotoxic medicinal products in dedicated cleanrooms. Firstly, cytotoxic medicinal products often follow an individual dosing scheme, based on body surface area and at or near the maximum tolerable dose. As a result, the therapeutic window is narrow, meaning that any calculation or medication errors during reconstitution can lead to excessive toxicity or reduced efficacy. Secondly, the patient population receiving this type of medication is vulnerable and prone to myelosuppression. Strict aseptic procedures are therefore essential to prevent microbiological contamination. Lastly, cytotoxic drugs pose inherent hazards to personnel involved in their preparation. Consequently, robust safety procedures are required to prevent occupational exposure and environmental contamination.

To ensure accurate dosing, various methods are employed. When a manual procedure is used, each calculation must be verified by a second person (the 'four-eye principle'). Additionally, validated software applications are used to calculate volumes or weights, guiding personnel through the compounding process and enabling electronic checks of in-process controls. When available, built-in cameras verify materials and drawn-up volumes. Gravimetric reconstitution, where either the syringe containing the fluid to be added to the final container is weighed, or the final container is weighed before and after addition, improves accuracy and reduces medication errors. Similarly, fully automated compounding robots (see Section 7.3.1) are employed in some Dutch hospital pharmacies, further enhancing dosing accuracy while minimising medication errors [116–119].

Over the past decades, specific safety measures have been continuously developed and improved in the Netherlands to protect staff and the environment from cytotoxic drug exposure [120,121]. The key safety principles applied during handling and reconstitution are summarised in Table 8. Longitudinal studies assessing these measures indicated that residual exposure or contamination, when present, remains below occupational safety alert levels [122]. Special attention must be given to handling vials containing commercial cytotoxic medicinal products because the majority are contaminated with trace residues of the cytotoxic drug they contain [123].

Personnel involved in the reconstitution, receipt and storage of cytotoxic medicinal products must be aware of all these risks. Secondary packaging should not be removed outside the designated preparation area. Personnel responsible for unpacking and/or disinfecting the vials must be adequately trained and protected by suitable clothing. In the Netherlands, a simple, effective method has been developed for this process. First, vials are not removed from their secondary packaging by hand, but are gently slid into a small plastic bag using tweezers. Second, disinfectant is sprayed in this bag to disinfect the vials. (see Figure 3). Third, the vials are transferred from the plastic bag placed into the biological safety cabinet, again without touching them [125].

Table 8. Occupational safety measures for handling and reconstitution of cytotoxic medicinal products in Dutch hospital pharmacies [124].

- Label all cytotoxic drugs with an adequate warning sign (a yellow hand or yellow hazard triangle).
- Never touch primary packaging without wearing protective gloves.
- Transport cytotoxic drugs in sealed secondary packaging.
- Compound in a separate, dedicated room with entry through a lock.
- Compound in a safety cabinet or isolator with negative pressure.
- Do not recirculate air from the safety cabinet or isolator into the room or hospital ventilation system (0% recirculation principle).
- Compound using spikes or other closed system transfer devices to limit aerosol development.
- Wear adequate gloves and gowns with full length sleeves and cuffs that have been tested and proven to protect against cytotoxic substances.
- Dispense compounded cytotoxic drugs with a barrier that prevents exposure of the administrating staff: a side-line or multi-way connector set filled with a neutral fluid.

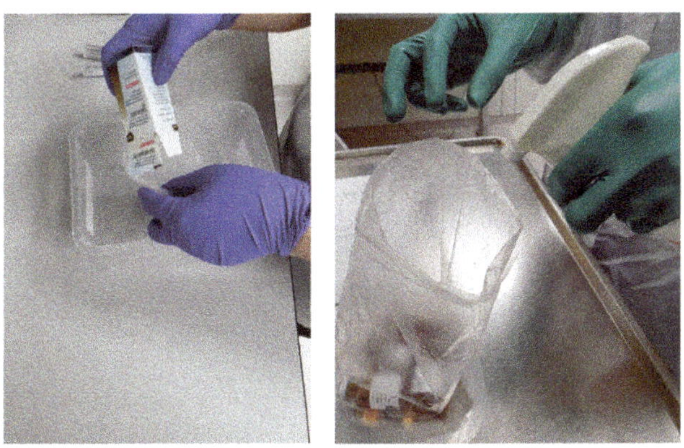

Figure 3. Unpacking (**left**) and disinfecting (**right**) of commercially obtained vials containing cytotoxic drugs without touching the outside of the primary packaging. Taken from [125] with permission.

Spillage requires special attention. Clear, written procedures must be in place, along with spill kits containing the necessary materials for safe clean-up. These kits should be readily available in the compounding room, adjacent storage areas, and any rooms where ready-to-administer cytotoxic medicinal products are checked and prepared for transport. All pharmacy personnel handling cytotoxic medicinal products must receive training on spill and incident management, with mandatory annual refresher courses [124]. The appropriate response for different types of incidents involving each cytotoxic medicinal product is detailed in the national crib sheet ('crash card oncolytics'), which is updated annually by the Working Conditions Committee of the NVZA [126].

In conclusion, the reconstitution of cytotoxic medicinal products constitutes a specific practice requiring strict precautions. The national framework of guidelines ensures the safety of both patients and healthcare workers.

7.2.2. Total Parenteral Nutrition (TPN)

TPN is a vital form of nutritional support for patients who are unable to meet their oral or enteral dietary needs. It is used in both hospital and home care settings and can be tailored to adult and paediatric patients.

Due to its microbiological vulnerability, TPN is primarily prepared in hospital pharmacies under strict aseptic conditions. Any contamination poses a significant risk to patients, particularly those with compromised immune systems. In the past, TPN was often prepared as a multicomponent formulation, sometimes using computerised pump systems to automate the process [127]. To enhance the safety and reliability of TPN preparation, this approach has largely been replaced by all-in-one multicomponent infusion bags. An additional advantage of this method is cost reduction [128]. At present, most TPN preparation processes typically begin with a commercially available three-chamber bag, which contain separate compartments: for a lipid emulsion, a glucose solution and an electrolyte solution. Once these compartments are combined, the TPN can be further customised to a patient's clinical needs by adding specific nutrients such as additional amino acids or lipids, electrolytes, vitamins, and trace elements.

To ensure compatibility and stability, pharmacists rely on information provided by the manufacturer. In some cases, TPN is entirely prepared from separate components, allowing for greater formulation flexibility. This approach is particularly useful for patients with complex nutritional needs or requiring highly individualised solutions. For example, paediatric patients with elevated liver enzymes may require customised lipid formulations to minimise hepatic stress. Similarly, patients with short bowel syndrome may need adjusted concentrations of electrolytes, additional amino acids, or fluids to compensate for altered absorption and metabolic demands [129–131].

Pharmacists' specialised knowledge and expertise are essential in precisely adjusting formulations while ensuring the highest standards of safety, stability, and compatibility. They also provide support in managing technical issues, such as a clogged infusion line caused by TPN administration. In the Netherlands, specialised (hospital) pharmacies are responsible for the compounding and distribution of TPN for home care patients.

7.2.3. Advanced Therapy Medicinal Products (ATMPs)

Advanced therapy medicinal products (ATMPs) have transformed the clinical landscape, demonstrating the potential to treat and even cure patients for whom conventional medicine is ineffective. According to the EMA, ATMPs are classified as either gene therapy, somatic-cell therapy, or tissue-engineered medicines. Additionally, an ATMP that includes one or more medical devices as an integral part of the medicinal product is designated as a combined ATMP. In the EU, ATMPs are considered biological medicinal products and are governed by Regulation 1394/2007 [132].

The manufacturing process of ATMPs should comply with GMP guidelines, specifically GMP Part IV—GMP Requirements for Advanced Therapy Medicinal Products [133]. Section 16 of GMP Part IV acknowledges that product reconstitution may be required after batch release, but before administration to the patient. It permits these activities to be carried out at the administration site outside a GMP-controlled environment. Examples of ATMP reconstitution include thawing, washing, centrifugation, dispersion, and dilution of the product. These handlings can take place in hospital pharmacies or dedicated facilities such as stem cell laboratories. As ATMPs may contain genetic material, viral vectors, genetically modified organisms (GMO), or cells or tissue of human origin, special cleaning and disinfection procedures may be required in the event of spillage.

Pharmacists and hospital pharmacies contribute to the research and development of ATMPs. Most Dutch academic centres have a GMP manufacturing license to produce clinical-grade ATMPs and can facilitate the translational research of in-house developed ATMPs. This also provides opportunities to conduct clinical trials for external parties. In-house manufactured ATMPs are manufactured at the hospital instead of a centralised production facility, which is typical for ATMPs with a marketing authorisation. Therefore, these products are referred to as point-of-care, place-of-care, or decentralised manufactured ATMPs.

A typical ATMP manufacturing process takes several days to weeks and consists mainly of biological processes. Compared to a conventional medicinal product, an ATMP is complex. ATMPs are inherently characterised by a considerable variability in product specifications as they are often produced using biological processes and analysed using biomolecular and biological assays. Additionally, for ATMPs manufactured from human donor material, considerable variability in the starting material is found, which may impact the final product specifications [134]. Pharmacists involved in the production, quality control testing and batch release of ATMPs should have the expertise to consider these inherent variabilities as well as the impact of deviations on the biological processes and analytical test results and, by extension, on the manufacturing process and the final drug product specification.

Pharmacists collaborate with preclinical and clinical researchers from different disciplines to facilitate the development and clinical translational research of ATMPs. During process development, pharmacists substantiate the use of non-compendial materials and processing aids. Besides supplier qualification, the materials are assessed for their suitability and the presence of impurities, mycoplasma, endotoxins, prions, and viruses by considering their origin, production processes and intended use during the ATMP manufacturing process. Furthermore, together with content experts from different disciplines, a stability study plan, risk assessments, validation protocols and reports, and batch records are compiled.

Currently, several ATMPs are being developed in Dutch academic hospitals (Table 9), with the ultimate goal of clinical application and patient access to novel therapies. To support this goal, the national consortium DARE-NL (Dutch infrastructure for cancer-specific ATMP Research) was established in 2022 and funded by the Dutch Cancer Society (KWF) [135].

Table 9. A selection of clinical-grade ATMPs that have been developed and investigated in clinical trials in the Netherlands.

ATMP	Indication	Institution	Manufacturing Process	Reference
Anti-CD19 CAR-T cells	Diffuse large B cell lymphoma	University Medical Center Groningen	CD4+ and CD8+ cells are enriched from leukapheresis material and ex vivo activated, transduced by a lentiviral vector, expanded, harvested, and formulated into the drug product.	[136]
Vvax-001	HPV-induced cancers	University Medical Center Groningen	RNA is produced from plasmid DNA and transfected into Vero cells that produce the Vvax-001 replicon particles, which, after purification, are formulated into the drug product.	[137]
Tumour-infiltrating lymphocytes (TIL)	Melanoma	Netherlands Cancer Institute	Melanoma lesion is surgically resected and enzymatic digested to harvest TILs, which are ex vivo expanded for 2–4 weeks, harvested, and formulated into the drug product.	[138]

Table 9. *Cont.*

ATMP	Indication	Institution	Manufacturing Process	Reference
Dendritic cell vaccination	Melanoma; prostate cancer	Radboud University Medical Center	Dendritic cells are isolated from apheresis material, matured, loaded with antigen, harvested, and formulated into the drug product.	[139,140]
Natural killer (NK) cells	Acute myeloid leukemia	Radboud University Medical Center	NK cells are ex vivo generated from umbilical cord blood-derived CD34+ progenitor cells using a mixture of cytokines and growth factors and are subsequently expanded, harvested, and formulated into the drug product.	[141,142]
ΔNPM1 T cell receptor (TCR)-engineered T cells	NPM1 mutated acute myeloid leukemia	Leiden University Medical Center	CD8+ cells are enriched from leukapheresis material and ex vivo activated, transduced by a lentiviral vector, expanded, harvested, and formulated into the drug product.	[143,144]
Vγ9Vδ2T cell receptor engineered T cells (TEG001)	Acute myeloid leukemia; multiple myeloma	University Medical Center Utrecht	T cells from leukapheresis material are ex vivo activated, transduced by a retroviral vector, expanded, purified, harvested, and formulated into the drug product.	[145,146]
MesoPher	Mesothelioma	Erasmus Medical Center	Monocytes are enriched from leukapheresis material and ex vivo cultured and differentiated into dendritic cells after which these dendritic cells are cultured in the presence of allogenic tumour lysate. Subsequently, the dendritic cells are matured, harvested, and formulated into the drug product.	[147]

7.2.4. Radiopharmaceuticals and Optical Tracers

Radiopharmaceuticals are medicinal products used in nuclear medicine for diagnostic and therapeutic purposes. They consist of a tracer molecule linked to a radionuclide. The tracer molecule localises the product in the body, while the radionuclide emits radiation that scanners can detect, or delivers a radiation dose to a target area. Radionuclides decay with a specific half-life, making the handling of radiopharmaceuticals time-dependent. Nuclear imaging using positron emission tomography (PET) and single-photon emission computed tomography (SPECT) are applied for diagnostic purposes.

As their shelf life is usually limited, radiopharmaceuticals must be prepared, often requiring reconstitution, shortly before the patient undergoes a nuclear medicine procedure or treatment. In addition, dosages of prepared radiopharmaceuticals, expressed in megabecquerels (MBq), need to be customised for each patient at a specific time. As a consequence of the unique aspects of radiopharmaceuticals, compounding pharmacies play an essential role in their supply [148].

In the Netherlands, radiopharmaceuticals are prepared in a number of specialised hospital pharmacies or in centralised radiopharmacies. Hospital pharmacies supplying radiopharmaceuticals have dedicated areas designed for their preparation, which may be for either in-house use or for use in other hospitals. Alternatively, nuclear departments in Dutch hospitals can order radiopharmaceuticals from centralised radiopharmacies, which specialise in the preparation, dispensing and distribution of radiopharmaceuticals. Furthermore, due to the relatively short distances, multiple shipments take place between the main production sites and various receiving hospitals, ensuring optimal availability of radiopharmaceuticals across the country. These features make the Netherlands well suited for conducting multicentre clinical trials involving radiopharmaceuticals.

Radiopharmaceuticals are prepared in biosafety cabinets situated in a cleanroom, according to GMP-Z Annex 3 and GMP, respectively [149]. The biosafety cabinets, typically fitted with additional lead glass, protect the operators from radiation while maintaining aseptic conditions. The classification of the cleanroom is usually class C or D, depending on the outcome of a risk analysis [150].

The prescription for a radiopharmaceutical comes from a nuclear medicine physician or a nuclear radiologist. In the Netherlands, this is nearly always carried out using a nuclear medicine information system. Prescriptions specify, among others, the dosage in MBq and the time of administration. For dispensing, radiopharmaceuticals can either be ordered as ready-to-use products or prepared in-house. Ready-to-use radiopharmaceuticals only require a volume containing the correct dosage to be drawn into an injection syringe. The syringes are labelled with dose information in MBq at the time of administration and a radioactivity symbol, in addition to the general information found on labels of prepared medicinal products.

The preparation of radiopharmaceuticals often involves the reconstitution of kits. These are vials containing the tracer molecule and other necessary ingredients to prepare a radiopharmaceutical, often for multiple doses. They are mostly licensed medicinal products, with their preparation and quality control described in the SmPC. Reconstitution begins with obtaining the desired radionuclide, which is often sourced from a radiopharmaceutical generator (such as a molybdenum/technetium generator) or sometimes purchased as a precursor. The radionuclide is then added in an adjusted volume to the kit. After incubation, sometimes requiring boiling or buffer addition, the radiopharmaceutical is obtained. Quality control of reconstituted radiopharmaceuticals includes a test for radiochemical purity, for which thin-layer chromatography is mostly applied. In addition to licensed kits, some compounding pharmacies use non-licensed kits or extemporaneous preparations. For these preparations, (sterile) starting materials are procured from commercial suppliers, but can also be obtained from other compounding pharmacies [149,150].

Some Dutch hospitals (mostly university medical centres) have their own cyclotron for the production of short-lived radioisotopes, such as ^{18}F, with a physical half-life of 110 min. In so-called hot cells, which are a lead-shielded GMP class C environments, radiopharmaceuticals for PET are synthesised, purified and formulated using automated synthesis modules. The final filtration step is performed in a GMP class A environment, ideally with a class B background. The preparations must comply with general and, where applicable, specific quality standards as described in the Ph. Eur. [151]. For small-scale production in the Netherlands, unlicensed diagnostic radiopharmaceuticals can, in principle, be produced in accordance with the regulations of other pharmaceutical preparations [149].

Once the preparation of the radiopharmaceutical is completed and the quality control results have been assessed, the product is released by a qualified pharmacist or a qualified person (QP). Due to the short half-life of radiopharmaceuticals, an exception is granted under GMP regulations, allowing for conditional release of the product under specific conditions before all tests (such as microbiological) are completed [152].

Following release, the radiopharmaceutical is delivered to the nuclear department in especially shielded containers to ensure safe handling. Specific transportation requirements apply to road transport, such as obtaining transport permits or notifying the Dutch nuclear safety authority [153].

Hospital pharmacists and radiopharmacists in the Netherlands are regularly consulted by nuclear medicine departments regarding preparations for special patient groups, adverse events, or drug interactions [154].

Currently, many new radiopharmaceuticals are being developed, also in (academic) hospitals, with an emerging role for theranostics. Theranostics use a single tracer molecule for both diagnostic and therapeutic purposes, enabling more precise patient selection and improved monitoring of treatment responses. Current examples include ^{68}Ga-DOTA-octreotide derivatives/^{177}Lu-DOTATE and ^{68}Ga-PSMA or ^{18}F-PSMA/^{177}Lu-PSMA. For the preparation of theranostics, an increasing role for specialised compounding pharmacies is anticipated [155]. Under the new EU clinical trial regulation, GMP is no longer required for diagnostic radiopharmaceuticals used as an investigational medicinal product (IMP). However, IMP radiopharmaceuticals for therapeutic purposes must still be manufactured in accordance with GMP regulations [156].

Another recent development, with the Netherlands as frontrunner, is the use of molecular imaging in drug development and to guide treatment with targeted therapies in oncology, specifically as biomarker imaging. Monoclonal antibodies or antibody derivatives are labelled with long-lived radioisotopes, such as ^{89}Zr, which matches the antibody's biological half-life. Typical handling steps are carried out in a shielded isolator in hospital pharmacies and include radiolabelling, purification, formulation, and sterile filtration steps, immediately followed by quality control testing. An example, also used in clinical patient care, is ^{89}Zr-trastuzumab for the detection of human epidermal growth factor receptor 2 (HER2)-positive tumour lesions [157]. Applications, challenges and future developments of molecular imaging in drug development and precision medicine are described in recent review papers [158,159]. In addition to labelling tracer molecules with isotopes, they can also be conjugated with optical dyes for near-infrared fluorescent molecular imaging to prepare fluorescent tracers. An advantage of this approach is the absence of radioactivity along with a generally longer shelf life, which allows for larger-scale manufacturing and stockpiling.

Fluorescent molecular imaging is complementary to nuclear imaging and provides more detailed information on the tissue and cellular level due to superior spatiotemporal resolution, whereas nuclear imaging provides the whole-body picture. Targeted tracers have been developed, based on antibodies, small molecules, peptides, nanoparticles, or proteins, and are used in various investigational applications, including image-guided surgery, pathology, endoscopy, and drug development [160]. Examples of monoclonal antibody-based optical tracers used in clinical studies are bevacizumab-800CW, cetuximab-800CW, trastuzumab-800CW, panitumumab-800CW, adalimumab-800CW, and vedolizumab-800CW [161].

The manufacturing process is performed under GMP conditions in hospital pharmacies and starts with a buffer exchange step to remove excipients, especially amino acids, from the original monoclonal antibody formulation. The dye is then coupled via direct conjugation to primary and secondary amines in the antibody, followed by removal of the free dye. The purified bulk solution is diluted in a formulation buffer and, after sterile filtration, vials are aseptically filled. After quality control, the final product is a ready-to-use solution for intravenous or topical administration [161].

A roadmap has been designed by a Dutch academic hospital for the development and clinical translation of optical tracers [162].

7.2.5. Clinical Trial Medication

Extemporaneous compounding is essential for the preparation of customised formulations required for clinical trials and investigational research or for the preparation of new products used in first-in-human studies. These studies are directed to drug development and aim to compare the safety and effects of different medicines and drug delivery systems [163]. For novel drug products, suitable formulations must be developed, taking their physicochemical properties and the route of administration into account. Study medication of other drug compounds may be unavailable in the desired dose or administration form, requiring the reformulation of existing products. In phase I-II clinical trials, the final product formulation is often not yet developed. Pharmacy preparations (such as capsules or liquid formulations) enable the execution of early-phase trials while development of the final product continues.

The preparation, handling, control and documentation of clinical trial medication, designated as IMPs, are strictly regulated in the Netherlands and Europe to ensure safety, quality and efficacy. The Dutch Medicines Act applies, while on a European level, the administration of IMPs to humans is regulated by the Clinical Trials Regulation No. 536/2014, which has been effective since 31 January 2022 [156].

Although the preparation of medication for a first-in-humans study remains costly, the ability to produce innovative medicines on a small scale within a hospital or compounding pharmacy offers a unique opportunity to conduct such studies within a limited time frame and with minimal investment in production infrastructure. This approach has been effectively applied. Spray-dried tobramycin powder was formulated into a newly developed inhalation device for pulmonary delivery, Cyclops®, in a tolerability and pharmacokinetics study in patients with non-cystic fibrosis bronchiectasis [164]. The performance of a newly developed colon delivery system, ColoPulse®, was tested in healthy volunteers and in Crohn's patients using a dual-label strategy with 13C-glucose and 15N-urea [165].

Many Dutch hospital and compounding pharmacies actively contribute to clinical studies and are generally well equipped to produce small-scale IMP batches. In addition to the examples above, their activities include the following:

- Re-labelling and encapsulation of licensed medicines for clinical trial use;
- Small-scale production of non-sterile medicines such as capsules, tablets, and dermal preparations;
- Sterile preparations, including reconstitution of trial medication produced by the pharmaceutical industry and small-scale in-house production of sterile products (e.g., biologicals, ATMPs, radiopharmaceuticals, other imaging agents, conjugated photodynamic therapy agents, and small-molecule products).

An example of support to a larger clinical study by a hospital pharmacy is the production of vitamin capsules designed for site-specific colon delivery [166]. However, for many larger clinical trial batches, production is typically carried out by specialised compounding facilities.

7.3. Technological Innovations

7.3.1. Robotisation in Reconstitution

Since many parenteral drugs are not marketed as RTA products, several handling steps are required before each administration. When performed manually on a larger scale, this process is labour-intensive and the repetitive nature of the movements may lead to hand and joint complaints [167,168]. In addition, the need for human checks, such as the four-eye principle for verifying drawn-up fluid volumes, raises concerns regarding patient safety [49]. These factors, combined with the national shortage of personnel, have led to an increasing interest in automated and robotic reconstitution methods.

Reconstitution robots first entered the market at the beginning of the 21st century, initially focusing on the reconstitution of cytotoxic medicinal products to reduce potential personnel exposure to harmful substances [169]. The first generation of robots achieved only moderate success due to their longer production times compared to manual processes. Second- and third-generation robots have demonstrated improved productivity [170].

As of 2024, there are four brands of reconstitution robots used in hospital pharmacies in the Netherlands: the Apoteca Chemo robot (Loccioni, Ancona, Italy), the RIVA robot (Arxium, Winnipeg, Canada), the Kiro robot (Kiro Grifols, Barcelona, Spain), and the IV Station robot (Health Robotics, Bolzano, Italy). These robots each have one or two robot arms that handle vials, bags and syringes, and feature a fully enclosed preparation area that meets GMP grade A requirements, alongside a loading and unloading area adjacent to the preparation area. The robots are capable of dissolving powders, drawing-up and adding fluids, and using gravimetric control, barcode scanning, or photo-recognition to ensure the correct medicinal product is prepared in the correct dose [167,170]. Depending on the model, the robots can either perform only individual reconstitution or a combination of individual and batch reconstitution. Additionally, some models feature automatic waste management, while others can also prepare elastomeric pumps. Figure 4 shows a reconstitution robot as operational in a Dutch hospital pharmacy.

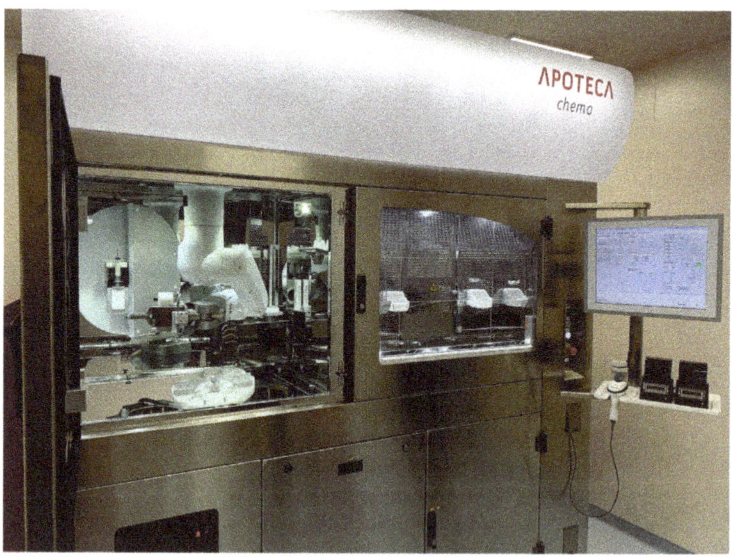

Figure 4. Reconstitution robot at the Department of Clinical Pharmacology and Pharmacy, Amsterdam University Medical Center, location Vrije Universiteit (photograph: MC).

In terms of productivity, there are no published data for RIVA or IV Station robots. Depending on the type of drug and the number of vials required per preparation, the Apoteca can compound up to 38 preparations per hour, while the Kiro can produce up to 13 preparations per hour [171,172]. Regarding dosing accuracy, robots perform as well as, or better than, manual reconstitution, with all models achieving an accuracy of 97–103% [167]. Finally, microbiological and chemical contamination performances are high, demonstrating that these robots are well suited for routine reconstitution in hospital pharmacies [173–177].

The number of hospital pharmacies implementing reconstitution robots is expected to increase over the coming years. Furthermore, although less advanced, several other robotic solutions are emerging to take over human tasks in compounding pharmacies.

For example, visual inspection of glass ampoules for particles and the integrity of blister packaging can now be automated.

7.3.2. Patient-Centric Solid Oral Dosage Forms

Currently, there is an increased demand for personalised medication and individualised therapies and a well-established lack of suitable medication with appropriate dosages and palatability for special patient groups, e.g., children. A promising approach in this context, to expand compounding capabilities, is the implementation of 3D printing technologies by which three-dimensional dosage forms are created in a layer-by-layer fashion. The size and shape of a dosage form are defined on an individual level in a computer programme that then generates a machine control code executed by a 3D printer.

Currently, different 3D printing technologies are extensively researched as manufacturing options for personalised medication. Most applicable for individual or small-scale manufacturing in pharmacies are extrusion-based technologies due to their small environmental footprint and low exposure risks. For larger-scale manufacturing, powder-based technologies such as binder jetting and selective laser sintering are used [178].

Three-dimensional printing of pharmaceutical dosage forms has multiple benefits, mainly for solid oral dosage forms. The size and shape of the dosage form can be readily modified in the computer without changing process parameters, thereby enabling personalisation of dosage and adjustment of release profiles [178]. Additionally, formulations with immediate- and sustained-release characteristics can also be developed and manufactured [179]. The technologies also enable the combination of multiple drugs in one dosage form ('polypills') [180,181]. Another benefit is the ability to use the same formulation irrespective of the intended dosage or shape, simplifying formulation development. This makes 3D printing a suitable technology for manufacturing clinical trial medication. Besides oral dosage forms, other solid dosage forms can be manufactured, such as suppositories [182]. Lastly, there is the possibility of incorporating commercial dosage forms into the formulation for a 3D printing process, enabling accurate individualisation of medicinal products that are still under patent protection [183].

The translation to clinical use in compounding and community pharmacies is facilitated by several companies founded in the past years providing workflows, printers, and dispensing systems.

The first hospitals and community pharmacies have acquired printing systems and are currently implementing them for use in everyday care or in clinical trials. The clinical translation of 3D printing is promising and accelerating. The first 3D printed medication as part of regular treatment will likely be provided to hospital patients in the Netherlands in 2025 and developments in community pharmacies indicate a similar timeline [184]. To ensure the highest quality standards for the future, close collaboration with the KNMP and national competent authorities is required.

Other patient-centric oral solid dosage forms that are currently receiving attention, are minitablets and orodispersible films.

With a diameter of 2–5 mm, minitablets are considerably smaller than regular-sized tablets. It has been demonstrated that minitablets are equally well accepted by neonates and children as syrup. Dose flexibility is easily achieved by administering a varying number of minitablets. As minitablets are industrially prepared for several drugs, efforts are made to develop extemporaneous compounded minitablets for a given patient, particularly in hospital settings [185].

Orodispersible films are thin films, measuring 1–2 cm by 1–2 cm, that readily dissolve or disintegrate in the mouth upon contact with saliva, after which they are easily swallowed. Three-dimensional printing of a drug substance onto a plain film appears to be the most suitable method for the extemporaneously produced, customised and patient-centred orodispersible films, although their production still has considerable limitations [186].

8. Conclusions, Perspectives and Challenges

Over the past decades, extemporaneous compounding has evolved from an artisan-based practice into a science grounded in knowledge and understanding. Mastery of this science is typically the domain of the pharmacist. Currently, pharmacy preparations constitute a relatively small proportion of the overall range of medicines but are indispensable to patient care. Due to their flexibility, pharmacy preparations are well suited to bridge the gap between industrially manufactured medicines and the specific needs of patients. Given the current rise in personalised medication, requiring individualised therapies based on, for example, genetic profiles, tailor-made pharmacy preparations, and the competencies to produce them, will remain a relevant and essential aspect of healthcare, providing a vital service to patients requiring tailored treatments.

New developments and perspectives have led to a resurgence of extemporaneous compounding with a renewed focus. Patient-centricity and individualised therapy are key to justifying extemporaneous compounding in (hospital) pharmacies. Additionally, patients are expected to demonstrate better adherence to tailor-made medication compared to less well-suited standard treatments, potentially leading to improved pharmacotherapeutic outcomes, reduced treatment costs, and reduced waste from unused products.

In the Netherlands, good practices include the standardisation of extemporaneously prepared medicines, continuous support from the national pharmacists' professional association for pharmaceutical product care, and stringent and robust regulations to ensure quality and safety. Customised GMP guidelines for hospital pharmacy in the form of GMP-Z are a unique feature. The Netherlands distinguishes itself from many other countries through the continuous development of pharmacy preparations based on clinical needs. This translational research is conducted in both hospital pharmacies and centralised compounding facilities.

In addition to extemporaneous preparations, several pharmacies also manufacture stock preparations. In recent years, stock manufacturing has become increasingly centralised in specialised pharmacies, driven by both economic and quality considerations. The delivery of unique products between pharmacies is currently permitted by the IGJ and is expected to be formally incorporated into legislation in the future. The way pharmacy-to-pharmacy delivery and outsourcing are organised and implemented in the Netherlands, along with the associated quality assurance, is unique both within Europe and globally.

Future challenges will include a stronger emphasis on sustainability and green compounding, as well as integrating environmentally friendly practices into pharmacy preparations. More focus will be on the role of the pharmacist in the preparation of high-tech products, like ATMPs, vaccines and biologicals. Artificial intelligence (AI) is expected to have an impact on extemporaneous compounding. It may be a valuable tool for optimising formulations, predicting stability, easing quality control, ensuring compliance with pharmaceutical standards, and automating compounding processes. Continuous education and life-long learning are of paramount importance.

Author Contributions: Conceptualisation, H.J.W., O.S.N.M.S., A.A.-D., J.M.M., K.J.M.S. and B.G.; methodology, H.J.W. and B.G.; writing—original draft preparation, H.J.W., B.v.B., C.O., O.S.N.M.S., A.A.-D., M.C., J.M.M., K.J.M.S., E.M.K., M.N.L.-d.H., N.S., M.E., A.S.R., R.B.L., J.Q., H.H.B., O.K., K.H.M.L.-B., P.P.H.L.B., R.J.K., R.C.A.S., O.B., H.W.F. and B.G.; writing—review and editing, H.J.W., B.v.B., C.O., O.S.N.M.S., A.A.-D., M.C., J.M.M., K.J.M.S., E.M.K., M.N.L.-d.H., N.S., M.E., A.S.R., R.B.L., J.Q., H.H.B., O.K., K.H.M.L.-B., P.P.H.L.B., R.J.K., R.C.A.S., O.B., H.W.F. and B.G.; supervision,

H.J.W. and B.G.; project administration, H.J.W. All authors have read and agreed to the published version of the manuscript.

Funding: This research received no external funding.

Data Availability Statement: Information on some websites cited is not publicly available, but only via paid subscription or membership. Specific detailed requests can be directed to the authors and will be granted on reasonable request.

Acknowledgments: The authors thank Sofieke de Wilde, Pauline Meij, Rosa de Groot, Paul de Jonge, Gerty Schreibelt, Mirjam Heemskerk and Jürgen Kuball for their input and feedback on Table 9 of this manuscript. The authors also thank Irene Renate den Toom for designing the figures.

Conflicts of Interest: The companies to which several authors are affiliated had no role in the design of this study; in the collection, analysis, or interpretation of data; in the writing of the manuscript; or in the decision to publish the results. The remaining authors declare that the research was conducted in the absence of any commercial or financial relationships that could be construed as a potential conflict of interest.

Abbreviations

The following abbreviations are used in this manuscript:

Abbreviation	Meaning	English Translation of Dutch (If Applicable)
AI	Artificial intelligence	
API	Active pharmaceutical ingredient	
ATMP	Advanced therapy medicinal product	
BP	British Pharmacopoeia	
BSc	Bachelor of Science	
CBG	College ter Beoordeling van Geneesmiddelen	Medicines Evaluation Board (MEB)
CEP	Certificate of suitability to the monographs of the European Pharmacopoeia	
CJI	Charlotte Jacobs Institute	
DAC/NRF	Deutscher Arzneimittel-Codex/Neues Rezeptur-Formularium	German Drug Codex/New German Formulary
EAHP	European Association of Hospital Pharmacists	
ECTS	European Credit Transfer System	
EDQM	European Directorate for the Quality of Medicines and HealthCare	
EMA	European Medicines Agency	
EU	European Union	
FDA	US Food and Drug Administration	
FNA	Formularium der Nederlandse Apothekers	Formulary of Dutch Pharmacists
GCP	Good Clinical Practice	
GMO	Genetically modified organism	
GMP	Good Manufacturing Practice	
GMP-Z	GMP-Ziekenhuisfarmacie	GMP-Hospital pharmacy
GW	Geneesmiddelenwet	Medicines Act
ICH	International Conference on Harmonisation	
IGJ	Inspectie Gezondheidszorg en Jeugd	Health and Youth Care Inspectorate
IMP	Investigational medicinal product	
KNMP	Koninklijke Nederlandse Maatschappij ter bevordering der Pharmacie	Royal Dutch Pharmacists Association

LNA	Laboratorium der Nederlandse Apothekers	Laboratory of Dutch Pharmacists
LU	Universiteit Leiden (UL)	Leiden University
MAA	Marketing Authorisation Application	
MAH	Marketing Authorisation Holder	
MIA	Manufacturing and Importation Authorisation	
MSc	Master of Science	
NVZA	Nederlandse Vereniging voor Ziekenhuisapothekers	Dutch Association of Hospital Pharmacists
OPAT	Outpatient parenteral antimicrobial therapy	
PET	Positron emission tomography	
PFSS	Prefilled sterilised syringe	
Ph. Eur.	European Pharmacopoeia	-
PIC/S	Pharmaceutical Inspection Convention/Pharmaceutical Inspection Co-operation Scheme	
PQS	Pharmaceutical quality system	
QA	Quality assurance	
QbD	Quality by design	
QP	Qualified person	
RiFaS	Risico instrument Farmaceutische Stoffen	Risk Instrument for Pharmaceutical Substances
RTA	Ready to administer	
RTU	Ready to use	
SIG	Special Interest Group	
SmPC	Summary of Product Characteristics	
SPECT	Single-photon emission computed tomography	
TPN	Total parenteral nutrition	
US(A)	United States (of America)	
USP	United States Pharmacopeia	
UG	Rijksuniversiteit Groningen (RUG)	University of Groningen
UU	Universiteit Utrecht (UU)	Utrecht University
VTGM	Voor toediening gereedmaken	Reconstitution (literally: Preparation for administration)
VU	Vrije Universiteit Amsterdam	
Wet BIG	Wet op de Beroepen in de Individuele Gezondheidszorg	Professions in Individual Health Care Act
WGBO	Wet op de Geneeskundige Behandelingsovereenkomst	Medical Treatment Contracts Act

References

1. Schalekamp, T.; Haisma, H.J. *Domeinspecifiek Referentiekader & Raamplan Farmacie 2016. [2016 Pharmacist Competency Framework & Domain-Specific Frame of Reference for the Netherlands]*; KNMP Medicijn Media: Den Haag, The Netherlands, 2016. Available online: https://www.knmp.nl/sites/default/files/2021-11/Referentiekader%20en%20Raamplan%202016%20def.pdf (accessed on 28 October 2024).
2. European Medicines Agency. Available online: https://www.ema.europa.eu/en/homepage (accessed on 12 December 2024).
3. College ter Beoordeling van Geneesmiddelen (CBG) (Dutch Medicines Evaluation Board). Available online: https://www.cbg-meb.nl (accessed on 12 December 2024).
4. Stichting Farmaceutische Kengetallen (SFK) (Foundation for Pharmaceutical Statistics). Data en Feiten 2021. Available online: https://www.sfk.nl/sites/sfk-nl/files/2025-01/Data_en_feiten_2021.pdf (accessed on 26 May 2025).
5. Stichting Farmaceutische Kengetallen (SFK). Aandeel generiek verder toegenomen. *Pharm. Weekbl.* **2024**, *159*, 7.
6. European Directorate for the Quality of Medicines & HealthCare (EDQM). Pharmaceutical Preparations. 07/2024: 2619. In *European Pharmacopoeia*, 11.5th ed.; EDQM Council of Europe: Strasbourg, France, 2023. Available online: https://pheur-online.edqm.eu/content/2619/en/current/ (accessed on 11 December 2024).
7. European Association of Hospital Pharmacists (EAHP). EAHP Position Paper on Pharmacy Preparations and Compounding. Making a Difference in Medication by Delivering Tailor-Made Medicines for the Benefit of Patients. October 2020. Available online: https://eahp.eu/wp-content/uploads/2024/03/eahp_position_paper_on_pharmacy_preparations_and_compounding_october_2020.pdf (accessed on 12 December 2024).

8. United States Food and Drug Administration (FDA). Human Drug Compounding. Available online: https://www.fda.gov/drugs/guidance-compliance-regulatory-information/human-drug-compounding (accessed on 28 October 2024).
9. Scheepers, H.P.A.; Langedijk, J.; Neerup Handlos, V.; Walser, S.; Schutjens, M.D.B.; Neef, C. Legislation on the preparation of medicinal products in European pharmacies and the Council of Europe Resolution. *Eur. J. Hosp. Pharm.* **2017**, *24*, 224–229. [CrossRef] [PubMed]
10. Council of Europe. Resolution CM/Res(2016)1 on Quality and Safety Assurance Requirements for Medicinal Products Prepared in Pharmacies for the Special Needs of Patients. Available online: https://search.coe.int/cm/Pages/result_details.aspx?ObjectID=090000168065c132 (accessed on 12 December 2024).
11. Koninklijke Nederlandse Maatschappij ter Bevordering der Pharmacie (KNMP) (Royal Dutch Pharmacists Association). KNMP Kennisbank. LNA-Mededeling Productzorg (January 2020). Available online: https://kennisbank.knmp.nl (upon subscription, accessed on 17 June 2025).
12. European Commission. The Rules Governing Medicinal Products in the European Union. EudraLex. Volume 4. Good Manufacturing Practice (GMP) Guidelines. Available online: https://health.ec.europa.eu/medicinal-products/eudralex/eudralex-volume-4_en (accessed on 11 December 2024).
13. U.S. Food and Drugs Administration (FDA). Current Good Manufacturing Practice (CGMP) Regulations. Available online: https://www.fda.gov/drugs/pharmaceutical-quality-resources/current-good-manufacturing-practice-cgmp-regulations (accessed on 12 December 2024).
14. World Health Organization (WHO). Health Products Policy and Standards. Good Manufacturing Practices. Available online: https://www.who.int/teams/health-product-policy-and-standards/standards-and-specifications/gmp (accessed on 12 December 2024).
15. International Council for Harmonisation of Technical Requirements for Pharmaceuticals for Human Use (ICH). Quality Guidelines. Available online: https://www.ich.org/page/quality-guidelines (accessed on 11 December 2024).
16. Pharmaceutical Inspection Convention. PIC/S Guide to Good Practices for the Preparation of Medicinal Products in Healthcare Establishments. PE 010-4. Available online: https://picscheme.org/docview/3443 (accessed on 11 December 2024).
17. Koster, A.S.; Mantel-Teeuwisse, A.K.; Woerdenbag, H.J.; Mulder, W.M.C.; Wilffert, B.; Schalekamp, T.; Buurma, H.; Wilting, I.; Westein, M.P.D. Alignment of CanMEDS-Based undergraduate and postgraduate Pharmacy curricula in The Netherlands. *Pharmacy* **2020**, *8*, 117. [CrossRef] [PubMed]
18. Koninklijke Nederlandse Maatschappij ter Bevordering der Pharmacie (KNMP) (Royal Dutch Pharmacists Association). Professionale Standaard Farmaceutische Zorg. Available online: https://www.knmp.nl/richtlijnen/professionele-standaard-farmaceutische-zorg (accessed on 29 November 2024).
19. Koninklijke Nederlandse Maatschappij ter Bevordering der Pharmacie (KNMP) (Royal Dutch Pharmacists Association). *Charter Professionalism of the Pharmacist. Foundation for Acting Professionally and Ethically. [Translation of 'Handvest van de Apotheker. Grondslag voor Professioneel en Ethisch Handelen' (2017)]*; KNMP: Den Haag, The Netherlands, 2018. Available online: https://www.knmp.nl/sites/default/files/2021-12/Charter%20Professionalism%20of%20the%20Pharmacist.pdf (accessed on 29 November 2024).
20. Nederlandse Vereniging voor Ziekenhuisapothekers (NVZA) (Dutch Association of Hospital Pharmacists). NVZA. Available online: https://nvza.nl (accessed on 16 December 2024).
21. Koninklijke Nederlandse Maatschappij ter Bevordering der Pharmacie (KNMP) (Royal Dutch Pharmacists Association). KNMP Kennisbank. Available online: https://kennisbank.knmp.nl/ (upon subscription, accessed on 23 January 2025).
22. Nederlandse Vereniging voor Ziekenhuisapothekers (NVZA) (Dutch Association of Hospital Pharmacists). *GMP-Z Richtlijn*; NVZA: Utrecht, The Netherlands. Available online: https://nvza.nl/voor-professionals/gmp/ (accessed on 29 October 2024).
23. Kennisinstituut V&VN. *Voor Toediening Gereed Maken (VTGM)*; V&VN: Utrecht, The Netherlands. Available online: https://kennisplatform.venvn.nl/onderwerp/vtgm/ (accessed on 23 January 2025).
24. Council of Europe. Resolution CM/Res(2016)2 on Good Reconstitution Practices in Health Care Establishments for Medicinal Products for Parenteral Use. Available online: https://www.edqm.eu/en/d/162941 (accessed on 28 November 2024).
25. Le Brun, P.; Crauste-Manciet, S.; Krämer, I.; Smith, J.; Woerdenbag, H. Chapter 1. Introduction. In *Practical Pharmaceutics. An International Guideline for the Preparation, Care and Use of Medicinal Products*, 2nd ed.; Le Brun, P., Crauste-Manciet, S., Krämer, I., Smith, J., Woerdenbag, H., Eds.; Springer Nature: Cham, Switzerland, 2023; pp. 1–5.
26. Watson, C.J.; Whitledge, J.D.; Siani, A.M.; Burns, M.M. Pharmaceutical compounding: A history, regulatory overview, and systematic review of compounding errors. *J. Med. Toxicol.* **2021**, *17*, 197–217. [CrossRef] [PubMed]
27. Falconer, J.R.; Steadman, K.J. Extemporaneously compounded medicines. *Aust. Prescr.* **2017**, *40*, 5–8. [CrossRef] [PubMed]
28. Breitkreutz, J.; Boos, J. Pediatric and geriatric drug delivery. *Exp. Opin. Drug Deliv.* **2007**, *4*, 37–45. [CrossRef]
29. Crommelin, D.J.A.; Bouwman-Boer, Y. Pharmacy preparations: Back in the limelight? Pharmacists make up your mind! *Int. J. Pharm.* **2016**, *514*, 11–14. [CrossRef]
30. Ofei, K. The role of compounding pharmacists during drug shortages. *Int. J. Pharm. Compd.* **2022**, *26*, 298–301. [PubMed]

31. Centraal Bureau voor de Statistiek (CBS) (Statistics Netherlands). Available online: https://opendata.cbs.nl/#/CBS/nl/dataset/03759ned/table?dl=39E0B (accessed on 11 June 2025).
32. Statista. Netherlands: Median Age of the Population 1950 to 2100. Available online: https://www.statista.com/statistics/276734/median-age-of-the-netherlands-population/ (accessed on 17 December 2024).
33. Koninklijke Nederlandse Maatschappij ter Bevordering der Pharmacie (KNMP) (Royal Dutch Pharmacists Association). Producten en Diensten. Available online: www.knmp.nl/over-de-knmp/producten-en-diensten/ (accessed on 16 December 2024).
34. Risico Instrument Farmaceutische Stoffen (RiFaS). Available online: https://www.rifas.nl (accessed on 16 December 2024).
35. Koninklijke Nederlandse Maatschappij ter Bevordering der Pharmacie (KNMP) (Royal Dutch Pharmacists Association). *Richtlijn Bereiden. (Directive Pharmacy Preparations)*; KNMP: Den Haag, The Netherlands, 2016. Available online: https://www.knmp.nl/richtlijnen/bereiden (accessed on 29 October 2024).
36. European Association of Hospital Pharmacists (EAHP). Available online: https://eahp.eu (accessed on 16 December 2024).
37. Inspectie Gezondheidszorg en Jeugd (IGJ) (Health and Youth Care Inspectorate). Geneesmiddelen. Available online: https://www.igj.nl/zorgsectoren/geneesmiddelen (accessed on 13 March 2025).
38. Stichting Farmaceutische Kengetallen (SFK) (Foundation for Pharmaceutical Statistics). Data en Feiten 2024. Available online: https://www.sfk.nl/publicaties/data-en-feiten/Dataenfeiten2024def.pdf (accessed on 11 December 2024).
39. Stichting Farmaceutische Kengetallen (SFK). Bereidingen: Aandeel orale preparaten daalt naar 33%. *Pharm. Weekbl.* **2024**, *159*, 6.
40. Koninklijke Nederlandse Maatschappij ter Bevordering der Pharmacie (KNMP) (Royal Dutch Pharmacists Association) (Alexanderstraat 11, 2514 JL Den Haag, The Netherlands). Personal communication, 7 January 2025.
41. Zorginstituut Nederland. Geneesmiddelen. Available online: https://www.zorginstituutnederland.nl/Verzekerde+zorg/geneesmiddelen-zvw (accessed on 17 June 2025).
42. Informatie over Volksgezondheid en Zorg (VZinfo). Ziekenhuiszorg. Aanbod. Instellingen. Available online: https://www.vzinfo.nl/ziekenhuiszorg/aanbod/instellingen (accessed on 20 June 2025).
43. Le Brun, P.P.J.; de Boer, A.H.; Frijlink, H.W.; Heijerman, H.G.M. A review of the technical aspects of drug nebulization. *Pharm. World. Sci.* **2000**, *22*, 75–81. [CrossRef]
44. Inspectie Gezondheidszorg en Jeugd (IGJ). Collegiaal Doorleveren van Eigen Bereidingen. Available online: https://www.igj.nl/zorgsectoren/geneesmiddelen/beschikbaarheid-van-geneesmiddelen/collegiaal-doorleveren (accessed on 28 April 2025).
45. CIBG. Ministry of Health, Welfare and Sport. Fabrikantenvergunning. Available online: https://www.farmatec.nl/vergunningen/fabrikantenvergunning#:~:text=De%20fabrikantenvergunning%20is%20verplicht%20voor,Noorwegen%2C%20IJsland%20en%20Liechtenstein (accessed on 12 December 2024).
46. Koninklijke Nederlandse Maatschappij ter Bevordering der Pharmacie (KNMP) (Royal Dutch Pharmacists Association). KNMP Kennisbank. LNA-Mededeling Organisatie Apotheekbereiding (October 2022). Available online: https://kennisbank.knmp.nl (upon subscription, accessed on 30 May 2025).
47. European Commission. *The Rules Governing Medicinal Products in the European Union. Annex 1. Manufacture of Sterile Medicinal Products*; Directorate-General for Health and Food Safety: Brussels, Belgium. Available online: https://health.ec.europa.eu/system/files/2022-08/20220825_gmp-an1_en_0.pdf (accessed on 16 December 2024).
48. Larmené-Beld, K.H.M.; Frijlink, H.W.; Taxis, K. A systematic review and meta-analysis of microbial contamination of parenteral medication prepared in a clinical versus pharmacy environment. *Eur. J. Clin. Pharmacol.* **2019**, *75*, 609–617. [CrossRef]
49. Hedlund, N.; Beer, I.; Hoppe-Tichy, T.; Trbovich, P. Systematic evidence review of rates and burden of harm of intravenous admixture drug preparation errors in healthcare settings. *BMJ Open* **2017**, *7*, e015912. [CrossRef] [PubMed]
50. Larmené-Beld, K.H.M.; Spronk, J.T.; Luttjeboer, J.; Taxis, K.; Postma, M.J. A cost minimization analysis of ready-to-administer prefilled sterilized syringes in a Dutch hospital. *Clin. Ther.* **2019**, *41*, 1139–1150. [CrossRef] [PubMed]
51. Wettenbank. Besluit Opleiding en Deskundigheidsgebied Apothekersassistent. Available online: https://wetten.overheid.nl/BWBR0008927/2023-01-01 (accessed on 2 April 2025).
52. Kwaliteitsregistratie en Accreditatie Beroepsbeoefenaren in de Zorg (Kabiz). Apothekersassistent. Available online: https://www.kabiz.nl/beroepen/beroep.aspx?onderwerp=apothekersassistent (accessed on 2 April 2025).
53. CIBG; Ministerie van Volksgezondheid en Sport (Ministry of Health, Welfare and Sport). BIG Register. Available online: https://bigregister.nl (accessed on 11 December 2024).
54. EduFarma. Available online: https://edufarma.nl/fv/ (accessed on 18 December 2024).
55. MediaVision. Available online: www.mediavision.nl (accessed on 18 December 2024).
56. Pharmatech. Available online: https://www.farmaceutische-educatie.nl/cursus/ (accessed on 18 December 2024).
57. Koninklijke Nederlandse Maatschappij ter Bevordering der Pharmacie (KNMP) (Royal Dutch Pharmacists Association). KNMP Kennisbank. LNA-Procedure P-06: Persoonsgebonden Kwalificatie bij Aseptische Handelingen (April 2012). Available online: https://kennisbank.knmp.nl (upon subscription, accessed on 2 April 2025).
58. Aleman, J.; Crul, M. Blijven werken aan bekwaamheid. *Pharm. Weekbl.* **2013**, *148*, 28–31.

59. Optima Farma. HBO Opleiding Farmakunde. Available online: https://optimafarma.nl/hbo-opleiding-farmaceutisch-consulent-en-farmakunde (accessed on 17 April 2025).
60. Wettenbank. Wet op de Beroepen in de Individuele Gezondheidszorg. Available online: https://wetten.overheid.nl/BWBR0006251/2024-07-01 (accessed on 12 December 2024).
61. European Commission. Reform of the EU Pharmaceutical Legislation. Available online: https://health.ec.europa.eu/medicinal-products/pharmaceutical-strategy-europe/reform-eu-pharmaceutical-legislation_en?prefLang=nl (accessed on 24 January 2025).
62. Wettenbank. Geneesmiddelenwet. Available online: https://wetten.overheid.nl/BWBR0021505/2024-01-01 (accessed on 12 December 2024).
63. Wettenbank. Wet op de Geneeskundige Behandelingsovereenkomst. Available online: https://wetten.overheid.nl/BWBR0007021/2006-02-01 (accessed on 12 December 2024).
64. European Union. Directive 2001/83/EC of the European Parliament and of the Council of 6 November 2001 on Community Code Relating to Medicinal Products for Human Use. Available online: https://eur-lex.europa.eu/legal-content/en/TXT/?uri=CELEX%3A32001L0083 (accessed on 29 October 2024).
65. European Commission. A pharmaceutical Strategy for Europe. Available online: https://health.ec.europa.eu/medicinal-products/pharmaceutical-strategy-europe_en (accessed on 12 December 2024).
66. Bruins, B.J. Letter of the Minister of Healthcare to the Parliament on April 8, 2019. Kamerstuk 29477, nr. 569. Available online: https://www.tweedekamer.nl/kamerstukken/brieven_regering/detail?id=2019Z07030&did=2019D14445 (accessed on 2 April 2025).
67. Bos, E. Doorleveren bereidingen: Alle voorwaarden zijn uitgewerkt. *Pharm. Weekbl.* **2017**, *152*, 8–10.
68. Inspectie Gezondheidszorg en Jeugd (IGJ) (Health and Youth Care Inspectorate). Circulaire Handhavend Optreden bij Collegiaal Doorleveren van Eigen Bereidingen Door Apothekers. Available online: https://www.igj.nl/publicaties/circulairen/2023/07/25/circulaire-handhavend-optreden-bij-collegiaal-doorleveren-van-eigen-bereidingen-door-apothekers-kopie (accessed on 29 October 2024).
69. Z-Index. *G-Standaard*; Z-Index BV: Utrecht, The Netherlands. Available online: https://www.z-index.nl/g-standaard (accessed on 29 October 2024).
70. Bijwerkingencentrum Lareb (Netherlands Pharmacovigilance Centre Lareb). Available online: https://www.lareb.nl (accessed on 13 December 2024).
71. Ministerie van Volksgezondheid en Sport (Ministry of Health, Welfare and Sport). Beleidsregel Collegiaal Doorleveren en ter Hand Stellen van Apotheekbereidingen. Staatscourant van het Koninkrijk der Nederlanden, 2024, 39917. 6 December 2024. Available online: https://officielebekendmakingen.nl/stcrt-2024-39917 (accessed on 24 March 2025).
72. Inspectie Gezondheidszorg en Jeugd (IGJ) (Health and Youth Care Inspectorate). Toezichtsdocument bij de Beleidsregel 'Collegiaal Doorleveren en ter Hand Stellen van Apotheekbereidingen'. Available online: https://www.igj.nl/publicaties/toetsingskaders/2024/12/09/toezichtsdocument-bij-de-beleidsregel-collegiaal-doorleveren-en-ter-hand-stellen-van-apotheekbereidingen (accessed on 24 March 2025).
73. Wettenbank. Beleidsregel Collegiaal Doorleveren en ter Hand Stellen van Apotheekbereidingen. Available online: https://wetten.overheid.nl/BWBR0050656/2025-02-01 (accessed on 24 March 2025).
74. European Medicines Agency (EMA). Reform of the EU Pharmaceutical Legislation. Available online: https://health.ec.europa.eu/medicinal-products/legal-framework-governing-medicinal-products-human-use-eu/reform-eu-pharmaceutical-legislation_en (accessed on 24 March 2025).
75. The New York Times. U.S. Races to Replenish Storm-Battered Supplies of iv Fluids at Hospitals. 10 October 2024. Available online: https://www.nytimes.com/2024/10/09/health/hurricane-helene-iv-shortages.html (accessed on 17 June 2025).
76. Medisch Contact. Tekort aan Infuuszakken Door Orkaan Helene nog niet Voorbij. 26 November 2024. Available online: https://www.medischcontact.nl/actueel/laatste-nieuws/artikel/tekort-aan-infuuszakken-door-orkaan-helene-nog-niet-voorbij (accessed on 18 June 2025).
77. Kiseļova, O.; Mauriņa, B.; Šidlovska, V.; Zvejnieks, J. The extent of extemporaneous preparation and regulatory framework of extemporaneous compounding in Latvia. *Medicina* **2019**, *55*, 531. [CrossRef]
78. Scheepers, H.P.A.; Neerup Handlos, V.; Walser, S.; Schutjens, M.D.B.; Neef, C. Impact of the Council of Europe resolution on quality and safety assurance requirements for medicinal products prepared in pharmacies for the special needs of patients. *Eur. J. Hosp. Pharm.* **2017**, *24*, 218–223. [CrossRef]
79. World Health Organization (WHO). *The Legal and Regulatory Framework for Community Pharmacies in the WHO European Region*; World Health Organization Regional Office for Europe: Copenhagen, Denmark, 2019. Available online: https://iris.who.int/bitstream/handle/10665/326394/9789289054249-eng.pdf (accessed on 2 April 2025).
80. Scope of DAC/NRF. Available online: https://dacnrf.pharmazeutische-zeitung.de/ueber-uns/english-version (accessed on 12 June 2025).

81. The FDA Group. 503A vs. 503B: A Quick-Guide to Compounding Pharmacy Designations & Regulations. 16 November 2021. Available online: https://www.thefdagroup.com/blog/503a-vs-503b-compounding-pharmacies (accessed on 2 April 2025).
82. U.S. Food and Drug Administration (FDA). Drugs. Available online: https://www.fda.gov/drugs (accessed on 17 June 2025).
83. European Medicines Agency (EMA). Quality by Design. Available online: https://www.ema.europa.eu/en/human-regulatory-overview/research-development/quality-design (accessed on 3 February 2025).
84. US Food & Drug Administration (FDA). Building Quality into the Design and Conduct of Clinical Studies: Integrating Quality by Design (QbD) and Risk-Based Monitoring (RBM) Approaches. Available online: https://www.fda.gov/drugs/news-events-human-drugs/building-quality-design-and-conduct-clinical-studies-integrating-quality-design-qbd-and-risk-based (accessed on 3 February 2025).
85. Koninklijke Nederlandse Maatschappij ter Bevordering der Pharmacie (KNMP) (Royal Dutch Pharmacists Association) (Alexanderstraat 11, 2514 JL Den Haag, The Netherlands). Personal communication, 27 May 2025.
86. Koninklijke Nederlandse Maatschappij ter Bevordering der Pharmacie (KNMP) (Royal Dutch Pharmacists Association). KNMP Kennisbank. LNA-Procedure Productdossier (December 2012). Available online: https://kennisbank.knmp.nl (upon subscription, accessed on 26 March 2025).
87. Koninklijke Nederlandse Maatschappij ter Bevordering der Pharmacie (KNMP) (Royal Dutch Pharmacists Association). Oralia.nl. Available online: https://www.oralia.nl (accessed on 26 March 2025).
88. European Directorate for the Quality of Medicines & HealthCare (EDQM). Substances for pharmaceutical use. 01/1024: 2034. In *European Pharmacopoeia*, 11.5th ed.; EDQM Council of Europe: Strasbourg, France, 2023. Available online: https://pheur-online.edqm.eu/content/2034/en/current/ (accessed on 5 January 2025).
89. European Medicines Agency (EMA). Guideline on Active Substance Master File Procedure. CHMP/QWP/227/02 Rev 4/ Corr. 8. EMA, Amsterdam, The Netherlands, 8 November 2018. Available online: https://www.ema.europa.eu/en/documents/report/final-guideline-active-substance-master-file-procedure-revision-4_en.pdf (accessed on 5 January 2025).
90. European Directorate for the Quality of Medicines & HealthCare (EDQM). *Certification of Suitability to the Monographs of the European Pharmacopoeia. How to Read CEP*; EDQM Certification of Substances Department: Strasbourg, France, 2018. Available online: https://www.edqm.eu/documents/52006/156629/Guidelines+-+Certification+of+suitability+to+the+Monographs+of+the+European+Pharmacopoeia+-+How+to+read+a+CEP.pdf/7461fefc-12cb-ee0f-8100-de16bee28a4b?t=1639142423648 (accessed on 5 January 2025).
91. Koninklijke Nederlandse Maatschappij ter Bevordering der Pharmacie (KNMP) (Royal Dutch Pharmacists Association). Beoordeling leveranciers (LNA). Available online: https://www.knmp.nl/over-de-knmp/producten-en-diensten/productzorg-bereiding-en-toediening/beoordeling-leveranciers (accessed on 30 May 2025).
92. Stichting Farmaceutische Kengetallen (SFK). Kwart meer Eerstejaars aan Farmaceutische Opleidingen. Available online: https://www.sfk.nl/publicatie/2025/pw-artikel/kwart-meer-eerstejaars-aan-farmaceutische-opleidingen (accessed on 3 March 2025).
93. Wettenbank. Besluit Opleidingseisen Apotheker. Available online: https://wetten.overheid.nl/BWBR0008895/2016-10-06 (accessed on 3 March 2025).
94. Royal College of Physicians and Surgeons of Canada. The CanMEDS Framework. Available online: https://www.royalcollege.ca/en/standards-and-accreditation/canmeds.html (accessed on 22 April 2025).
95. Koninklijke Nederlandse Maatschappij ter Bevordering der Pharmacie (KNMP) (Royal Dutch Pharmacists Association). Specialisten Registratie Commissie—Openbare Farmacie. Available online: https://www.knmp.nl/beroepsontwikkeling/colleges-en-commissies/specialisten-registratie-commissie-openbare-farmacie (accessed on 3 March 2025).
96. Koninklijke Nederlandse Maatschappij ter Bevordering der Pharmacie (KNMP) (Royal Dutch Pharmacists Association). Inhoud Opleiding Openbaar Apotheker. Available online: https://www.knmp.nl/beroepsontwikkeling/opleidingen/inhoud-opleiding-openbaar-apotheker (accessed on 3 March 2025).
97. Koninklijke Nederlandse Maatschappij ter Bevordering der Pharmacie (KNMP) (Royal Dutch Pharmacists Association). Inhoud Opleiding Ziekenhuisapotheker. Available online: https://www.knmp.nl/beroepsontwikkeling/opleidingen/inhoud-opleiding-ziekenhuis-apotheker (accessed on 3 March 2025).
98. Koninklijke Nederlandse Maatschappij ter Bevordering der Pharmacie (KNMP) (Royal Dutch Pharmacists Association). Nascholingen en Accreditatie. Available online: https://www.knmp.nl/beroepsontwikkeling/nascholingen-en-accreditatie (accessed on 3 March 2025).
99. Bouwman-Boer, Y.; Fenton-May, V.; Le Brun, P. Preface. In *Practical Pharmaceutics. An International Guideline for the Preparation, Care and Use of Medicinal Products*; Bouwman-Boer, Y., Fenton-May, V., Le Brun, P., Eds.; Springer International Publishing: Cham, Switzerland, 2015; pp. v–vi.
100. Le Brun, P.; Crauste-Manciet, S.; Krämer, I.; Smith, J.; Woerdenbag, H. (Eds.) *Practical Pharmaceutics. An International Guideline for the Preparation, Care and Use of Medicinal Products*, 2nd ed.; Springer Nature: Cham, Switzerland, 2023.

101. Van Riet-Nales, D.A.; De Jager, K.E.; Schobben, A.F.A.M.; Egberts, T.C.G.; Rademaker, C.M.A. The availability and age-appropriateness of medicines authorized for children in the Netherlands. *Br. J. Clin. Pharmacol.* **2011**, *72*, 1365–2125. [CrossRef]
102. Fadda, H.M.; Weiler, H.; Carvalho, M.; Lee, Y.Z.; Dassouki, H.; AbuBlan, R.; Iurian, S.; Hamid, A.; Şeremet, G.; Li, Z.; et al. Pediatric oral extemporaneous preparations and practices: International Pharmaceutical Federation (FIP) global study. Pediatric oral extemporaneous preparations and practices: International Pharmaceutical Federation (FIP) global study. *Eur. J. Pharm. Biopharm.* **2024**, *204*, 114483. [CrossRef]
103. Khan, D.; Kirby, D.; Bryson, S.; Shah, A.M.; Rahman Mohammed, R. Paediatric specific dosage forms: Patient and formulation considerations. *Int. J. Pharm.* **2022**, *616*, 121501. [CrossRef]
104. Rouaz, K.; Chiclana-Rodríguez, B.; Nardi-Ricart, A.; Suñé-Pou, M.; Mercadé-Frutos, D.; Suñé-Negre, J.M.; Pérez-Lozano, P.; García-Montoya, E. Excipients in the paediatric population: A review. *Pharmaceutics* **2021**, *13*, 387. [CrossRef]
105. European Medicines Agency (EMA). *Reflection Paper: Formulations of Choice for the Paediatric Population*; EMEA: London, UK, 2006. Available online: https://www.ema.europa.eu/en/documents/scientific-guideline/reflection-paper-formulations-choice-paediatric-population_en.pdf (accessed on 24 January 2025).
106. Kinderformularium. Available online: www.kinderformularium.nl (accessed on 25 May 2025).
107. Woerdenbag, H.J.; Visser, J.C.; Leferink op Reinink, M.P.A.M.; van Orsoy, R.R.; Eissens, A.C.; Hagedoorn, P.; Dijkstra, H.; Allersma, D.P.; Ng, S.W.; Smeets, O.S.N.M.; et al. Performance of tablet splitters, crushers, and grinders in relation to personalised medication with tablets. *Pharmaceutics* **2022**, *14*, 320. [CrossRef]
108. Hamad, Y.; Dodda, S.; Frank, A.; Beggs, J.; Sleckman, C.; Kleinschmidt, G.; Lane, M.A.; Burnett, Y. Perspectives of patients on outpatient parenteral antimicrobial therapy: Experiences and adherence. *Open Forum Infect. Dis.* **2020**, *7*, ofaa205. [CrossRef]
109. Psaltikidis, E.M.; Silva, E.N.D.; Bustorff-Silva, J.M.; Moretti, M.L.; Resende, M.R. Economic evaluation of outpatient parenteral antimicrobial therapy: A systematic review. *Expert Rev. Pharmacoecon. Outcomes Res.* **2017**, *17*, 355–375. [CrossRef] [PubMed]
110. Mohammed, S.A.; Roberts, J.A.; Cotta, M.O.; Rogers, B.; Pollard, J.; Assefa, G.M.; Erku, D.; Sime, F.B. Safety and efficacy of outpatient parenteral antimicrobial therapy: A systematic review and meta-analysis of randomized clinical trials. *Int. J. Antimicrob. Agents* **2024**, *64*, 107263. [CrossRef] [PubMed]
111. Williams, D.N.; Baker, C.A.; Kind, A.C.; Sannes, M.R. The history and evolution of outpatient parenteral antibiotic therapy (OPAT). *Int. J. Antimicrob. Agents* **2015**, *46*, 307–312. [CrossRef] [PubMed]
112. Wolie, Z.T.; Roberts, J.A.; Gilchrist, M.; McCarthy, K.; Sime, F.B. Current practices and challenges of outpatient parenteral antimicrobial therapy: A narrative review. *J. Antimicrob. Chemother.* **2024**, *79*, 2083–2102. [CrossRef]
113. Stichting Werkgroep Antibioticabeleid (SWAB). Praktijkgids. Implementatie van een OPAT-Programma in Het Ziekenhuis. Available online: https://swab.nl/nl/exec/file/download/263 (accessed on 9 June 2025).
114. European Union. Directive 2004/37/EC of the European Parliament and of the Council of 29 April 2004 on the Protection of Workers from the Risks Related to Exposure to Carcinogens or Mutagens at Work. Available online: https://eur-lex.europa.eu/legal-content/EN/TXT/?uri=celex%3A32004L0037 (accessed on 12 December 2024).
115. Nederlandse Vereniging van Ziekenhuis Apothekers (NVZA) (Dutch Association of Hospital Pharmacists). GMP-Z Herziening 2013 Z4: Handelingen Met Risicovolle Stoffen en Preparaten. Available online: https://nvza.nl/wp-content/uploads/gmpz_z4_herziening_2013_handelingen_met_risicovolle_stoffen_en_preparaten.pdf (accessed on 12 December 2024).
116. Carrez, L.; Bouchoud, L.; Fleury-Souverain, S.; Combescure, C.; Falaschi, L.; Sadeghipour, F.; Bonnabry, P. Reliability of chemotherapy preparation processes: Evaluating independent double-checking and computer-assisted gravimetric control. *J. Oncol. Pharm. Pract.* **2017**, *23*, 83–92. [CrossRef]
117. Terkola, R.; Czejka, M.; Bérubé, J. Evaluation of real-time data obtained from gravimetric preparation of antineoplastic agents shows medication errors with possible critical therapeutic impact: Results of a large-scale, multicentre, multinational, retrospective study. *J. Clin. Pharm. Ther.* **2017**, *42*, 446–453. [CrossRef]
118. Benizri, F.; Dalifard, B.; Zemmour, C.; Henriquet, M.; Fougereau, E.; Le Franc, B. DrugCam®—An intelligent video camera system to make safe cytotoxic drug preparations. *Int. J. Pharm.* **2016**, *502*, 198–207. [CrossRef]
119. Geersing, T.H.; Klous, M.G.; Franssen, E.J.F.; van den Heuvel, J.J.G.; Crul, M. Robotic compounding versus manual compounding of chemotherapy: Comparing dosing accuracy and precision. *Eur. J. Pharm. Sci.* **2020**, *155*, 105536. [CrossRef]
120. Integraal Kankercentrum Nederland (IKNL) (Netherlands Comprehensive Cancer Organisation). Available online: https://iknl.nl (accessed on 12 December 2024).
121. Crul, M.; Breukels, O. Safe handling of cytostatic drugs: Recommendations from independent science. *Eur. J. Hosp. Pharm.* **2024**, *31*, 191–196. [CrossRef]
122. Crul, M.; Hilhorst, S.; Breukels, O.; Bouman-d'Onofrio, J.R.C.; Stubbs, P.; van Rooij, J.G. Occupational exposure of pharmacy technicians and cleaning staff in Dutch hospitals. *J. Occup. Environ. Hyg.* **2020**, *17*, 343–352. [CrossRef] [PubMed]
123. Hilliquin, D.; Tanguay, C.; Bussières, J.F. External contamination of commercial containers by antineoplastic agents: A literature review. *Eur. J. Hosp. Pharm.* **2020**, *27*, 313–314. [CrossRef] [PubMed]

124. Ministerie van Sociale Zaken en Werkgelegenheid. Arboportaal, Cytostatica. Available online: https://www.arboportaal.nl/onderwerpen/cytostatica (accessed on 14 May 2025).
125. Van den Berg, R.B.; de Poot, S.; Swart, E.L.; Crul, M. Assessment of occupational exposure to nebulized isopropyl alcohol as disinfectant during aseptic compounding of parenteral cytotoxic drugs in cleanrooms. *J. Occup. Environ. Hyg.* **2021**, *18*, 361–368. [CrossRef] [PubMed]
126. Nederlandse Vereniging van Ziekenhuis Apothekers (NVZA) (Dutch Association of Hospital Pharmacists). Crashkaart Oncolytica. Available online: https://nvza.nl/wp-content/uploads/Crashkaart-NVZA-versie-8_26112023-final.xls (accessed on 2 April 2025).
127. Gonnermann, C.; Maier, L. Computer-assisted compounding of TPN-solutions. *Krankenhauspharmazie* **1998**, *19*, 67–70.
128. Pichard, C.; Schwarz, G.; Frei, A.; Kyle, U.; Jolliet, P.; Morel, P.; Romand, J.A.; Sierro, C. Economic investigation of the use of three-compartment total parenteral nutrition bag: Prospective randomized unblinded controlled study. *Clin. Nutr.* **2000**, *19*, 245–251. [CrossRef]
129. Mays, A.; Ayers, P.; Monczka, R.D.; Cober, M.P. Safety in parenteral nutrition compounding. *Nutr. Clin. Pract.* **2023**, *38*, 1253–1262. [CrossRef]
130. Berlana, D. Parenteral nutrition overview. *Nutrients* **2022**, *14*, 4480. [CrossRef]
131. Riskin, A.; Picaud, J.C.; Shamir, R. ESPGHAN/ESPEN/ESPR/CSPEN Working Group on Pediatric Parenteral Nutrition. ESPGHAN/ESPEN/ESPR/CSPEN Guidelines on Pediatric Parenteral Nutrition: Standard Versus Individualized Parenteral Nutrition. *Clin. Nutr.* **2018**, *37*, 2409–2417. [CrossRef]
132. European Medicines Agency (EMA). Advanced Therapy Medicinal Products: Overview. Available online: https://www.ema.europa.eu/en/human-regulatory-overview/advanced-therapy-medicinal-products-overview (accessed on 6 February 2025).
133. European Commission. The Rules Governing Medicinal Products in the European Union. Volume 4. Guidelines on Good Manufacturing Practice Specific to Advanced Therapy Medicinal Products. Available online: https://health.ec.europa.eu/document/download/ad33d9dd-03f0-4bef-af53-21308ce2187d_en?filename=2017_11_22_guidelines_gmp_for_atmps.pdf (accessed on 6 February 2025).
134. Mastrobatista, E.; Doevendans, E.; van Tol, N.P.; Kemp, V.; de Vrij, J.; Hoogendoorn, K. *Pharmaceutical Biotechnology*, 6th ed.; Crommelin, D.J.A., Sindelar, R.D., Meiboom, B., Eds.; Springer Nature: Cham, Switzerland, 2024; pp. 323–399.
135. DARE-NL. Available online: https://www.dare-nl.nl (accessed on 18 June 2025).
136. European Clinical Trial Database. HOVON 161: A Phase II Non-Inferiority Study Comparing Point-of-Care Produced CAR T-Cell to Commercial CAR T-Cells in Patients with Relapsed/Refractory Non-Hodgkin Lymphoma. Available online: https://euclinicaltrials.eu/search-for-clinical-trials/?lang=en&EUCT=2024-511979-15-00 (accessed on 6 February 2025).
137. Eerkens, A.L.; Esajas, M.D.; Brummel, K.; Vledder, A.; van Rooij, N.; Plat, A.; Avalos Haro, S.B.; Paijens, S.T.; Slagter-Menkema, L.; Schuuring, E.; et al. Vvax001, a therapeutic vaccine for patients with HPV16-positive high-grade cervical intraepithelial neoplasia: A phase II trial. *Clin. Cancer Res.* **2025**, *31*, 1016–1026. [CrossRef]
138. Rohaan, M.W.; Borch, T.H.; van den Berg, J.H.; Met, Ö.; Kessels, R.; Geukes Foppen, M.H.; Stoltenborg Granhøj, J.; Nuijen, B.; Nijenhuis, C.; Jedema, I.; et al. Tumor-infiltrating lymphocyte therapy or ipilimumab in advanced melanoma. *N. Engl. J. Med.* **2022**, *387*, 2113–2125. [CrossRef] [PubMed]
139. Westdorp, H.; Creemers, J.H.A.; van Oort, I.M.; Schreibelt, G.; Gorris, M.A.J.; Mehra, N.; Simons, M.; de Goede, A.L.; van Rossum, M.M.; Croockewit, A.J.; et al. Blood-derived dendritic cell vaccinations induce immune responses that correlate with vlinical outcome in patients with chemo-naive castration-resistant prostate cancer. *J. Immunother. Cancer* **2019**, *7*, 302. [CrossRef] [PubMed]
140. De Jonge, P.K.J.D.; van Hauten, P.M.M.; Janssen, L.D.; de Goede, A.L.; Berrien-Elliott, M.M.; van der Meer, J.M.R.; Mousset, C.M.; Roeven, M.W.H.; Foster, M.; Blijlevens, N.; et al. Good manufacturing practice production of CD34+ progenitor-derived NK cells for adoptive immunotherapy in acute myeloid leukemia. *Cancer Immunol. Immunother.* **2023**, *72*, 3323–3335. [CrossRef] [PubMed]
141. Dolstra, H.; Roeven, M.W.H.; Spanholtz, J.; Hangalapura, B.N.; Tordoir, M.; Maas, F.; Leenders, M.; Bohme, F.; Kok, N.; Trilsbeek, C.; et al. Successful transfer of umbilical cord blood CD34+ hematopoietic stem and progenitor-derived NK cells in older acute myeloid leukemia patients. *Clin. Cancer Res.* **2017**, *23*, 4107–4118. [CrossRef]
142. Yonezawa Ogusuku, I.E.; Herbel, V.; Lennartz, S.; Brandes, C.; Argiro, E.; Fabian, C.; Hauck, C.; Hoogstraten, C.; Veld, S.; Hageman, L.; et al. Automated manufacture of ΔNPM1 TCR-engineered T cells for AML therapy. *Mol. Ther. Methods Clin. Dev.* **2024**, *32*, 101224. [CrossRef]
143. European Clinical Trial Database. A Study of the Safety and Efficacy of MB-dNPM-1-TCR.1 in Patients with Relapsed or Refractory AML. Available online: https://euclinicaltrials.eu/search-for-clinical-trials/?lang=en&EUCT=2023-505806-41-00 (accessed on 6 February 2025).
144. Straetemans, T.; Kierkels, G.J.J.; Doorn, R.; Jansen, K.; Heijhuurs, S.; dos Santos, J.M.; van Muyden, A.D.D.; Vie, H.; Clemenceau, B.; Raymakers, R.; et al. GMP-grade manufacturing of T cells engineered to express a defined ΓδTCR. *Front. Immunol.* **2018**, *9*, 1062. [CrossRef]

145. De Witte, M.; Scheepstra, J.; Weertman, N.; Daudeij, A.; van der Wagen, L.; Oostvogels, R.; de Haar, C.; Prins, H.-J.; Dohmen, W.; Bartels-Wilmer, C.; et al. First in human clinical responses and persistence data on TEG001: A next generation of engineered Aβ T cells targeting AML and MM with a high affinity Γ9δ2TCR. *Blood* **2022**, *140* (Suppl. S1), 12737–12739. [CrossRef]
146. Bol, K.F.; Schreibelt, G.; Bloemendal, M.; van Willigen, W.W.; Hins-de Bree, S.; de Goede, A.L.; de Boer, A.J.; Bos, K.J.H.; Duiveman-de Boer, T.; Olde Nordkamp, M.A.M.; et al. Adjuvant dendritic cell therapy in stage IIIB/C melanoma: The MIND-DC randomized phase III trial. *Nat. Commun.* **2024**, *15*, 1632. [CrossRef]
147. Aerts, J.G.; Belderbos, R.; Baas, P.; Scherpereel, A.; Bezemer, K.; Enninga, I.; Meijer, R.; Willemsen, M.; Berardi, R.; Fennell, D.; et al. Dendritic cells loaded with allogeneic tumour cell lysate plus best supportive care versus best supportive care alone in patients with pleural mesothelioma as maintenance therapy after chemotherapy (DENIM): A multicentre, open-label, randomised, phase 2/3 study. *Lancet Oncol.* **2024**, *25*, 865–878. [CrossRef]
148. Weatherman, K.D.; Kowalsky, R.J. Radiopharmaceuticals, nuclear medicine, and nuclear pharmacy: An overview. In *Radiopharmaceuticals in Nuclear Pharmacy and Nuclear Medicine*, 4th ed.; Kowalsky, R.J., Weatherman, K.D., Eds.; American Pharmacists Association: Washington, DC, USA, 2020; pp. 3–18.
149. Nederlandse Vereniging van Ziekenhuisapothekers (NVZA) (Dutch Association of Hospital Pharmacists). GMP-Z Annex 3. Bereiding van Radiofarmaca, Herziening 2021. Available online: https://nvza.nl/wp-content/uploads/GMP-Z-herziening-2021-Annex-3-Bereiding-van-radiofarmaca.pdf (accessed on 8 April 2025).
150. Lange, R.; Schreuder, N.; Hendrikse, H. Radiopharmaceuticals. In *Practical Pharmaceutics. An International Guideline for the Preparation, Care and Use of Medicinal Products*, 2nd ed.; Le Brun, P., Crauste-Manciet, S., Krämer, I., Smith, J., Woerdenbag, H., Eds.; Springer Nature: Cham, Switzerland, 2023; pp. 531–550.
151. European Directorate for the Quality of Medicines & HealthCare (EDQM). Radiopharmaceutical preparations. (0125). In *European Pharmacopoeia*, 11.5th ed.; EDQM Council of Europe: Strasbourg, France, 2023. Available online: https://pheur-online.edqm.eu/content/0125/en/current/ (accessed on 21 October 2024).
152. European Commission. Eudralex. The Rules Governing Medicinal Products in the European Union. Volume 4. EU Guidelines to Good Manufacturing Practice Medicinal Products for Human and Veterinary Use. Annex 3. Manufacture of Radiopharmaceuticals. Available online: https://health.ec.europa.eu/document/download/bf281e1f-4897-469a-ba60-18d867b14a94_en?filename=2008_09_annex3_en.pdf (accessed on 21 October 2024).
153. United Nations. Agreement Concerning the International Carriage of Dangerous Goods by Road. Available online: https://unece.org/transport/standards/transport/dangerous-goods/adr-2023-agreement-concerning-international-carriage (accessed on 21 October 2024).
154. Schreuder, N.; Jacobs, N.A.; Jager, P.L.; Kosterink, J.G.W.; van Puijenbroek, E.P. Patient-reported adverse events of radiopharmaceuticals: A prospective study of 1002 patients. *Drug Saf.* **2021**, *44*, 211–222. [CrossRef]
155. Baum, R.P.; Rösch, F. (Eds.) *Theranostics, Gallium-68, and Other Radionuclides: A Pathway to Personalized Diagnosis and Treatment*, 1st ed.; Springer: New York, NY, USA, 2013.
156. European Medicines Association (EMA). Clinical Trials Regulation. Available online: https://www.ema.europa.eu/en/human-regulatory-overview/research-development/clinical-trials-human-medicines/clinical-trials-regulation (accessed on 24 January 2025).
157. Bensch, F.; Brouwers, A.H.; Lub-de Hooge, M.N.; de Jong, J.R.; van der Vegt, B.; Sleijfer, S.; de Vries, E.G.E.; Schröder, C.P. ^{89}Zr-trastuzumab PET supports clinical decision making in breast cancer patients, when HER2 status cannot be determined by standard work up. *Eur. J. Nucl. Med. Mol. Imaging* **2018**, *45*, 2300–2306. [CrossRef] [PubMed]
158. de Vries, E.G.E.; Kist de Ruijter, L.; Lub-de Hooge, M.N.; Dierckx, R.A.; Elias, S.G.; Oosting, S.F. Integrating molecular nuclear imaging in clinical research to improve anticancer therapy. *Nat. Rev. Clin. Oncol.* **2019**, *16*, 241–255. [CrossRef] [PubMed]
159. de Groot, D.J.A.; Lub-de Hooge, M.N.; van Meerten, T.; Brouwers, A.H.; de Vries, E.G.E. Facts and hopes for PET imaging-derived immunotherapy biomarkers. *Clin. Cancer Res.* **2024**, *30*, 5252–5259. [CrossRef] [PubMed]
160. van Dam, G.M.; Themelis, G.; Crane, L.M.; Harlaar, N.J.; Pleijhuis, R.G.; Kelder, W.; Sarantopoulos, A.; de Jong, J.S.; Arts, H.J.; van der Zee, A.G.; et al. Intraoperative tumor-specific fluorescence imaging in ovarian cancer by folate receptor-α targeting: First in-human results. *Nature Med.* **2011**, *17*, 1315–1319. [CrossRef]
161. Schouw, H.M.; Huisman, L.A.; Janssen, Y.F.; Slart, R.H.J.A.; Borra, R.J.H.; Willemsen, A.T.M.; Brouwers, A.H.; van Dijl, J.M.; Dierckx, R.A.; van Dam, G.M.; et al. Targeted optical fluorescence imaging: A meta-narrative review and future perspectives. *Eur. J. Nucl. Med. Mol. Imaging* **2021**, *48*, 4272–4292. [CrossRef]
162. Linssen, M.D.; ter Weele, E.J.; Allersma, D.P.; Lub-de Hooge, M.N.; van Dam, G.M.; Jorritsma-Smit, A.; Nagengast, W.B. Roadmap for the development and clinical translation of optical tracers cetuximab-800CW and trastuzumab-800CW. *J. Nucl. Med.* **2019**, *60*, 418–423. [CrossRef]
163. Allen, L.V., Jr. Compounding for investigational and clinical studies. *Int. J. Pharm. Compd.* **2022**, *26*, 201–209. [PubMed]

164. Hoppentocht, M.; Akkerman, O.W.; Hagedoorn, P.; Alffenaar, J.W.; van der Werf, T.S.; Kerstjens, H.A.; Frijlink, H.W.; de Boer, A.H. Tolerability and pharmacokinetic evaluation of inhaled dry powder tobramycin free base in non-cystic fibrosis bronchiectasis patients. *PLoS ONE* **2016**, *11*, e0149768. [CrossRef]
165. Maurer, J.M.; Schellekens, R.C.A.; van Rieke, H.M.; Stellaard, F.; Wutzke, K.D.; Buurman, D.J.; Dijkstra, G.; Woerdenbag, H.J.; Frijlink, H.W.; Kosterink, J.G.W. ColoPulse tablets perform comparably in healthy volunteers and Crohn's patients and show no influence of food and time of food intake on bioavailability. *J. Control. Release* **2013**, *172*, 618–624. [CrossRef]
166. Ahmed, A.A.; Otten, A.T.; Gareb, B.; Huijmans, J.E.; Eissens, A.C.; Rehman, A.; Dijkstra, G.; Kosterink, J.G.W.; Frijlink, H.W.; Schellekens, R.C.A. Capsules with ileocolonic-targeted release of vitamin B_2, B_3, and C (ColoVit) intended for optimization of gut health: Development and validation of the production process. *Pharmaceutics* **2023**, *15*, 1354. [CrossRef]
167. Batson, S.; Mitchell, S.A.; Lau, D.; Canobbio, M.; de Goede, A.; Singh, I.; Loesch, U. Automated compounding technology and workflow solutions for the preparation of chemotherapy: A systematic review. *Eur. J. Hosp. Pharm. Sci. Pract.* **2020**, *27*, 330–336. [CrossRef]
168. Zamani, M.; Chan, K.; Wilcox, J. Pharmacy technicians' perceptions of risk reduction strategies implemented in response to the repetitive strain injury associated with sterile compounding. *Int. J. Pharm. Compd.* **2021**, *25*, 182–186. [PubMed]
169. European Commission. Guidance for the Safe Management of Hazardous Medicinal Products at Work. Available online: https://osha.europa.eu/sites/default/files/documents/guidance%20for%20the%20safe%20management%20of%20hazardous%20medicinal-KE0723274ENN.pdf (accessed on 15 November 2024).
170. Cerutti, A.; Ledoux, T.; Vantard, N.; Cerfon, M.A.; Kimbidima, R.; Larbre, V.; Herledan, C.; Lattard, C.; Baudouin, A.; Caffin, A.G.; et al. Comparing different robots available in the European market for the preparation of injectable chemotherapy and recommendations to users. *J. Oncol. Pharm. Pract.* **2023**, *29*, 1599–1612. [CrossRef] [PubMed]
171. Masini, C.; Nanni, O.; Antaridi, S.; Gallegati, D.; Marri, M.; Paolucci, D.; Minguzzi, M.; Altini, M. Automated preparation of chemotherapy: Quality improvement and economic sustainability. *Am. J. Health Syst. Pharm.* **2014**, *7*, 579–585. [CrossRef]
172. Deljehier, T.; Bouguéon, G.; Heloury, J.; Moreno, V.; Berroneau, A.; Crauste-Manciet, S. Simulation program of a cytotoxic compounding robot for monoclonal antibodies and anti-infectious sterile drug preparation. *J. Oncol. Pharm. Pract.* **2019**, *25*, 1873–1890. [CrossRef]
173. Jobard, M.; Brandely-Piat, M.L.; Chast, F.; Batista, R. Qualification of a chemotherapy-compounding robot. *J. Oncol. Pharm. Pract.* **2020**, *26*, 312–324. [CrossRef]
174. Geersing, T.H.; Franssen, E.J.F.; Pilesi, F.; Crul, M. Microbiological performance of a robotic system for aseptic compounding of cytostatic drugs. *Eur. J. Pharm. Sci.* **2019**, *130*, 181–185. [CrossRef]
175. Krämer, I.; Federici, M.; Schierl, R. Environmental and product contamination during the preparation of antineoplastic drugs with robotic systems. *Pharm. Technol. Hosp. Pharm.* **2018**, *3*, 153–164. [CrossRef]
176. Schierl, R.; Masini, C.; Groeneveld, S.; Fischer, E.; Böhlandt, A.; Rosini, V.; Paolucci, D. Environmental contamination by cyclophosphamide preparation: Comparison of conventional manual production in biological safety cabinet and robot-assisted production by APOTECAchemo. *J. Oncol. Pharm. Pract.* **2016**, *22*, 37–45. [CrossRef]
177. Werumeus Buning, A.; Geersing, T.H.; Crul, M. The assessment of environmental and external cross-contamination in preparing ready-to-administer cytotoxic drugs: A comparison between a robotic system and conventional manual production. *Int. J. Pharm. Pract.* **2020**, *28*, 66–74. [CrossRef]
178. Lyousoufi, M.; Lafeber, I.; Kweekel, D.; de Winter, B.C.M.; Swen, J.J.; Le Brun, P.P.H.; Bijleveld-Olierook, E.C.M.; van Gelder, T.; Guchelaar, H.J.; Moes, D.J.A.R.; et al. Development and bioequivalence of 3D-printed medication at the point-of-care: Bridging the gap toward personalized medicine. *Clin. Pharmacol. Ther.* **2023**, *113*, 1125–1131. [CrossRef]
179. Korte, C.; Quodbach, J. Formulation development and process analysis of drug-loaded filaments manufactured via hot-melt extrusion for 3D-printing of medicines. *Pharm. Develop. Technol.* **2018**, *23*, 1117–1127. [CrossRef] [PubMed]
180. Windolf, H.; Chamberlain, R.; Breitkreutz, J.; Quodbach, J. 3D printed mini-floating-polypill for Parkinson's disease: Combination of levodopa, benserazide, and pramipexole in various dosing for personalized therapy. *Pharmaceutics* **2022**, *14*, 931. [CrossRef]
181. Anaya, B.J.; Cerda, J.R.; D'Atri, R.M.; Yuste, I.; Luciano, F.C.; Kara, A.; Ruiz, H.K.; Ballesteros, M.P.; Serrano, D.R. Engineering of 3D printed personalized polypills for the treatment of the metabolic syndrome. *Int. J. Pharm.* **2023**, *642*, 123194. [CrossRef] [PubMed]
182. Kocabas, L.I.; Ayyoubi, S.; Tajqurishi, M.; Quodbach, J.; Vermonden, T.; Kok, R.J. 3D-printed prednisolone phosphate suppositories with tunable dose and rapid release for the treatment of inflammatory bowel disease. *Int. J. Pharm.* **2024**, *649*, 123639. [CrossRef]
183. Levine, V.R.; Paulsson, M.; Strømme, M.; Quodbach, J.; Lindh, J. Off-the-shelf medication transformed: Custom-dosed metoprolol tartrate tablets via semisolid extrusion additive manufacturing and the perception of this technique in a hospital context. *Int. J. Pharm. X* **2024**, *8*, 100277. [CrossRef]
184. Bos, E. Apotheker kan met 3D-printer maatwerk leveren voor kind of kwetsbare oudere. *Pharm. Weekbl.* **2025**, *160*, 8–9.

185. Meruva, S.; Singaraju, A.B.; Vinjamuri, B.P.; Ternik, R.; Stagner, W.C. Current state of minitablet product design: Review. *J. Pharm. Sci.* **2024**, *113*, 1123–1154. [CrossRef]
186. Tian, Y.; Orlu, M.; Woerdenbag, H.J.; Scarpa, M.; Kiefer, O.; Kottke, D.; Sjöholm, E.; Öblom, H.; Sandler, N.; Hinrichs, W.L.J.; et al. Oromucosal films: From patient centricity to production by printing techniques. *Expert Opin. Drug Deliv.* **2019**, *16*, 981–993. [CrossRef]

pharmaceutics

MDPI

Review

^{68}Ga Extemporaneous Preparations in Radiopharmacy

Marzia Rizzello [1,2], Anna Pacelli [1], Maria Domenica De Bari [1], Annalisa Cutrignelli [2], Rosa Maria Iacobazzi [2], Antonio Lopalco [2,*] and Nunzio Denora [2]

1 BeForPharma S.r.l., Volga Street c/o Fiera del Levante Pad. 129, 70132 Bari, Italy; m.rizzello@beforpharma.com (M.R.); a.pacelli@beforpharma.com (A.P.); m.debari@beforpharma.com (M.D.D.B.)

2 Department of Pharmacy-Pharmaceutical Sciences, University of Bari Aldo Moro, 4, E. Orabona Street, 70125 Bari, Italy; annalisa.cutrignelli@uniba.it (A.C.); rosamaria.iacobazzi@uniba.it (R.M.I.); nunzio.denora@uniba.it (N.D.)

* Correspondence: antonio.lopalco@uniba.it; Tel.: +39-0805442764

Abstract

Gallium-68 (^{68}Ga) radiopharmaceuticals are increasingly used in nuclear medicine due to their rapid production capabilities and exceptional specificity in molecular imaging applications. Several of these tracers have demonstrated remarkable clinical efficacy across various oncological conditions, including prostate cancer, neuro-endocrine tumours, and cancers expressing fibroblast activation protein. Commercial kits allow the use of the standardised production protocol, but extemporaneous preparations are the economic and flexible alternatives, particularly within hospital-based radiopharmacy settings. However, such preparations need meticulous conformity to quality control measures and regulation to ensure safety and effectiveness. This review provides an analysis of current methodologies employed in ^{68}Ga extemporaneous preparations and examines pertinent regulatory frameworks. Further clinical validation trials and technical advancement remain essential to facilitate the routine clinical practice's widespread usage and long-term feasibility of such preparations.

Keywords: gallium-68; PSMA; DOTATOC; FAPI; extemporaneous preparations; radiopharmaceuticals; nuclear medicine; NBP; GMP

1. Introduction

Nuclear medicine has transformed modern healthcare by significantly enhancing disease diagnosis and treatment methodologies. Central to this progress is the implementation of radiopharmaceuticals: compounds that integrate radioactive isotopes with biologically active molecules to target specific physiological or pathological processes. Among the diverse radionuclides employed in nuclear medicine, gallium-68 (^{68}Ga) is particularly noteworthy for its distinctive properties. With a brief half-life of approximately 68 min and positron emission capabilities, ^{68}Ga demonstrates exceptional efficacy for positron emission tomography (PET) imaging applications [1]; furthermore, the overall versatility of this radionuclide is reinforced by a supply chain that includes multiple readily available sources, simple radiochemical handling, and several routes for GMP-compliant radiopharmaceutical production. This unique combination of features is unmatched by any other PET radionuclide [2].

In recent years, ^{68}Ga applications have expanded significantly, especially in prostate cancer and neuroendocrine tumour imaging. Some of the most commonly used ^{68}Ga radiopharmaceuticals include prostate-specific membrane antigen (PSMA) [3] ligands and somatostatin receptor (SSTR2)-targeting tracers like DOTA-TOC [4]. More recently, fibroblast activation protein inhibitor (FAPI) tracers have emerged as promising agents for diagnosing a broader spectrum of malignancies beyond prostate and neuroendocrine tumours [5]. Beyond these established radiopharmaceuticals, it is noteworthy that numerous novel ^{68}Ga-labelled tracers are currently under investigation. These include [^{68}Ga]Ga-NeoB, a DOTA-coupled gastrin releasing peptide receptor (GRPR) antagonist with high affinity for GRPR and demonstrated good in vivo stability [6]. Additionally, [^{68}Ga]Ga-PentixaFor, a PET agent targeting CXCR4, is emerging as a versatile radiotracer with promising applications across oncology, cardiology, and inflammatory diseases [7]. Furthermore, αvβ6-integrin has emerged as a promising molecular target for both oncological and non-oncological conditions [8], expanding the potential scope of ^{68}Ga-based imaging agents, such as [^{68}Ga]Ga-Trivehexin. These compounds (Figure 1) have transformed tumour detection, allowing for precise localisation, earlier diagnosis, and better treatment planning. Indeed, in the field of oncology, the early detection of small lesions remains a critical factor. Compared to conventional imaging modalities, PET radiotracers, particularly those labelled with ^{68}Ga, offer the distinct advantage of noninvasively mapping and quantifying molecular and biochemical processes in vivo. These tracers distribute systemically, enabling high-resolution, three-dimensional visualisation of specific biological targets, and allow for the rapid acquisition of dynamic tomographic data, facilitating efficient whole-body assessments. This functional imaging capability significantly exceeds the purely anatomical information provided by techniques such as CT or MRI [2].

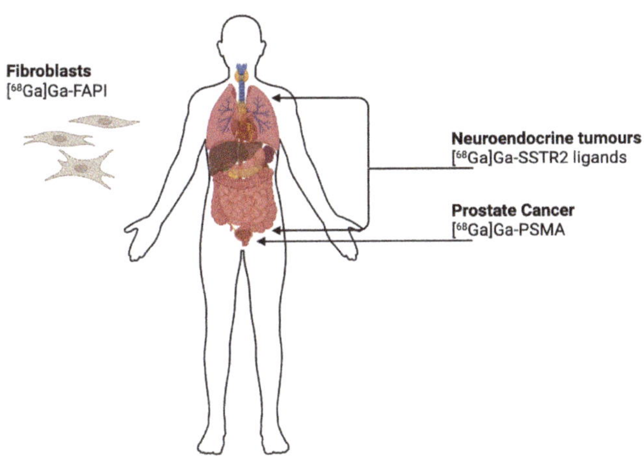

Figure 1. Schematic overview of the principal molecular targets of ^{68}Ga-labelled radiopharmaceuticals used in clinical imaging: [^{68}Ga]Ga-PSMA targets prostate-specific membrane antigen used in the diagnosis and staging of prostate cancer; [^{68}Ga]Ga-SSTR2 ligands bind to somatostatin receptors expressed by neuroendocrine tumours; [^{68}Ga]Ga-FAPI targets fibroblast activation protein (FAP) overexpressed in cancer-associated fibroblasts, allowing visualisation of the tumour stroma in a variety of malignancies.

Given the short physical half-life of ^{68}Ga-radiopharmaceuticals, small-scale production at non-industrial facilities, such as hospital-based radiopharmacies, is often essential. Simultaneously, there is an increasing demand for personalised or precision medicine, with treatments specifically tailored to the individual clinical needs of each patient [9].

This review delineates the current landscape of extemporaneous ^{68}Ga-labelled radiopharmaceutical preparation, encompassing the radiochemical characteristics, production methodologies, clinical applications, and regulatory frameworks governing their use. By integrating technical insights with regulatory considerations, it addresses the unique challenges inherent to small-scale, hospital-based manufacturing, emphasising the critical importance of standardised procedures and stringent quality control.

2. ^{68}Ga in Nuclear Medicine

2.1. Chemical and Physical Properties of ^{68}Ga

Out of the 40 identified Ga radioisotopes, three—^{66}Ga, ^{67}Ga, and ^{68}Ga—have found applications in nuclear medicine. Among these, ^{68}Ga is particularly valuable due to its positron emission properties, making it an ideal candidate for molecular imaging using PET [10], as summarised in Table 1. In contrast, ^{67}Ga, most commonly administered as ^{67}Ga-citrate, has been widely used for infection and inflammation imaging. ^{66}Ga has also been explored for similar diagnostic purposes and has been employed as an alternative to ^{68}Ga in PET imaging of radioligands with slower pharmacokinetics [11]. However, its clinical use remains limited due to its relatively short half-life and higher positron energy, which may compromise image resolution and dosimetry profiles [12].

Table 1. Comparison of the physical characteristics of clinically relevant Ga radioisotopes, including half-life, maximum energy, and principal type of radiation emitted.

Radionuclide	Half-Life	E_{max} (keV)	Radiation
^{66}Ga	9.5 h	4153	β^+ (56%)
^{67}Ga	78.3 min	91, 93, 185, 296, 388	γ
^{68}Ga	67.7 min	1899, 770	β^+ (89%)

Indeed, ^{68}Ga is a positron-emitting radionuclide with a physical half-life of 67.7 min. It decays predominantly by β^+ emission ($\approx$89%), with a maximum positron energy (E_{max}) of 1899 keV and an average positron energy of approximately 770 keV. The emitted positrons undergo annihilation with electrons, resulting in the production of two 511 keV photons that are detected by PET scanners [1]. One of the main advantages of ^{68}Ga is this short physical half-life, which is compatible with the pharmacokinetics and biological half-lives of numerous radiopharmaceuticals, including peptides, oligonucleotides, and affibody molecules [8]. ^{68}Ga rapid decay kinetics enable efficient imaging within a clinically relevant timeframe. Although such a short half-life might be perceived as a limitation, it offers important clinical benefits by allowing adequate time for radiolabelling, quality control, and image acquisition, while minimising radiation exposure to patients [9]. Moreover, the [^{68}Ga]Ga^{3+} cation can form stable complexes with a wide range of ligands containing donor atoms such as oxygen and nitrogen [1], further expanding its applicability in molecular imaging.

2.2. Production of ^{68}Ga

The main source of ^{68}Ga in many nuclear medicine radiopharmaceuticals is the ^{68}Ge/^{68}Ga generator. This device relies on the principle of radioactive decay coupled with chemical separation, enabling the continuous on-site availability of ^{68}Ga derived from its long-lived parent isotope, ^{68}Ge. In this system, ^{68}Ge is immobilised on a solid chromatographic matrix and undergoes electronic capture (EC) decay to form ^{68}Ga, as illustrated in Figure 2.

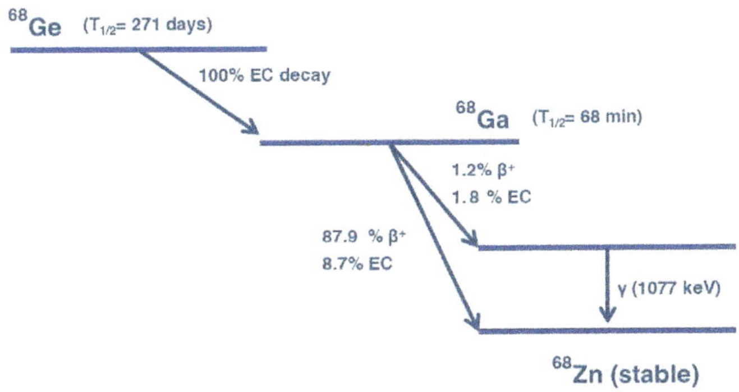

Figure 2. Decay scheme of ^{68}Ge into ^{68}Ga. ^{68}Ge decays via EC with a half-life of 271 days to ^{68}Ga. ^{68}Ga subsequently decays with a half-life of 68 min through multiple pathways: predominantly via positron emission (β^+, 87.9%) and electron capture (EC, 8.7%) to the ground state of stable Zinc-68 (^{68}Zn), and to a lesser extent via β^+ (1.2%) and EC (1.8%) to an excited state of ^{68}Zn, followed by gamma emission (γ, 1077 keV).

Since ^{68}Ge has a half-life of approximately 271 days, it continuously generates ^{68}Ga over an extended period. The ^{68}Ga produced remains trapped in the generator until it is extracted through an elution process [13]. To collect ^{68}Ga, a small volume of HCl solution is passed through the generator column, selectively dissolving the accumulated ^{68}Ga while leaving the parent ^{68}Ge behind. The resulting solution, which contains [^{68}Ga]GaCl$_3$, can then be used directly for radiopharmaceutical preparations (Figure 3). After each elution, the generator begins accumulating ^{68}Ga again; within approximately 68 min (one half-life of ^{68}Ga), about 50% of the total radioactivity is restored, and 4 h later, it is over 91% [14], allowing multiple dose extractions per day. Elution conditions vary according to the generator's resin composition and radiochemical purity specifications. For example, the GalliaPharm® generator (Eckert & Ziegler Radiopharma, GmbH, Berlin, Germany). is typically eluted with 10 mL of 0.1 M HCl over 5 min [15]. The IRE ELiT generator (IRE ELiT S.A., Fleurus, Belgium) employs 7 mL of 0.1 M HCl at a controlled flow rate of 1 mL/min [16], while the GalliAd® generator (IRE ELiT S.A., Fleurus, Belgium). is eluted with 1.1 mL of 0.05 M HCl over a minimum of 3 min [16].

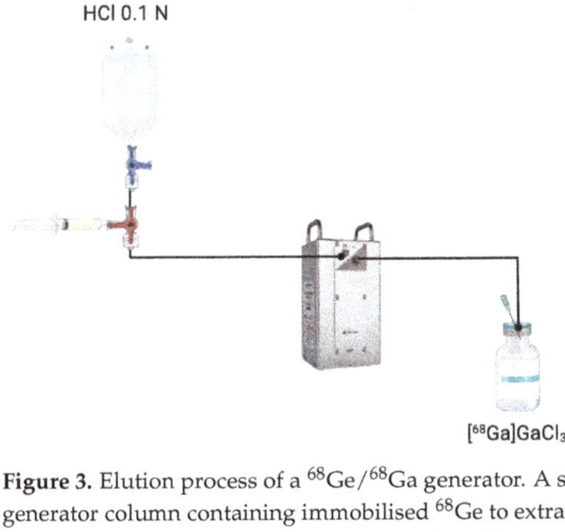

Figure 3. Elution process of a ^{68}Ge/^{68}Ga generator. A solution of HCl 0.1 N is passed through the generator column containing immobilised ^{68}Ge to extract [^{68}Ga]GaCl$_3$. This eluate is collected and subsequently used for radiopharmaceutical applications.

Metal impurities commonly present in the ^{68}Ga generator eluate can negatively impact the radiolabelling efficiency of bifunctional chelator-derived radiopharmaceuticals by competing with gallium ions during complexation. These impurities may lead to reduced yield, lower radiochemical purity, and potential instability of the final product [17]. To mitigate these effects, it is essential to implement strict measures during reagent preparation and handling. Contact with metallic surfaces should be avoided throughout the process, and the use of plastic-based disposable materials is strongly recommended. Additionally, reagents should be prepared using trace-metal grade chemicals and ultrapure deionised water with minimal metal content. Standard laboratory glassware is discouraged, as it may introduce contaminating ions or adsorb gallium. In some radiopharmacy settings, working areas such as hot cells or fume hoods are lined with adhesive plastic films to minimise corrosion and prevent iron-based contamination, further preserving the quality of the radiolabelling process [18].

Over the years, different types of ^{68}Ge/^{68}Ga generators have been developed, utilising various solid-phase supports such as titanium dioxide, tin dioxide, silica, nano-zirconia, and modified polymer-based materials; these supports retain the long-lived parent nuclide ^{68}Ge within the column and enable the elution of ^{68}Ga in a chemical form suitable for direct radiolabelling [19]. The ^{68}Ge/^{68}Ga generator has several advantages for medical centres that are located far from ^{68}Ga distribution facilities. Generators do not require specialised infrastructure, high energy consumption, or highly trained personnel for operation and maintenance, making them an attractive choice for many nuclear medicine centres [14]. Additionally, when compared to other PET radionuclides such as fluorine-18 (^{18}F), ^{68}Ga generators provide greater operational autonomy and simplicity. The production of ^{18}F, indeed, depends on a cyclotron and involves more complex radiochemical synthesis, which often confines its use to centralised radiopharmacies or necessitates a well-established distribution system [20]. The technical characteristics of commercially available ^{68}Ge/^{68}Ga generators, including elution yield, initial ^{68}Ge activity, ^{68}Ge breakthrough, and operational differences such as the use of built-in versus external eluents, have been comprehensively reviewed in other publications [14,19,21]. To avoid redundancy, these comparative aspects are not discussed in detail in this review.

In recent years, researchers have been exploring cyclotron-based production as an alternative strategy to diversify the supply of ^{68}Ga beyond generator-based systems and to provide higher activity levels. This approach is based on the ^{68}Zn (p, n) ^{68}Ga nuclear reaction and can be implemented using either solid or liquid targets [22]. In the solid target method, enriched ^{68}Zn is employed in different forms, such as electroplated, pressed, foil, or molten targets. The process involves proton irradiation of the solid target using medical cyclotrons [23]. The target is then dissolved using either concentrated HCl or HNO_3. The separation and purification of ^{68}Ga are achieved through one-, two-, or three-column chromatography techniques, maximising the apparent molar activity (AAm) and ensuring high-purity ^{68}Ga suitable for radiopharmaceutical applications [24]. Studies using the GE PETtrace cyclotron have shown promising results, with end-of-purification (EOP) activity exceeding 3.7 GBq, and could be distributed to other nuclear medicine centres [25]. The highest end-of-bombardment (EOB) activity reported was over 370 GBq [24].

Recent advances have led to the development of liquid target production of ^{68}Ga, which offers an alternative for facilities without solid target infrastructure. Instead of irradiating a solid material, a liquid solution of enriched [^{68}Zn]Zn$(NO_3)_2$ in HNO_3 is used as the target medium [26]. This approach minimises target preparation time and simplifies the process by eliminating the need for complex target dissolution steps. Liquid target production has demonstrated promising results, with studies reporting EOB activities exceeding 9 GBq when using optimised concentrations of Zn$(NO_3)_2$ and HNO_3 [27]. To achieve high-purity ^{68}Ga, the irradiated solution undergoes a two-column purification process, typically using Zr resin and TK200 resin. After separation, the final ^{68}Ga is formulated as [^{68}Ga]$GaCl_3$, which can then be used for radiosynthesis [24].

2.3. ^{68}*Ga Chelators*

Chelators play a fundamental role in the development of ^{68}Ga radiopharmaceuticals. Ga^{3+} is a hard Lewis acid that preferentially forms coordination complexes with oxygen, nitrogen, and sulphur donor atoms. The most stable ^{68}Ga complexes adopt an octahedral geometry, meaning that six donor atoms are ideally involved in the chelation process. Functional groups commonly used for Ga^{3+} coordination include amines, carboxylates, hydroxamates, and phenolates [28]. Choosing the right chelating agent is essential to ensure that ^{68}Ga remains stably bound to the radiopharmaceutical throughout imaging. Chelators must exhibit strong thermodynamic stability, fast complexation kinetics, and minimal dissociation under physiological conditions [29]. The first clinically relevant ^{68}Ga complexes were based on EDTA (ethylenediaminetetraacetic acid) (Figure 4a). In the early days of ^{68}Ga imaging, EDTA was used to form ^{68}Ga complexes directly in generator eluates, which were then administered for perfusion imaging [30]. However, EDTA chelates exhibited poor in vivo stability, leading to transchelation with endogenous metal ions such as Fe^{3+} and Zn^{2+}, reducing their clinical applicability [31]. Building upon EDTA, DTPA (diethylenetriaminepentaacetic acid, Figure 4b) emerged as a more effective chelator for ^{68}Ga. DTPA derivatives have been widely used in radiopharmaceutical chemistry for various radioisotopes, but when applied to ^{68}Ga, they still demonstrated moderate in vivo stability concerns [30]. Their acyclic nature makes them more prone to metal exchange and dissociation in physiological conditions.

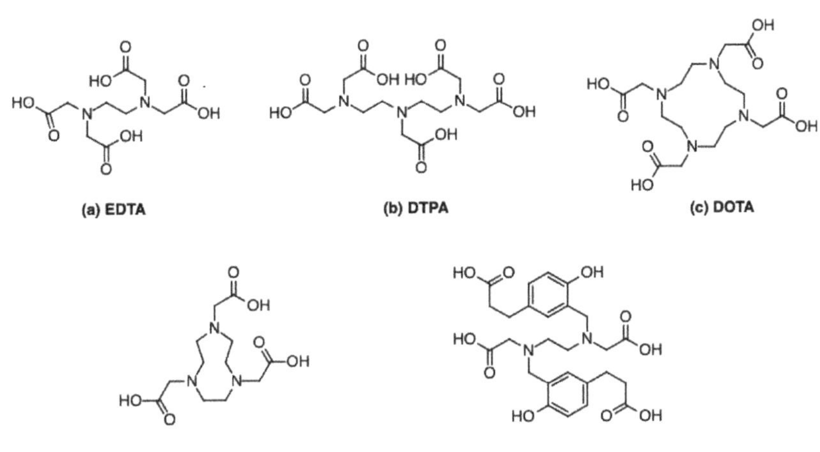

Figure 4. Chemical structure of several ^{68}Ga chelators: (**a**) EDTA; (**b**) DTPA; (**c**) DOTA; (**d**) NOTA; (**e**) HBED-CC.

To overcome these limitations, macrocyclic chelators were introduced. Some of the most widely used macrocyclic chelators include the following:

- DOTA (1,4,7,10-Tetraazacyclododecane-1,4,7,10-tetraacetic acid, Figure 4c), which forms exceptionally stable ^{68}Ga complexes in vivo, preventing dissociation or transmetallation under physiological conditions [32]. For instance, the study performed by Oehlke and colleagues analysed the stability of [^{68}Ga]Ga-DOTATATE towards transmetallation with Cu^{2+}, Fe^{3+}, Pb^{2+}, and Zn^{2+}, and found that only the addition of

Cu^{2+} at 95 °C leads to noticeable transmetallation [33].

DOTA radiolabelling requires high temperatures (~90 °C) for approximately 10 min. This heating step is crucial, due the rigidity of its macrocyclic structure, which must undergo conformational rearrangement to accommodate the Ga^{3+} ion within its coordination cavity [30]. The ideal pH range for DOTA chelation is 3.5–4.0. At lower pH, DOTA becomes overly protonated, while at higher pH, Ga^{3+} may form insoluble species [34]. Structurally, DOTA provides an octadentate N_4O_4 coordination environment and a relatively large macrocyclic cavity that may lead to slower complexation kinetics and reduced resistance to transchelation due to imperfect fitting with the ionic radius of Ga^{3+} [35].

- NOTA (1,4,7-Triazacyclononane-1,4,7-triacetic acid), which forms highly stable complexes at room temperature [30]. This property is attributed to the intrinsic structural features of NOTA (Figure 4d): its compact macrocyclic geometry, hexadentate N_3O_3 coordination, and smaller cavity size, which better matches the ionic radius of Ga^{3+}, facilitating faster complex formation and superior kinetic stability [36]. Ga^{3+}-NOTA complexes exhibit an exceptionally high stability constant (logK = 30.98), significantly higher than that of Ga^{3+}-DOTA (logK = 21.33), highlighting NOTA's stronger affinity for Ga^{3+} and more favourable thermodynamics [32]. Structurally, NOTA forms slightly distorted octahedral complexes with facially arranged donors, allowing the formation of multiple five-membered chelate rings with minimal strain, unlike DOTA. This lower energetic barrier enables efficient complexation even at mild conditions [37]. In terms of in vivo stability, although NOTA forms more inert complexes with Ga^{3+} than DOTA, the overall biological performance of the radiopharmaceutical also depends on the charge, hydrophilicity, and pharmacokinetics of the resulting bioconjugate. For example, DOTA-based vectors may display more favourable biodistribution in certain contexts, despite their lower thermodynamic stability [32]. Similarly to DOTA, NOTA has shown strong resistance to transmetallation, particularly against biologically relevant cations such as Zn^{2+} and Ca^{2+}; additionally [33]. NOTA, provides enhanced kinetic inertness even under physiological conditions [32,38].

Meanwhile, efforts have continued to refine non-macrocyclic chelators that offer faster labelling kinetics at room temperature. The most notable example is HBED-CC (N,N′-bis(2-hydroxy-5-(carboxyethyl)benzyl)ethylenediamine-N,N′-diacetic acid, Figure 4e), an acyclic hexadentate ligand that coordinates Ga^{3+} through phenolic, amine, and carboxylate donor atoms to form stable complexes. Despite lacking a macrocyclic structure, HBED-CC achieves high thermodynamic stability and kinetic inertness due to the optimal spatial arrangement and strong coordinating ability of its donor groups, allowing it to efficiently chelate ^{68}Ga at room temperature and at pH ~4 [39].

2.4. Conditions of ^{68}Ga Complexation

The production of ^{68}Ga-labelled radiopharmaceuticals requires rigorous control over reaction conditions to ensure efficient complexation and full compliance with regulatory standards. This is particularly crucial given the short half-life of the radionuclide, which imposes significant time constraints on the production process.

In aqueous solutions, Ga^{3+} ions exhibit acid–base behaviour that results in the formation of multiple hydrolysed species [39]. At pH values below 3, Ga predominantly exists as the fully hydrated complex $[Ga(H_2O)_6]^{3+}$. As the pH increases, progressive deprotonation occurs, leading to the formation of hydroxo complexes such as $[Ga(OH)]^{2+}$, $[Ga(OH)_2]^+$, $[Ga(OH)]_3$, and $[Ga(OH)_4]^-$. The speciation is also temperature dependent. At 25 °C, $[Ga(OH)]^{2+}$ is the main species between pH 3 and 5, whereas at 100 °C, $[Ga(OH)_2]^+$ predominates. Above pH 5, $[Ga(OH)_4]^-$ becomes the dominant form, regardless of temperature. These equilibria highlight the importance of maintaining an appropriate pH to ensure optimal Ga availability for complexation [40].

The efficiency of the labelling process is also critically dependent on the choice of chelating agent [41]. An ideal chelator should form a stable complex with the radiometal under mild conditions and at very low (nano- to micromolar) concentrations of the radiometal. It should also be capable of quantitatively binding the radionuclide even when used in low molar amounts, ensuring high molar activity of the final product. This is essential to prevent competition between the unlabelled precursor and the radiolabelled molecule for target receptors in vivo, which could compromise the specificity of the radiopharmaceutical. Furthermore, the complex must be sufficiently stable under physiological conditions to avoid premature release of the radiometal, which would result in undesirable accumulation in non-target tissues [41].

Another critical component of the synthesis is the selection of an appropriate buffer system [42]. Buffers are selected based on their pKa and ability to maintain the pH between 3.5 and 5.0, the optimal range for Ga complexation. Clinically suitable buffers must be pharmaceutically approved and not form themselves strong complexes with Ga, thus interfering with the labelling. For instance, citrate binds Ga^{3+} strongly and is unsuitable as a buffer for ^{68}Ga radiolabelling, as proved by its clinical use in inflammation imaging [43]. Alternatives like HEPES, succinate, glutamate, and oxalate offer good pH control and can enhance labelling yields [42], but many lack pharmacopoeial approval. HEPES improves labelling efficiency by reducing precursor mass requirements. However, its use is limited by the European Pharmacopoeia's strict 200 μg per dose limit for intravenous administration [44], based on limited toxicity data. Yet, studies have shown that much higher doses are well tolerated [45], and HEPES is found in approved drugs, indicating its safety at levels exceeding those used in radiopharmacy. These findings suggest that a reassessment of current regulatory limits may be warranted, potentially expanding the clinical applicability of HEPES-buffered ^{68}Ga radiopharmaceuticals without compromising patient safety [46].

3. Regulatory Guidelines of ^{68}Ga Radiopharmaceuticals

3.1. Regulatory Guidelines and Radiation Protection Regulations

In the field of radiopharmaceutical production, a distinction must be made among the following:

- Industrial-scale ready-to-use radiopharmaceuticals, produced under full GMP and subject to centralised marketing authorisation procedures;
- Radiopharmaceutical precursors, manufactured under GMP and intended for subsequent radiolabelling in healthcare facilities;
- Small-scale extemporaneous radiopharmaceutical preparations, compounded within hospital or academic radiopharmacy settings under national exemptions and pharmacopoeial standards [47].

This review primarily focuses on the third category, which includes magistral and officinal preparations of ^{68}Ga-labelled radiopharmaceuticals produced onsite in nuclear medicine departments, often under time-sensitive and patient-specific conditions.

The regulatory framework for radiopharmaceuticals in the European Union was first introduced with Directive 89/343/EEC, which primarily focused on radiation protection measures and compliance with pharmacopoeial standards [48]. Since 1989, radiopharmaceuticals have been formally recognised as medicinal products and their current legal basis is established by Directive 2001/83/EC, the Community Code relating to medicinal products for human use [49]. This Directive provides exemptions from the requirement for marketing authorisation (MA) under Articles 3 and 5(1), which allow the use of magistral and officinal formulas, as well as preparations authorised under national provisions, including extemporaneously radiopharmaceutical preparations [49]. This exemption plays a key role for radiopharmaceuticals, as small-scale preparations at non-industrial sites, such as nuclear medicine departments, are often necessary due to the short physical half-life of many radionuclides, including ^{68}Ga [50]. Extemporaneously radiopharmaceutical preparations are commonly prepared on-site, often as single-dose formulations customised to specific clinical needs. They typically include magistral preparations, compounded in a pharmacy in accordance with an individual medical prescription, and officinal preparations, produced in line with a pharmacopoeial monograph. In both cases, the radiopharmaceuticals are intended for direct administration to patients [51]. However, the evolution of nuclear medicine practices and the increasing complexity of radiopharmaceutical production have highlighted critical limitations in the current regulatory framework. As outlined by the European Association of Nuclear Medicine (EANM), Directive 2001/83/EC remains largely focused on traditional kit-based preparations and fails to adequately address the regulatory needs of novel, in-house, and complex radiopharmaceutical formulations. This regulatory gap results in inconsistencies across Member States, disproportionate administrative burdens, and potential barriers to innovation and patient access [52].

In Italy, Directive 2001/83/EC has been transposed into national law through Legislative Decree No. 219 of 24 April 2006 [53]. Within this framework, the preparation of magistral and officinal radiopharmaceuticals is permitted under the exemption provided by Article 3 of the Directive. The quality requirements for magistral formulations are defined in the "Norme di buona preparazione in medicina nucleare" (Good compounding practice in nuclear medicine, NBP-MN) published in the Official Pharmacopeia of the Italian Republic [54]. In parallel, radioprotection aspects related to the extemporaneous preparation and clinical use of radiopharmaceuticals are regulated by Legislative Decree No. 101 of 31 July 2020 [55], which transposes the European Directive 2013/59/Euratom [56] into national law. This decree establishes the basic safety standards for protection against the risks associated with exposure to ionising radiation, covering all activities involving radioactive substances, including those performed within nuclear medicine departments. Among its provisions, the decree assigns key responsibilities to the Radiation Protection Expert (Esperto di Radioprotezione, ERP), who must ensure that shielding, handling protocols, and monitoring systems are appropriate to minimise occupational and environmental exposure [57]. For small-scale preparations, the legislation requires dedicated infrastructure, including containment systems (e.g., hot cells), dose calibrators, contamination control measures, and personal dosimetry devices [57].

3.2. European Pharmacopoeia

The European Pharmacopoeia (Eur. Ph.) establishes official standards for the qualitative and quantitative composition of medicinal products, as well as for the analytical procedures applicable to both finished pharmaceuticals and raw materials used in their manufacture [58]. In the field of radiopharmaceutical production, the General Monograph 0125 "Radiopharmaceutical Preparations" [59], provides a comprehensive regulatory framework outlining the fundamental quality requirements applicable to all radiopharmaceuticals. In addition to this general guidance, the Eur. Ph. includes approximately 70 individual monographs covering radiolabelled preparations and radioactive precursors. Among these, specific monographs have been established for [^{68}Ga]Ga-PSMA-11 (Monograph 3109) [60] and [^{68}Ga]Ga-DOTATOC, also known as edotreotide (Monograph 3098) [61], which define the quality specifications for the identity, content, purity, and radiochemical characteristics of these extemporaneous radiopharmaceuticals. These monographs are distinct from those intended for ready-to-use industrial radiopharmaceuticals and reflect the specific constraints and operational realities of extemporaneous preparation in hospital settings. In particular, they often allow for adapted quality testing strategies due to the short half-life and immediate-use nature of ^{68}Ga-labelled products.

In the case of commercially available kits, the Eur. Ph. allows partial exemptions from certain tests, provided that the preparation is compliant with a marketing authorisation and the generator specified in the approved documentation is used. However, if a licensed kit is used outside of its intended specifications, or with a non-authorised generator, a full analytical release profile is required [62].

3.3. Good Manufacturing Practice Guidelines

Good Manufacturing Practice (GMP) refers to a set of internationally recognised standards that ensure the consistent production and control of medicinal products according to quality standards appropriate for their intended use [63]. In the European Union, GMP principles are codified in EudraLex Volume 4, which is structured into three main parts:

- Part I, Basic Requirements for Medicinal Products, outlines the GMP standards applicable to the manufacture and control of finished pharmaceutical products for both human and veterinary use. It is organised into nine chapters: Chapter 1 defines the Pharmaceutical Quality System necessary to consistently produce medicines that meet regulatory and patient expectations; Chapter 2 specifies the responsibilities, qualifications, and training requirements for personnel involved in GMP activities; Chapter 3 outlines the design, maintenance, and control standards for premises and equipment; Chapter 4 addresses documentation management, including procedures, records, and batch documentation; Chapter 5 describes principles for production operations, contamination control, and process validation; Chapter 6 establishes the requirements for sampling, testing, release, and stability studies; Chapter 7 regulates the management of outsourced activities; Chapter 8 defines procedures for handling complaints, investigating quality defects, and executing product recalls; and Chapter 9 covers the requirements for self-inspections to ensure ongoing GMP compliance.
- Part II, Basic Requirements for Active Substances used as Starting Materials, defines the GMP framework for the production of active pharmaceutical ingredients (APIs), focusing on quality, purity, and traceability throughout the manufacturing process.
- Part III, GMP-related Documents, compiles complementary guidelines, such as ICH Q9 on Quality Risk Management and ICH Q10 on Pharmaceutical Quality Systems, which extend and reinforce the broader quality framework necessary for maintaining GMP compliance.

GMP principles are not fully applicable to extemporaneously prepared radiopharmaceuticals, due to their intrinsic characteristics such as short physical half-lives, the need for aseptic handling, and time-critical preparation. To address these specific challenges and ensure consistent quality and regulatory compliance, targeted technical annexes have been developed to guide production practices across all stages [50].

Annex 1 of EudraLex Volume 4 ("Manufacture of Sterile Medicinal Products"), focused on sterile manufacturing, is particularly applicable to radiopharmacy [64]. It provides detailed guidance on environmental classifications (Grades A to D), cleanroom standards, personnel training, and environmental monitoring, all essential for maintaining aseptic conditions during critical steps like sterile filtration and final dose preparation [64]. The 2023 revision of Annex 1 of EudraLex Volume 4 introduced significant changes compared to the previous version, reflecting the evolving regulatory expectations for sterile manufacturing. A key advancement is the formal incorporation of a contamination control strategy (CCS), which requires manufacturers to establish a holistic, documented, and proactive approach to contamination risk assessment and mitigation across the entire lifecycle of the product. Unlike the previous version, which provided more prescriptive guidance focused on individual aspects of sterility assurance, the current Annex emphasises an integrated quality-by-design philosophy, risk-based decision-making, and continuous process verification. Greater attention is also given to topics such as environmental monitoring, personnel gowning qualification, and the use of barrier technologies (e.g., Restricted Access Barrier Systems and isolators) to minimise contamination risks.

Annex 3 of EudraLex Volume 4 ("Manufacture of Radiopharmaceuticals") specifically provides recommendations for the preparation of radiopharmaceuticals, including those prepared extemporaneously [65]. It serves as a key regulatory reference for aligning hospital-based radiopharmaceutical preparation with the broader principles of pharmaceutical quality and patient safety. The Annex mandates compliance with GMP Parts I and II and emphasises the importance of a robust quality assurance system, including contamination control, aseptic production practices, and specialised training in both GMP and radiation protection. It also accommodates the unique operational constraints of radiopharmaceuticals by allowing specific concessions to standard GMP practices such as permitting most container labelling to occur prior to manufacturing to reduce radiation exposure and by authorising conditional batch release when full quality control results are not available before administration. For radiopharmaceuticals with short half-lives such as ^{68}Ga-labelled preparations, microbiological testing (e.g., sterility) is typically completed only after the product has already been administered to the patient. Therefore, Annex 3 explicitly permits the release of the product prior to the availability of sterility test results, provided that all other critical quality attributes (e.g., radiochemical purity, pH, radionuclidic identity, endotoxins) are compliant and that a validated aseptic process is in place. Furthermore, Annex 3 incorporates additional GMP elements by referring to Annex 11 for computerised systems and Annex 13 for investigational medicinal products. Annex 3, therefore, introduces a more rigorous and harmonised framework, bringing radiopharmaceutical manufacturing closer to mainstream pharmaceutical GMP standards while still recognising the specific needs of nuclear medicine.

Across the European Union, however, the degree of GMP application in radiopharmaceutical preparation varies by Member State. In countries such as France and Italy, a tailored approach known as Good Compounding Practice has been adopted, adapting GMP principles to the specific context of hospital-based preparation. In contrast, Member States including Belgium, Austria, and Finland apply the standards defined in PIC/S Annex 3, which is specifically designed for the preparation of medicinal products in healthcare establishments. In other jurisdictions, such as Germany, Spain, Denmark, and the United Kingdom, compliance with the full scope of GMP requirements is mandatory, regardless of the production scale or setting. A detailed review on how different European countries approach this topic can be found on [66].

3.4. *International Council for Harmonisation Guidelines*

The validation of analytical procedures in pharmaceutical development is regulated by the International Council for Harmonisation (ICH) guidelines, notably, ICH Q2 (R2) [67]. Although this framework is widely applied to conventional pharmaceutical products, its direct implementation in the context of extemporaneous radiopharmaceutical preparations raises several challenges due to the distinctive nature of these compounds.

Radiopharmaceuticals, particularly those involving short-lived radionuclides, as ^{68}Ga, are characterised by rapid radioactive decay and the frequent unavailability of isolated reference standards for radioactive components [68]. These peculiarities are not fully addressed by the ICH Q2 (R2) guidelines. Furthermore, the radioactive drug substance is often inseparable from the formulation matrix, necessitating either significant adaptations to conventional validation protocols or the implementation of alternative strategies. As a result, although ICH Q2 (R2) offers a valuable framework, it must be complemented by radiopharmacy-specific methodologies [69].

Recognising these limitations, the European Association of Nuclear Medicine (EANM) has issued specialised guidance tailored to the validation of analytical methods for radiopharmaceuticals [69]. These documents incorporate parameters critical to radiopharmaceutical quality, including radionuclidic identity and radiochemical purity, and promoted their formal consideration as exceptions to conventional ICH procedures [47].

In alignment with ICH Q2 (R2), the validation of analytical methods for extemporaneously prepared radiopharmaceuticals must still address core attributes such as accuracy, precision, specificity, detection and quantification limits, linearity, and range. However, these parameters must be reinterpreted considering the distinct characteristics of radiopharmaceuticals. Due its short half-life, ^{68}Ga presents significant challenges related to its decay kinetics, the time-sensitivity of quality control procedures, and the limited availability of reference materials for radiolabelled impurities.

Moreover, an analytical method should undergo re-validation whenever significant changes occur that could impact its reliability or performance. These changes include the following:

- Modifications in the radiopharmaceutical preparation process that may introduce new or different impurities not previously considered, such as a change in purification strategy or the use of an alternative precursor;
- Alterations in the final product composition, including increased radioactivity levels or the introduction of different excipients;
- Substantial adjustments to the analytical procedure itself, for instance, the replacement of the HPLC column with one featuring a different stationary phase, or major changes to the mobile phase composition [69].

Additional regulatory guidelines relevant to radiopharmaceuticals include ICH Q3C (R9) "Residual solvents" [70] and ICH Q3D (R2) "Guideline for Elemental Impurities" [71]. According to ICH Q3C (R9), solvents commonly used in radiosynthesis, such as ethanol and acetic acid, are classified as Class 3 solvents, characterised by low toxic potential. However, their residual content must be carefully monitored. ICH Q3D (R2), on the other hand, establishes permissible daily exposure limits for elemental impurities. For [^{68}Ga]$GaCl_3$ solutions eluted from ^{68}Ge/^{68}Ga generators, zinc and iron are recognised as the principal elemental impurities, with their acceptable limits defined in the corresponding European Pharmacopoeia monograph [72]. In the case of cyclotron-produced $^{68}GaCl_3$, additional elements such as nickel and copper must also be considered and appropriately controlled to ensure product safety [73].

4. Overview of Main ^{68}Ga Tracers Extemporaneously Prepared

4.1. PSMA Tracers

Prostate-specific membrane antigen (PSMA) is a type II transmembrane glycoprotein predominantly expressed in prostatic tissue, with expression levels significantly increased in prostate cancer cells [74], particularly in high-grade, metastatic, and hormone-refractory tumours [75]. This expression profile makes PSMA an ideal molecular target for both diagnostic and therapeutic applications in prostate cancer.

Among the various radiolabelled compounds developed for PSMA-targeted imaging, three low-molecular-weight ligands, PSMA-11, PSMA-617, and PSMA-I&T, have gained prominence. Their chemical structures, along with the conserved PSMA-binding motif, are illustrated in Figure 5.

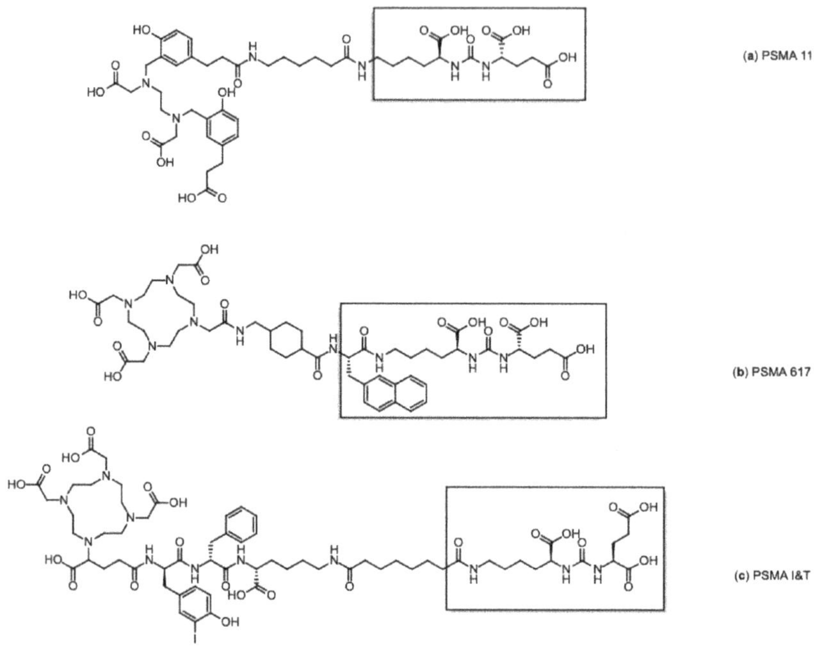

Figure 5. Chemical structures of PSMA ligands: (**a**) PSMA-11, (**b**) PSMA-617, and (**c**) PSMA I&T. The PSMA binding motif is in brackets.

[^{68}Ga]Ga-PSMA-11 (Glu-NH-CO-NH-Lys(Ahx)-[^{68}Ga(HBED-CC)]) (Figure 5a), the first ^{68}Ga-labelled radiopharmaceutical approved by the FDA for PET imaging in prostate cancer, was developed by the Heidelberg group [76]. Eder et al. demonstrated its high affinity for human PSMA and its efficient internalisation in PSMA-positive tumour cells. Its biodistribution closely mirrors the physiological and pathological expression of PSMA, supporting its clinical use for accurate tumour localisation and staging. Other PSMA-directed radiotracers, including [^{68}Ga]Ga-PSMA-617 (Figure 5b) and [^{68}Ga]Ga-PSMA-I&T (Figure 5c), exhibit comparable pharmacokinetic and imaging characteristics, further validating the robustness of PSMA as a target for prostate cancer imaging [77]. However, despite their diagnostic capability, these two compounds are primarily employed in therapeutic contexts, as their structural design is compatible with therapeutic radionuclides such as ^{177}Lu, making them more suitable for radioligand therapy than for routine PET imaging [78]. Accordingly, PSMA-617 has only been approved by FDA/EMA in its therapeutic form labelled with ^{177}Lu, while [^{68}Ga]Ga-PSMA-I&T and [^{177}Lu]Lu PSMA-I&T remain investigational and are currently limited to clinical studies.

4.2. DOTATOC and Somatostatin Receptor Tracers

Three main types of [^{68}Ga]Ga-DOTA-conjugated peptides are routinely employed in clinical practice: [^{68}Ga]Ga-DOTA-TOC ([Ga-DOTA-D-Phe^1-Tyr^3]octreotide, Figure 6a), [^{68}Ga]Ga-DOTA-NOC ([Ga-DOTA-D-Phe^1-1NaI^3]octreotide, Figure 6b), and [^{68}Ga]Ga-DOTA-TATE ([Ga-DOTA-D-Phe^1-Tyr^3]octreotate, Figure 6c). These radiolabelled somatostatin analogues are SSTR agonists, specifically developed to target somatostatin receptors (SSRs), which are overexpressed on the surface of neuroendocrine tumour (NET) cells [79]. They are capable of binding to the receptor and triggering internalisation, a key feature that facilitates intracellular accumulation of the radiotracer and enables both effective imaging and targeted radionuclide therapy. Internalisation into tumour cells is considered a hallmark of the diagnostic and therapeutic efficacy of these compounds [80].

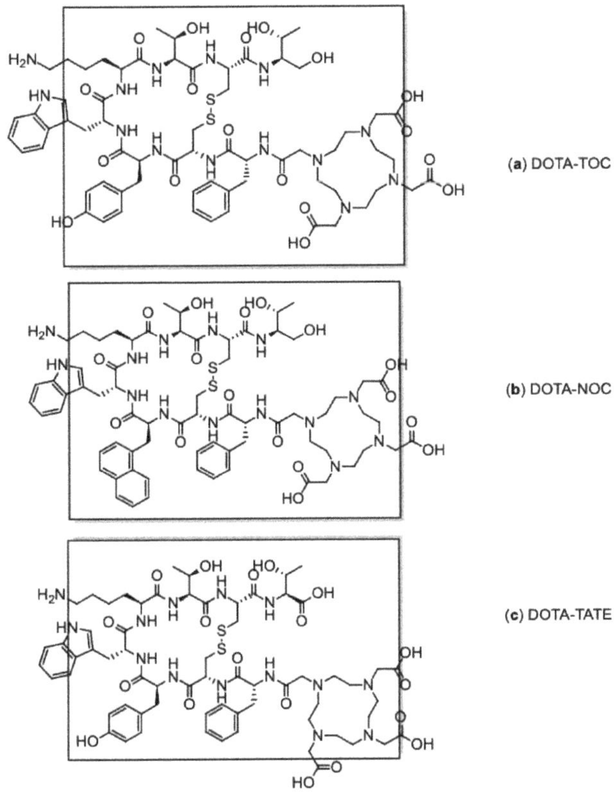

Figure 6. Chemical structures of SSR ligands: (**a**) DOTA-TOC, (**b**) DOTA-NOC, and (c) DOTA TATE. The SSR binding motif is in brackets.

Each compound exhibits high binding affinity for distinct SSR subtypes: Both DOTA-TOC and DOTA-TATE predominantly target SSR2 and show moderate affinity for SSR5 [81], whereas DOTA-NOC also demonstrates binding to SSR3 [82]. Among them, [^{68}Ga]Ga-DOTA-TOC is the most widely used in routine clinical practice due to its strong affinity for SSR2 and favourable interaction with SSR5, offering an optimal balance between diagnostic sensitivity and receptor coverage.

4.3. FAPI Tracers

While most diagnostic and therapeutic strategies have traditionally focused on targeting tumour cells, increasing attention is now being directed toward the tumour microenvironment (TME). The TME is a complex environment composed of immune cells, vasculature, extracellular matrix components, and cancer-associated fibroblasts (CAFs). Among the limited number of available biomarkers for CAFs, the fibroblast activation protein (FAP) has emerged as one of the most promising. FAP is a membrane-bound serine protease and transmembrane glycoprotein that is selectively overexpressed on activated fibroblasts within the stroma of various solid tumours [83].

Preliminary evidence has generated interest in FAP as the next target in the field of nuclear medicine [84]. A range of radiolabelled fibroblast activation protein inhibitors

(FAPI) are currently under investigation as PET imaging agents across multiple tumour types, with several compounds also showing potential for theranostic applications. Notable examples include FAPI-04 and FAPI-46, as illustrated in Figure 7.

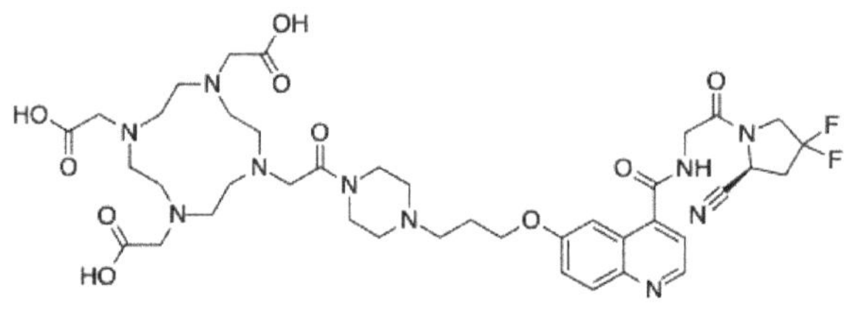

(a) FAPI-04

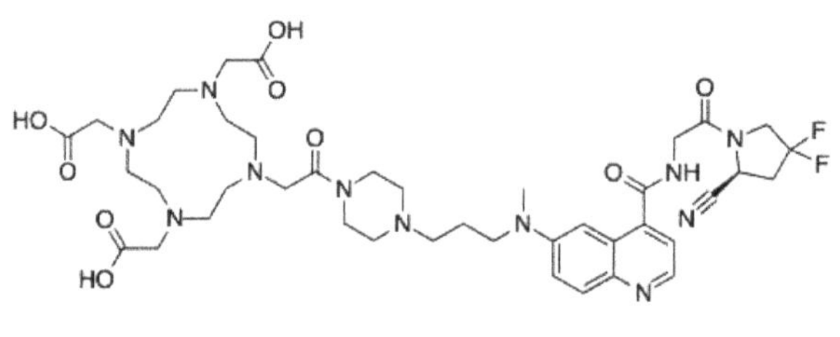

(b) FAPI-46

Figure 7. Chemical structures of FAPI compounds: (**a**) FAPI-04, (**b**) FAPI-46.

5. Extemporaneous Formulations and Quality Control of ^{68}Ga Radiopharmaceuticals

5.1. Production of Extemporaneous Formulations of ^{68}Ga Radiopharmaceuticals for Clinical Uses

According to the Eur. Ph. [85], the preparation of extemporaneous radiopharmaceuticals involves a series of critical operations, including the purchasing of raw materials, the production or elution of the radionuclide, radiolabelling, formulation, purification (where applicable), sterilisation, quality control analysis, dispensing, and final product release to the patients (Figure 8). Each of these steps must be performed within a structured quality management system, guided by principles of risk assessment and aligned with current Good Radiopharmacy Practice (cGRPP) [47], as well as relevant national and European regulatory frameworks.

The process typically begins with the elution of [^{68}Ga]GaCl$_3$ from a ^{68}Ge/^{68}Ga generator or via cyclotron-based production, as described in Section 2.2 and according to the Eur. Ph. monograph 2464 [86]. Manual radiolabelling synthesis is performed within a Grade A laminar flow isolator, whereas automated synthesis is typically carried out inside a shielded Grade C hotcell. Following sterilisation, the dispensing of the final product takes place within a shielded Grade A environment to ensure sterility [87]. Overall, these activities are carried out within a Grade C or D cleanroom, depending on the sterility requirements and the complexity of the radiopharmaceutical preparation process.

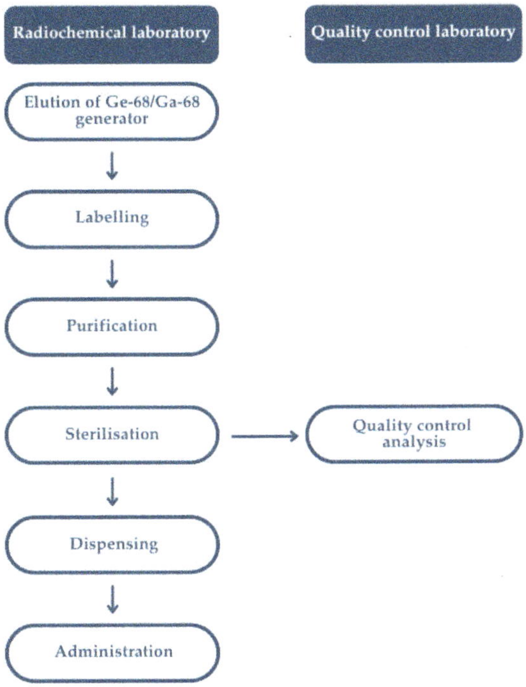

Figure 8. Flowchart of a multistep extemporaneous preparation of ^{68}Ga-labelled radiopharmaceuticals, including radiolabelling, purification, formulation, and sterile filtration to yield an injectable product suitable for clinical administration.

Ensuring the sterility of radiopharmaceutical preparations is a fundamental prerequisite for patient safety. In the case of ^{68}Ga-labelled radiopharmaceuticals, achieving sterility poses particular challenges due to the physicochemical properties of the compounds and the short half-life of the radionuclide, which necessitate rapid preparation, quality control, and release within tight time constraints. Terminal sterilisation by autoclaving is considered the gold standard for sterile drug products; however, it typically involves exposure to steam at 121 °C for at least 15 min and, therefore, this method is not feasible for ^{68}Ga-radiopharmaceuticals. These formulations are highly sensitive to heat; elevated temperatures can induce molecular degradation, loss of radiochemical purity, and the formation of impurities. Additionally, the time associated with autoclaving would result in significant radioactive decay, thereby compromising the clinical utility of the product [88,89]. For this reason, sterilisation is typically achieved through sterile filtration, unless the nature of the compound precludes it, in which case strict aseptic techniques become critical. Consequently, sterile filtration followed by aseptic handling is the preferred approach to ensure both the microbiological safety and the preservation of the chemical and radiochemical integrity of ^{68}Ga-radiopharmaceuticals. In European radiopharmacy practice, sterile filtration is widely implemented as a standard procedure, in compliance with Eur. Ph. and national regulations [90]. When properly integrated into an aseptic workflow and supported by validated integrity testing, it ensures microbiological safety even in time-sensitive, small-scale extemporaneous preparations. However, the selection of the filter membrane is a critical factor, as certain materials may interact with the radiopharmaceutical compound, potentially leading to reduced radiochemical yield. Therefore, compatibility studies are essential to ensure that the filter does not adsorb the radiolabelled product or alter its chemical integrity.

5.1.1. Manual Production

Radiolabelling with ^{68}Ga can be carried out manually through a simple process. Initially, the reaction mixture is prepared by combining [^{68}Ga]GaCl$_3$ with a suitable buffer, the precursor molecule, and any required additives. The solution is then incubated for a defined period under specific temperature conditions to enable efficient complexation of the radiometal. Following incubation, purification may be performed using a solid-phase extraction (SPE) cartridge. The purified product is then eluted and passed through a sterile filter, yielding the final injectable formulation [62].

This method can be adapted to accommodate different precursors and formulation needs. A practical example of this approach is implemented at the Nuclear Medicine Department of the Policlinico di Bari, where [^{68}Ga]Ga-PSMA-11 is routinely prepared. In this protocol, 5 mL of [^{68}Ga]GaCl$_3$ in 0.1 N HCl is incubated at room temperature for 7.5 min with 60 mg of acetic acid buffer and 20 µg of PSMA-11 precursor. Upon completion of the radiolabelling reaction, the solution is reformulated by adding 5 mL of 0.9% NaCl, then it is filtered through a 0.22 µm sterile filter to obtain the final product, ready for administration. Radiochemical purity consistently exceeds 99% as assessed by HPLC, and the overall radiolabelling yield approaches 100% decay corrected.

5.1.2. Automated Production

The increasing clinical demand for ^{68}Ga radiopharmaceuticals has accelerated the adoption of automated synthesis platforms, which provide clear advantages in terms of process reproducibility, radiochemical yield, operator safety, and compliance with GMP standards [91]. Most commercially available systems in use employ cassette-based technology (Figure 9). In these platforms, single-use disposable cassettes are replaced after each synthesis run, ensuring sterility, minimising cross-contamination, and facilitating batch-to-batch standardisation [62]. The use of disposable, pre-sterilised cassettes is considered best practice to reduce microbial risk and radiation exposure, while also simplifying cleaning procedures and minimising operator intervention [68].

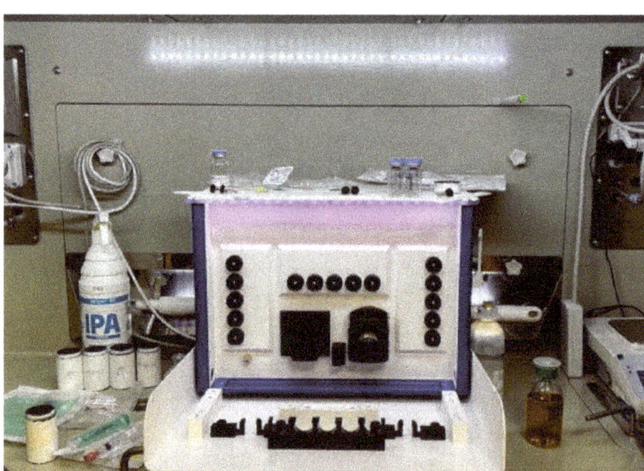

Figure 9. Example of a synthesis module for the preparation of ^{68}Ga radiopharmaceuticals, installed within a shielded hot cell in a hospital radiopharmacy. The module is equipped with pre-defined positions for reagents, cassettes, and waste containers, enabling standardised and operator-independent execution of radiolabelling procedures under aseptic and radiologically safe conditions.

Similar to manual procedures, automated ^{68}Ga-labelling processes comprises four key steps: (1) production of ^{68}Ga from a generator or a cyclotron; (2) SPE purification to concentrate the eluate and remove metallic or ionic impurities; (3) preparation of the reaction mixture containing the precursor, buffer, and optional additives; and (4) final purification of the labelled product prior to sterile filtration and formulation for clinical use (Figure 10).

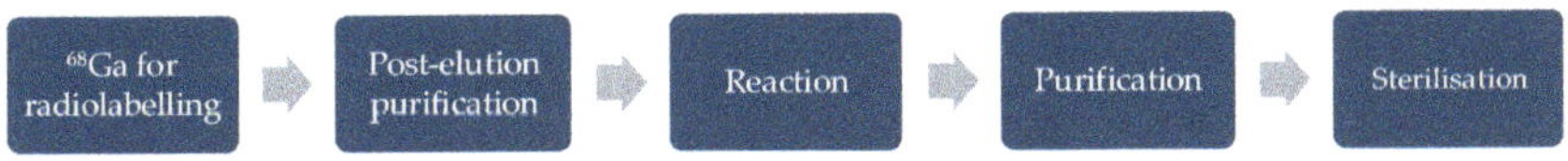

Figure 10. Schematic overview of the general workflow for the preparation of ^{68}Ga-labelled radiopharmaceuticals.

A common challenge in automated workflows is the relatively large elution volume (5–10 mL), which may require post-[^{68}Ga]GaCl$_3$ production processing to concentrate the activity and remove metallic or ionic impurities prior to the radiolabelling step. Three purification strategies are commonly employed:

- Fractionation, which isolates the most active portion of the eluate, although this approach may lead to activity losses and requires higher precursor amounts [79];
- Anion-exchange chromatography, which traps the anionic $[GaCl_4]^-$ complex formed at HCl concentrations > 5.5 M and releases Ga^{3+} upon elution with water [34];
- Cation-exchange chromatography, which retains Ga^{3+} while removing metal impurities (e.g., ^{68}Ge, Zn^{2+}, Fe^{3+}) using acetone/HCl or alternative eluents such as HCl/NaCl. As acetone is not suitable for injection, its presence must be quantified by gas chromatography prior to clinical use [62].

Following purification, the [^{68}Ga]GaCl$_3$ solution is introduced into a reaction vessel containing the reaction mixture: buffer, precursor, and any required additives. After the radiolabelling step, a purification procedure may be performed if required. In most cases, reversed-phase C18 cartridges are employed to retain the labelled product. Unreacted ^{68}Ga species, typically in ionic form, do not bind to the cartridge and are flushed into the waste stream. The radiolabelled compound, along with any colloidal forms of ^{68}Ga, is retained on the stationary phase. Subsequently, the final product is eluted using an ethanol/water mixture, passed through a 0.22 µm sterile filter, and collected in the final product vial. Colloidal gallium species remain adsorbed on the C18 phase, thereby improving the radiochemical purity of the final formulation.

Several examples illustrate the versatility of automated production:

- Fuscaldi et al. [92] described the synthesis of [^{68}Ga]Ga-PSMA-11 using the Modular-Lab PharmTracer module. In this protocol, PSMA-11 (10–20 µg) is dissolved in 1.0 mL of 0.1 M sodium acetate buffer (pH 4.5). ^{68}Ga is eluted from a ^{68}Ge/^{68}Ga generator with 0.1 M HCl, purified via cation exchange, and transferred into the reaction vial. Labelling occurs at 85 °C for 3–5 min, followed by C18 cartridge purification and sterile filtration, completing the process in approximately 25 min. The final product exhibits >99% radiochemical purity and is clinically suitable.
- Fouillet et al. [93] developed a method transposable to PSMA I&T and PSMA-617 using the GAIA® synthesis module (Elysia-Raytest, GmbH, Straubenhardt, Germany). Here, 10 µg of PSMA-11 is dissolved in 2.8 mL of 0.08 M ammonium acetate buffer (pH 4.6), with ^{68}Ga eluted and concentrated via SCX cartridge, then labelled at 97 °C for 8 min. Purification through a C18 cartridge and sterile filtration yields a product meeting GMP clinical-grade standards with >91% radiochemical purity within 27 min.

- The Nuclear Medicine Department of Policlinico di Bari routinely synthesises [^{68}Ga]Ga-DOTATOC using the GAIA® synthesis module. In this method, 5 mL of [^{68}Ga]GaCl_3 is labelled with 50 µg of DOTATOC at 90 °C for 10 min. The formulation uses a buffer system of acetic acid, ammonium acetate, and HCl, followed by C18 purification and sterile filtration to obtain the injectable product.
- Spreckelmeyer et al. [94] described the semi-automated production of [^{68}Ga]Ga-FAPI-46 using the Modular Lab PharmTracer and Modular Lab eazy systems. After SCX purification and radiolabelling at 95–98 °C for 10 min, the product is purified with a CM cartridge and sterile-filtered. As the CM cartridge traps unreacted ^{68}Ga species and flushes [^{68}Ga]Ga-FAPI-46 directly in the product vial, this method avoids the use of ethanol, thereby eliminating the need for residual solvent testing.

A comparative overview of different manual and automated ^{68}Ga-radiopharmaceutical production methods is shown in Table 2.

Table 2. Summary of ^{68}Ga-radiopharmaceutical production methods.

Method	Precursor	Reaction Buffer	Incubation	Purification	Final Processing	Time (min)
Manual [^{68}Ga]Ga-PSMA-11 (Policlinico Bari)	20 µg PSMA-11	Sodium acetate buffer	7.5 min, RT	None	NaCl addition + Filtration	~15
Automated [^{68}Ga]Ga-PSMA-11 (Fuscaldi et al. [92])	10–20 µg PSMA-11	0.1 M Sodium acetate	85 °C, 3–5 min	C18 Cartridge	Sterile Filtration	~25
Automated [^{68}Ga]Ga-PSMA-11 (Fouillet et al. [93])	10 µg PSMA-11	0.08 M Ammonium acetate	97 °C, 8 min	C18 Cartridge	Sterile Filtration	~27
Automated [^{68}Ga]Ga-DOTATOC (Policlinico Bari)	50 µg DOTATOC	Acetic acid, Ammonium acetate, HCl	90 °C, 10 min	C18 Cartridge	Sterile Filtration	~30
Semi-Automated [^{68}Ga]Ga-FAPI-46 (Spreckelmeyer et al. [94])	50 µg FAPI-46	Acetate/Sodium ascorbate	95–98 °C, 10 min	CM Cartridge	Sterile Filtration	~30

5.1.3. Cold Kit

Similarly to the long-established use of ^{99m}Tc cold kits in SPECT imaging, cold kit formulations for ^{68}Ga-radiolabelling have become a practical and efficient solution for PET applications. These kits typically contain a lyophilised precursor along with excipients such as buffering agents and stabilisers, facilitating the streamlined preparation of ^{68}Ga-labelled radiopharmaceuticals in hospital. Among the commercially available options are kits targeting PSMA (e.g., Locametz® by Novartis (Novartis AG, Basel, Switzerland), Illumet™ or Illuccix® by Telix Pharmaceuticals (Telix Pharmaceuticals Ltd., Melbourne, VIC, Australia) and Isoprotrace® by Isotopia (Isotopia Molecular Imaging Ltd., Ramat Gan, Israel), all containing PSMA-11, and GalliProst® by ROTOP (ROTOP Pharmaka GmbH, Dresden, Germany), containing THP-PSMA), somatostatin receptors (e.g., DOTA-TATE, marketed as Netspot® by Novartis), and DOTA-TOC (Somakit-TOC® by Novartis) [18].

An overview of current kit-based formulations is provided by Satpati et al. [95]. For instance, Somakit-TOC® contains 40 µg of DOTA-TOC and is designed to be radiolabelled with 5 mL of ^{68}Ga eluate (0.1 N HCl), supporting a maximum activity of up to 1100 MBq. Similarly, GalliProst® includes 40 µg of THP-PSMA along with sodium bicarbonate, mannitol, and phosphate buffer, providing a mixture suitable for rapid complexation under mild conditions [96].

5.2. Quality Control Analysis

According to current guidelines, quality control of ^{68}Ga extemporaneous formulations of radiopharmaceuticals must include the following tests [59,90]:

- Appearance: Radiopharmaceuticals must be clear, colourless solutions, free of visible particulate matter or turbidity. Visual inspection is typically performed under a calibrated light source using a clean glass inspection station or white background panel.
- pH: The final formulation, intended for intravenous administration, should exhibit a pH compatible with parenteral use, typically within the range of 3.5 to 8.5. For generator eluates, the pH is expected to be below 2 to prevent the precipitation of gallium hydroxide. Measurements are performed using benchtop pH meters with microelectrodes.
- Radionuclidic identity: established via half-life measurement (acceptable range: 62–74 min) and γ-emission spectrum, with characteristic peaks at 511 and 1077 keV. This requires a γ spectrometry system with energy-calibrated sodium iodide scintillation crystals or high-purity Germanium detectors.
- Radionuclidic purity: The level of long-lived impurities, particularly ^{68}Ge breakthrough, must be below 0.001% of total radioactivity. Additional limits are set for any other unintended radionuclidic species. γ spectroscopy with shielding and spectral analysis software is used to quantify breakthrough and confirm compliance. Since ^{68}Ge has a much longer half-life than ^{68}Ga, this analysis must be performed after product release, once the sample has decayed sufficiently, in order to avoid interference from ^{68}Ga and allow accurate quantification of long-lived contaminants.
- Radiochemical purity: Defined as the percentage of radioactivity bound to the intended compound, radiochemical purity must exceed 95%, as unbound ^{68}Ga (e.g., free Ga^{3+} or colloidal species) could compromise diagnostic quality. Analytical procedures include thin-layer chromatography (iTLC) and high-performance liquid chromatography (HPLC), both equipped with radiometric detectors.
- Residual solvents: If organic solvents are used during synthesis (e.g., ethanol, acetic acid), their presence in the final formulation must be quantified by gas chromatography equipped at least with a flame ionisation detector (GC-FID), typically with headspace injection to comply with ICH guidelines.
- Bacterial endotoxins: evaluated using the Limulus Amebocyte Lysate (LAL) assay. Endotoxin quantification is commonly performed with portable or benchtop systems using kinetic chromogenic or turbidimetric methods (e.g., Endosafe® or similar), with an acceptance limit of $\leq$175 EU per total volume of the radiopharmaceutical.
- Sterility: While sterility testing is performed retrospectively in accordance to Ph. Eur. 2.6.1), integrity testing of the sterile filter (e.g., bubble point test) must be completed prior to batch release using validated integrity testers; sterility testing and sterile filtration are conducted in Grade A environments with Grade B background, typically inside shielded isolators or laminar flow hot cells.
- Radioactivity content and concentration: measured using ionisation chamber-based dose calibrators routinely cross-calibrated with secondary standards to ensure correct activity per administered volume.
- Specific or molar activity: Although not always required, the (apparent) specific activity (e.g., MBq/µg) or molar activity (e.g., MBq/nmol) can be reported, acknowledging the presence of excess unlabelled precursor or ligand in most preparations.

These extensive controls are not necessary when radiopharmaceuticals are prepared using a kit with a marketing authorisation. In this case, pre-release quality control analyses are detailed in the Summary of Product Characteristics (SmPC) of the marketing authorisation. These typically encompass several standardised assessments:

- Visual inspection for particulate matter and colour changes;
- pH determination using either a pH meter or indicator strips;
- Radiolabelling efficiency evaluation through iTLC;
- Radioactivity measurement using a dose calibrator.

An illustrative example of such standardised quality control protocols is found in the Locametz® kit preparation procedures.

6. Conclusions

The extemporaneous preparation of ^{68}Ga-labelled radiopharmaceuticals plays a key role in expanding access to personalised diagnostic agents in nuclear medicine. This flexible and efficient approach allows for the rapid, on-demand production of radiopharmaceuticals tailored to specific clinical indications, ensuring timely patient management and optimising the use of short-lived radionuclides such as ^{68}Ga [97].

As the field continues to evolve, one of the most promising future directions is extending extemporaneous preparation beyond diagnostic applications to include therapeutic radiopharmaceuticals. The increasing interest in theranostic approaches and the development of novel therapeutic radionuclides suggest the feasibility of preparing radiopharmaceutical therapies directly in-house [98]. This would represent a significant step forward in the personalisation of nuclear medicine, enabling truly patient-specific treatment strategies to be implemented rapidly and efficiently.

The continued advancement of this practice will depend on the refinement of synthesis protocols, the development of reliable automated systems, and the strengthening of multidisciplinary collaborations. Extemporaneous preparations are not only a practical solution for today's diagnostic challenges, but they also represent a strategic framework toward the future of individualised radiopharmaceutical therapy.

Author Contributions: Conceptualisation, A.L. and A.C.; software, R.M.I. and N.D.; writing—original draft preparation, M.R.; writing—review and editing, A.L. and A.P.; visualisation, M.R., A.L., A.C., R.M.I., N.D., A.P. and M.D.D.B.; supervision, A.L. and M.D.D.B. All authors have read and agreed to the published version of the manuscript.

Funding: This research received no external funding.

Conflicts of Interest: Authors Marzia Rizzello, Anna Pacelli and Maria Domenica De Bari were employed by the Company BeForPharma S.r.l. The remaining authors declare that the research was conducted in the absence of any commercial or financial relationships that could be construed as potential conflicts of interest.

References

1. Martiniova, L.; Palatis, L.; Etchebehere, E.; Ravizzini, G. Gallium-68 in Medical Imaging. *Curr. Radiopharm.* **2016**, *9*, 187–207. [CrossRef] [PubMed]
2. Kleynhans, J.; Ebenhan, T.; Sathekge, M.M. Expanding Role for Gallium-68 PET Imaging in Oncology. *Semin. Nucl. Med.* **2024**, *54*, 778–791. [CrossRef] [PubMed]
3. Bois, F.; Noirot, C.; Dietemann, S.; Mainta, I.C.; Zilli, T.; Garibotto, V.; Walter, M.A. [$^{(68)}$Ga]Ga-PSMA-11 in prostate cancer: A comprehensive review. *Am. J. Nucl. Med. Mol. Imaging* **2020**, *10*, 349–374. [PubMed]
4. Graham, M.M.; Gu, X.; Ginader, T.; Breheny, P.; Sunderland, J.J. $^{(68)}$Ga-DOTATOC Imaging of Neuroendocrine Tumors: A Systematic Review and Metaanalysis. *J. Nucl. Med.* **2017**, *58*, 1452–1458. [CrossRef]
5. Prive, B.M.; Boussihmad, M.A.; Timmermans, B.; van Gemert, W.A.; Peters, S.M.B.; Derks, Y.H.W.; van Lith, S.A.M.; Mehra, N.; Nagarajah, J.; Heskamp, S.; et al. Fibroblast activation protein-targeted radionuclide therapy: Background, opportunities, and challenges of first (pre)clinical studies. *Eur. J. Nucl. Med. Mol. Imaging* **2023**, *50*, 1906–1918. [CrossRef]
6. Pretze, M.; Reffert, L.; Diehl, S.; Schonberg, S.O.; Wangler, C.; Hohenberger, P.; Wangler, B. GMP-compliant production of [$^{(68)}$Ga]Ga-NeoB for positron emission tomography imaging of patients with gastrointestinal stromal tumor. *EJNMMI Radiopharm. Chem.* **2021**, *6*, 22. [CrossRef]

7. Lindenberg, L.; Ahlman, M.; Lin, F.; Mena, E.; Choyke, P. Advances in PET Imaging of the CXCR4 Receptor: [$^{(68)}$Ga]Ga-PentixaFor. *Semin. Nucl. Med.* **2024**, *54*, 163–170. [CrossRef]
8. Urso, L.; Napolitano, R.; Speltri, G.; Tuncel, M.; Badrane, I.; Uccelli, L.; Porto, F.; Martini, P.; Niorettini, A.; Cittanti, C.; et al. $^{(68)}$Ga-Trivehexin: Current Status of alphavbeta6-Integrin Imaging and Perspectives. *Cancers* **2025**, *17*, 1504. [CrossRef]
9. Mirnezami, R.; Nicholson, J.; Darzi, A. Preparing for precision medicine. *N. Engl. J. Med.* **2012**, *366*, 489–491. [CrossRef]
10. Holden, N.E. Table of the Isotopes. In *Handbook of Chemistry and Physics*, 85th ed.; CRC Press: Boca Raton, FL, USA, 2004.
11. Amor-Coarasa, A.; Kelly, J.M.; Ponnala, S.; Nikolopoulou, A.; Williams, C., Jr.; Babich, J.W. (66)Ga: A Novelty or a Valuable Preclinical Screening Tool for the Design of Targeted Radiopharmaceuticals? *Molecules* **2018**, *23*, 2575. [CrossRef]
12. Jalilian, A.R. An overview on Ga-68 radiopharmaceuticals for positron emission tomography applications. *Iran. J. Nucl. Med.* **2016**, *24*, 1–10.
13. Greene, M.; Tucker, W. An Improved Gallium-68 cow. *Radiat. Isot.* **1961**, *12*, 62–63. [CrossRef]
14. Velikyan, I. ^{68}Ga-Based radiopharmaceuticals: Production and application relationship. *Molecules* **2015**, *20*, 12913–12943. [CrossRef] [PubMed]
15. Eckert & Ziegler Radiopharma GmbH. *GalliaPharm 68Ge/^{68}Ga Generator—Summary of Product Characteristics*; Eckert & Ziegler Radiopharma GmbH: Berlin, Germany, 2024.
16. IRE ELiT, S.A. *GalliAd® 68Ge/^{68}Ga Generator—Riassunto delle Caratteristiche del Prodotto*; IRE ELiT S.A.: Fleurus, Belgium, 2018.
17. Cusnir, R.; Cakebread, A.; Cooper, M.S.; Young, J.D.; Blower, P.J.; Ma, M.T. The effects of trace metal impurities on Ga-68-radiolabelling with a tris(3-hydroxy-1,6-dimethylpyridin-4-one) (THP) chelator. *RSC Adv.* **2019**, *9*, 37214–37221. [CrossRef]
18. Nelson, B.J.B.; Andersson, J.D.; Wuest, F.; Spreckelmeyer, S. Good practices for $^{(68)}$Ga radiopharmaceutical production. *EJNMMI Radiopharm. Chem.* **2022**, *7*, 27. [CrossRef]
19. Dash, A.; Chakravarty, R. Radionuclide generators: The prospect of availing PET radiotracers to meet current clinical needs and future research demands. *Am. J. Nucl. Med. Mol. Imaging* **2019**, *9*, 30–66.
20. Eberl, S.; Eriksson, T.; Svedberg, O.; Norling, J.; Henderson, D.; Lam, P.; Fulham, M. High beam current operation of a PETtrace cyclotron for 18F- production. *Appl. Radiat. Isot.* **2012**, *70*, 922–930. [CrossRef]
21. Lepareur, N. Cold Kit Labeling: The Future of $^{(68)}$Ga Radiopharmaceuticals? *Front. Med.* **2022**, *9*, 812050. [CrossRef]
22. Kumar, K. The Current Status of the Production and Supply of Gallium-68. *Cancer Biother. Radiopharm.* **2020**, *35*, 163–166. [CrossRef]
23. Svedjehed, J.; Parnaste, M.; Gagnon, K. Demystifying solid targets: Simple and rapid distribution-scale production of [$^{(68)}$Ga]GaCl$^{(3)}$ and [$^{(68)}$Ga]Ga-PSMA-11. *Nucl. Med. Biol.* **2022**, *104–105*, 1–10. [CrossRef]
24. Thisgaard, H.; Kumlin, J.; Langkjaer, N.; Chua, J.; Hook, B.; Jensen, M.; Kassaian, A.; Zeisler, S.; Borjian, S.; Cross, M.; et al. Multi-curie production of gallium-68 on a biomedical cyclotron and automated radiolabelling of PSMA-11 and DOTATATE. *EJNMMI Radiopharm. Chem.* **2021**, *6*, 1. [CrossRef] [PubMed]
25. Nelson, B.J.B.; Wilson, J.; Richter, S.; Duke, M.J.M.; Wuest, M.; Wuest, F. Taking cyclotron $^{(68)}$Ga production to the next level: Expeditious solid target production of $^{(68)}$Ga for preparation of radiotracers. *Nucl. Med. Biol.* **2020**, *80–81*, 24–31. [CrossRef] [PubMed]
26. Riga, S.; Cicoria, G.; Pancaldi, D.; Zagni, F.; Vichi, S.; Dassenno, M.; Mora, L.; Lodi, F.; Morigi, M.P.; Marengo, M. Production of Ga-68 with a General Electric PETtrace cyclotron by liquid target. *Phys. Med.* **2018**, *55*, 116–126. [CrossRef] [PubMed]
27. Pandey, M.K.; Byrne, J.F.; Schlasner, K.N.; Schmit, N.R.; DeGrado, T.R. Cyclotron production of $^{(68)}$Ga in a liquid target: Effects of solution composition and irradiation parameters. *Nucl. Med. Biol.* **2019**, *74–75*, 49–55. [CrossRef]
28. Velikyan, I. Positron emitting [^{68}Ga]Ga-based imaging agents: Chemistry and diversity. *Med. Chem.* **2011**, *7*, 345–379. [CrossRef]
29. Martell, A.E.; Motekaitis, R.J.; Clarke, E.T.; Delgado, R.; Sun, Y.; Ma, R. Stability constants of metal complexes of macrocyclic ligands with pendant donor groups. *Supramol. Chem.* **1996**, *6*, 353–363. [CrossRef]
30. Spang, P.; Herrmann, C.; Roesch, F. Bifunctional Gallium-68 Chelators: Past, Present, and Future. *Semin. Nucl. Med.* **2016**, *46*, 373–394. [CrossRef]
31. Hofman, M.S.; Hicks, R.J. Gallium-68 EDTA PET/CT for Renal Imaging. *Semin. Nucl. Med.* **2016**, *46*, 448–461. [CrossRef]
32. Price, E.W.; Orvig, C. Matching chelators to radiometals for radiopharmaceuticals. *Chem. Soc. Rev.* **2014**, *43*, 260–290. [CrossRef]
33. Seemann, J.; Waldron, B.P.; Parker, D. Influence of metal ions on the ^{68}Ga-labeling of DOTATATE. *Appl. Radiat. Isot.* **2013**, *82*, 63–68. [CrossRef]
34. Meyer, G.J.; Macke, H.; Schuhmacher, J.; Knapp, W.H.; Hofmann, M. ^{68}Ga-labelled DOTA-derivatised peptide ligands. *Eur. J. Nucl. Med. Mol. Imaging* **2004**, *31*, 1097–1104. [CrossRef] [PubMed]
35. Ray Banerjee, S.; Chen, Z.; Pullambhatla, M.; Lisok, A.; Chen, J.; Mease, R.C.; Pomper, M.G. Preclinical Comparative Study of $^{(68)}$Ga-Labeled DOTA, NOTA, and HBED-CC Chelated Radiotracers for Targeting PSMA. *Bioconjug Chem.* **2016**, *27*, 1447–1455. [CrossRef] [PubMed]
36. Roesch, F.; Riss, P.J. The Renaissance of the 68Ge/^{68}Ga Radionuclide Generator Initiates New Developments in ^{68}Ga Radiopharmaceutical Chemistry. *Curr. Top. Med. Chem.* **2010**, *10*, 1633–1668. [CrossRef] [PubMed]

37. Velikyan, I.; Maecke, H.; Langstrom, B. Convenient preparation of ^{68}Ga-based PET-radiopharmaceuticals at room temperature. *Bioconjug Chem.* **2008**, *19*, 569–573. [CrossRef]
38. Martell, A.E.; Smith, R.M. Critical Stability Constants. In *Coordination Chemistry Reviews*; Plenum Press: New York, NY, USA, 1977; Volume 1–4.
39. Tsionou, M.I.; Knapp, C.E.; Foley, C.A.; Munteanu, C.R.; Cakebread, A.; Imberti, C.; Eykyn, T.R.; Young, J.D.; Paterson, B.M.; Blower, P.J.; et al. Comparison of macrocyclic and acyclic chelators for gallium-68 radiolabelling. *RSC Adv.* **2017**, *7*, 49586–49599. [CrossRef]
40. Wood, S.; Samson, I. The aqueous geochemistry of gallium, germanium, indium and scandium. *Ore Geol. Rev.* **2006**, *28*, 57–102. [CrossRef]
41. Blower, J.E.; Cooper, M.S.; Imberti, C.; Ma, M.T.; Marshall, C.; Young, J.D.; Blower, P.J. The Radiopharmaceutical Chemistry of the Radionuclides of Gallium and Indium. In *Radiopharmaceutical Chemistry*; Lewis, J.S., Windhorst, A.D., Zeglis, B.M., Eds.; Springer International Publishing: Cham, Switzerland, 2019; pp. 255–271.
42. Bauwens, M.; Chekol, R.; Vanbilloen, H.; Bormans, G.; Verbruggen, A. Optimal buffer choice of the radiosynthesis of $^{(68)}$Ga-Dotatoc for clinical application. *Nucl. Med. Commun.* **2010**, *31*, 753–758. [CrossRef]
43. Weiner, R.E.; Thakur, M.L. Chemistry of gallium and indium radiopharmaceuticals. In *Handbook of Radiopharmaceuticals: Radiochemistry and Applications*; Welch, M.J., Redvanly, C.S., Eds.; John Wiley & Sons: New York, NY, USA, 2003; pp. 363–399.
44. Council of Europe. *European Pharmacopoeia*, 11th ed.; Council of Europe: Strasbourg, France, 2023; Volume Supplement 11.3, pp. 2990–2991.
45. Antunes, I.F.; Franssen, G.M.; Zijlma, R.; Laverman, P.; Boersma, H.H.; Elsinga, P.H. New sensitive method for HEPES quantification in $^{(68)}$Ga-radiopharmaceuticals. *EJNMMI Radiopharm. Chem.* **2020**, *5*, 12. [CrossRef]
46. le Roux, J.; Kleynhans, J.; Rubow, S. The use of HEPES-buffer in the production of gallium-68 radiopharmaceuticals—Time to reconsider strict pharmacopoeial limits? *EJNMMI Radiopharm. Chem.* **2021**, *6*, 15. [CrossRef]
47. Gillings, N.; Hjelstuen, O.; Ballinger, J.; Behe, M.; Decristoforo, C.; Elsinga, P.; Ferrari, V.; Kolenc Peitl, P.; Koziorowski, J.; Laverman, P.; et al. Guidance on current good radiopharmacy practice (cGRPP) for the small-scale preparation of radiopharmaceuticals. *Eur. J. Nucl. Med. Mol. Imaging* **2012**, *39*, 82–84.
48. European Union. Council Directive 89/343/EEC of 3 May 1989 amending Directive 65/65/EEC as regards medicinal products derived from human blood or human plasma. *Off. J. Eur. Communities* **1989**, *142*, 16–18.
49. European Union. Directive 2001/83/EC of the European Parliament and of the Council of 6 November 2001 on the Community code relating to medicinal products for human use. *Off. J. Eur. Communities* **2001**, *311*, 67–128.
50. Gillings, N.; Hjelstuen, O.; Behe, M.; Decristoforo, C.; Elsinga, P.H.; Ferrari, V.; Kiss, O.C.; Kolenc, P.; Koziorowski, J.; Laverman, P.; et al. EANM guideline on quality risk management for radiopharmaceuticals. *Eur. J. Nucl. Med. Mol. Imaging* **2022**, *49*, 3353–3364. [CrossRef] [PubMed]
51. Hendrikse, H.; Kiss, O.; Kunikowska, J.; Wadsak, W.; Decristoforo, C.; Patt, M. EANM position on the in-house preparation of radiopharmaceuticals. *Eur. J. Nucl. Med. Mol. Imaging* **2022**, *49*, 1095–1098. [CrossRef]
52. European Association of Nuclear Medicine (EANM Executive Office). *Statement of the European Association of Nuclear Medicine (EANM) for a Better Inclusion of the Particularities of Radiopharmaceuticals Within the Review of Directive 2001/83/EC on Pharmaceutical Legislation*; EANM Executive Office: Vienna, Austria, 2021.
53. Republic of Italy. Legislative Decree No. 219 of 24 April 2006: Implementation of Directive 2001/83/EC and subsequent amendments, relating to medicinal products for human use. In *Gazzetta Ufficiale della Repubblica Italiana, No. 142, 21 June 2006—Supplemento Ordinario No. 153*; Istituto Poligrafico e Zecca dello Stato: Rome, Italy, 2006.
54. Ministero della Salute. *Farmacopea Ufficiale Della Repubblica Italiana, XII Edizione—Supplemento: Norme di Buona Preparazione dei Radiofarmaci in Medicina Nucleare (NBP-MN)*; Istituto Poligrafico e Zecca dello Stato: Rome, Italy, 2010.
55. Republic of Italy. Legislative Decree No 101 of 31 July 2020: Implementation of Directive 2013/59/Euratom, establishing basic safety standards for protection against the dangers arising from exposure to ionising radiation. In *Gazzetta Ufficiale Della Repubblica Italiana, No. 201, 12 August 2020—Supplemento Ordinario No. 29*; Istituto Poligrafico e Zecca dello Stato: Rome, Italy, 2020.
56. European Union. Council Directive 2013/59/Euratom of 5 December 2013: Laying down basic safety standards for protection against the dangers arising from exposure to ionising radiation, and repealing Directives 89/618/Euratom, 90/641/Euratom, 96/29/Euratom, 97/43/Euratom and 2003/122/Euratom. *Off. J. Eur. Union* **2013**, *13*, 1–73.
57. Republic of Italy. Legislative Decree No. 101 of 31 July 2020: Implementation of Directive 2013/59/Euratom, establishing basic safety standards for protection against the dangers arising from exposure to ionising radiation. Articles 130–131 (Radiation Protection Expert), Article 146, Annex XXIII. In *Gazzetta Ufficiale Della Repubblica Italiana, No. 201, 12 August 2020—Supplemento Ordinario No. 29*; Istituto Poligrafico e Zecca dello Stato: Rome, Italy, 2020.
58. European Directorate for the Quality of Medicines and HealthCare. *European Pharmacopoeia*, 11th ed.; Council of Europe: Strasbourg, France, 2023.

59. European Directorate for the Quality of Medicines and HealthCare. Monograph 0125—Radiopharmaceutical Preparations. In *European Pharmacopoeia*, 11th ed.; Council of Europe: Strasbourg, France, 2023.
60. European Directorate for the Quality of Medicines and HealthCare. Monograph 3109—Gallium (^{68}Ga) PSMA-11 Injection. In *European Pharmacopoeia*, 11th ed.; Council of Europe: Strasbourg, France, 2023.
61. European Directorate for the Quality of Medicines and HealthCare. Monograph 3098—Gallium (^{68}Ga) Edotreotide Injection. In *European Pharmacopoeia*, 11th ed.; Council of Europe: Strasbourg, France, 2023.
62. Meisenheimer, M.; Saenko, Y.; Eppard, E. Gallium-68: Radiolabeling of Radiopharmaceuticals for PET Imaging—A Lot to Consider. Chapter 2. In *Medical Isotopes*; 2019; pp. 1–22.
63. European Commission. EudraLex—Volume 4—Good Manufacturing Practice (GMP) Guidelines. 2022. Available online: https://health.ec.europa.eu/medicinal-products/eudralex/eudralex-volume-4_en (accessed on 21 March 2025).
64. European Commission. EudraLex Volume 4, Annex 1: Manufacture of Sterile Medicinal Products. In *The Rules Governing Medicinal Products in the European Union*; European Commission: Brussels, Belgium, 2022.
65. PIC/S Guide to Good Practices for the Preparation of Medicinal Products in Healthcare Establishments—Annex 3: Preparation of Radiopharmaceuticals. In *Pharmaceutical Inspection Convention Pharmaceutical Inspection Co-Operation Scheme*; PIC/S: Geneva, Switzerland, 2014.
66. Moya, E.; Cerrato, C.; Bedoya, L.M.; Guerra, J.A. Radiopharmaceutical small-scale preparation in Europe: Will we be able to harmonize the situation? *EJNMMI Radiopharm. Chem.* **2024**, *9*, 64. [CrossRef]
67. International Council for Harmonisation (ICH). *ICH Harmonised Guideline: Validation of Analytical Procedures Q2(R2)*; ICH: Geneva, Switzerland, 2022.
68. Velikyan, I. Prospective of ^{68}Ga-Radiopharmaceutical Development. *Theranostics* **2014**, *4*, 47–80. [CrossRef]
69. Gillings, N.; Todde, S.; Behe, M.; Decristoforo, C.; Elsinga, P.; Ferrari, V.; Hjelstuen, O.; Peitl, P.K.; Koziorowski, J.; Laverman, P.; et al. EANM guideline on the validation of analytical methods for radiopharmaceuticals. *EJNMMI Radiopharm. Chem.* **2020**, *5*, 7. [CrossRef]
70. International Council for Harmonisation (ICH Secretariat). *ICH Harmonised Guideline Q3C(R9): Impurities: Guideline for Residual Solvents*; ICH Secretariat: Geneva, Switzerland, 2021.
71. International Council for Harmonisation (ICH Secretariat). *ICH Harmonised Guideline Q3D(R2): Guideline for Elemental Impurities*; ICH Secretariat: Geneva, Switzerland, 2022.
72. European Commission. Gallium (^{68}Ga) chloride solution for radiolabelling. In *European Pharmacopoeia*, 11th ed.; Council of Europe: Strasbourg, France, 2023; p. 3051.
73. European Commission. Gallium (^{68}Ga) chloride solution produced by cyclotron. In *European Pharmacopoeia*, 11th ed.; Council of Europe: Strasbourg, France, 2023; p. 3052.
74. Silver, D.A.; Pellicer, I.; Fair, W.R.; Heston, W.D.; Cordon-Cardo, C. Prostate-specific membrane antigen expression in normal and malignant human tissues. *Clin. Cancer Res.* **1997**, *3*, 81–85.
75. Mannweiler, S.; Amersdorfer, P.; Trajanoski, S.; Terrett, J.A.; King, D.; Mehes, G. Heterogeneity of prostate-specific membrane antigen (PSMA) expression in prostate carcinoma with distant metastasis. *Pathol. Oncol. Res.* **2009**, *15*, 167–172. [CrossRef]
76. Hennrich, U.; Eder, M. [$^{(68)}$Ga]Ga-PSMA-11: The First FDA-Approved $^{(68)}$Ga-Radiopharmaceutical for PET Imaging of Prostate Cancer. *Pharmaceuticals* **2021**, *14*, 713. [CrossRef] [PubMed]
77. Fendler, W.P.; Eiber, M.; Beheshti, M.; Bomanji, J.; Ceci, F.; Cho, S.; Giesel, F.; Haberkorn, U.; Hope, T.A.; Kopka, K.; et al. $^{(68)}$Ga-PSMA PET/CT: Joint EANM and SNMMI procedure guideline for prostate cancer imaging: Version 1.0. *Eur. J. Nucl. Med. Mol. Imaging* **2017**, *44*, 1014–1024. [CrossRef] [PubMed]
78. Schuchardt, C.; Zhang, J.; Kulkarni, H.R.; Chen, X.; Muller, D.; Baum, R.P. Prostate-Specific Membrane Antigen Radioligand Therapy Using $^{(177)}$Lu-PSMA I&T and $^{(177)}$Lu-PSMA-617 in Patients with Metastatic Castration-Resistant Prostate Cancer: Comparison of Safety, Biodistribution, and Dosimetry. *J. Nucl. Med.* **2022**, *63*, 1199–1207. [CrossRef] [PubMed]
79. Breeman, W.A.; de Jong, M.; de Blois, E.; Bernard, B.F.; Konijnenberg, M.; Krenning, E.P. Radiolabelling DOTA-peptides with ^{68}Ga. *Eur. J. Nucl. Med. Mol. Imaging* **2005**, *32*, 478–485. [CrossRef]
80. Fani, M.; Nicolas, G.P.; Wild, D. Somatostatin Receptor Antagonists for Imaging and Therapy. *J. Nucl. Med.* **2017**, *58*, 61S–66S. [CrossRef]
81. Reubi, J.C.; Waser, B. Concomitant expression of several peptide receptors in neuroendocrine tumours: Molecular basis for in vivo multireceptor tumour targeting. *Eur. J. Nucl. Med. Mol. Imaging* **2003**, *30*, 781–793. [CrossRef]
82. Antunes, P.; Ginj, M.; Zhang, H.; Waser, B.; Baum, R.P.; Reubi, J.C.; Maecke, H. Are radiogallium-labelled DOTA-conjugated somatostatin analogues superior to those labelled with other radiometals? *Eur. J. Nucl. Med. Mol. Imaging* **2007**, *34*, 982–993. [CrossRef]
83. Garin-Chesa, P.; Old, L.J.; Rettig, W.J. Cell surface glycoprotein of reactive stromal fibroblasts as a potential antibody target in human epithelial cancers. *Proc. Natl. Acad. Sci. USA* **1990**, *87*, 7235–7239. [CrossRef]
84. Calais, J. FAP: The Next Billion Dollar Nuclear Theranostics Target? *J. Nucl. Med.* **2020**, *61*, 163–165. [CrossRef]

85. European Directorate for the Quality of Medicines and HealthCare. *5.19. Extemporaneous Preparation of Radiopharmaceuticals*, 11th ed.; Council of Europe: Strasbourg, France, 2022.
86. Council of Europe. Monograph: Gallium (^{68}Ga) chloride (accelerator-produced). In *European Pharmacopoeia*, 11th ed.; Council of Europe: Strasbourg, France, 2023; Volume Supplement 11.3.
87. Lange, R.; ter Heine, R.; Decristoforo, C.; Penuelas, I.; Elsinga, P.H.; van der Westerlaken, M.M.; Hendrikse, N.H. Untangling the web of European regulations for the preparation of unlicensed radiopharmaceuticals: A concise overview and practical guidance for a risk-based approach. *Nucl. Med. Commun.* **2015**, *36*, 414–422. [CrossRef]
88. Hasanain, F.; Guenther, K.; Mullett, W.M.; Craven, E. Gamma sterilization of pharmaceuticals--a review of the irradiation of excipients, active pharmaceutical ingredients, and final drug product formulations. *PDA J. Pharm. Sci. Technol.* **2014**, *68*, 113–137. [CrossRef] [PubMed]
89. DeCollibus, D.P.; Searcy, J.; Tivesten, A.; Akhtar, N.; Lindenberg, C.; Abarrou, N.; Pradhan, S.; Fiandaca, M.; Franklin, J.; Govindan, G.; et al. Considerations for the Terminal Sterilization of Oligonucleotide Drug Products. *Nucleic Acid. Ther.* **2023**, *33*, 159–177. [CrossRef] [PubMed]
90. International Atomic Energy Agency. *Quality Control in the Production of Radiopharmaceuticals*; International Atomic Energy Agency: Vienna, Austria, 2018.
91. Decristoforo, C. Gallium-68—A new opportunity for PET available from a long shelf-life generator—Automation and applications. *Curr. Radiopharm.* **2012**, *5*, 212–220. [CrossRef] [PubMed]
92. Fuscaldi, L.L.; Sobral, D.V.; Durante, A.C.R.; Mendonca, F.F.; Miranda, A.C.C.; da Cunha, M.L.; Malavolta, L.; Mejia, J.; de Barboza, M.F. Standardization of the [$^{(68)}$Ga]Ga-PSMA-11 Radiolabeling Protocol in an Automatic Synthesis Module: Assessments for PET Imaging of Prostate Cancer. *Pharmaceuticals* **2021**, *14*, 385. [CrossRef]
93. Fouillet, J.; Donze, C.; Deshayes, E.; Santoro, L.; Rubira, L.; Fersing, C. "One Method to Label Them All": A Single Fully Automated Protocol for GMP-Compliant $^{(68)}$Ga Radiolabeling of PSMA-11, Transposable to PSMA-I&T and PSMA-617. *Curr. Radiopharm.* **2024**, *17*, 285–301. [CrossRef]
94. Spreckelmeyer, S.; Balzer, M.; Poetzsch, S.; Brenner, W. Fully-automated production of [$^{(68)}$Ga]Ga-FAPI-46 for clinical application. *EJNMMI Radiopharm. Chem.* **2020**, *5*, 31. [CrossRef]
95. Satpati, D. Recent Breakthrough in $^{(68)}$Ga-Radiopharmaceuticals Cold Kits for Convenient PET Radiopharmacy. *Bioconjug Chem.* **2021**, *32*, 430–447. [CrossRef]
96. Derlin, T.; Schmuck, S.; Juhl, C.; Teichert, S.; Zorgiebel, J.; Wester, H.J.; Schneefeld, S.M.; Walte, A.C.A.; Thackeray, J.T.; Ross, T.L.; et al. Imaging Characteristics and First Experience of [$^{(68)}$Ga]THP-PSMA, a Novel Probe for Rapid Kit-Based Ga-68 Labeling and PET Imaging: Comparative Analysis with [$^{(68)}$Ga]PSMA I&T. *Mol. Imaging Biol.* **2018**, *20*, 650–658. [CrossRef]
97. Decristoforo, C.; Patt, M. Are we "preparing" radiopharmaceuticals? *EJNMMI Radiopharm. Chem.* **2017**, *1*, 12. [CrossRef]
98. Weber, W.A.; Barthel, H.; Bengel, F.; Eiber, M.; Herrmann, K.; Schafers, M. What Is Theranostics? *J. Nucl. Med.* **2023**, *64*, 669–670. [CrossRef]

pharmaceutics

MDPI

Article

Metronidazole Suspension for Paediatric Use in Developing Countries: Formulation, Quality, and Stability

Francesca Baratta [1,2,*], Chiara Zingarelli [1], Federica Fanton [1], Editson Lamy [3], Gaetano Di Lascio [2] and Paola Brusa [1,2]

1 Department of Drug Science and Technology, University of Turin, Via Pietro Giuria 9, 10125 Turin, Italy; chiara.zingarelli@unito.it (C.Z.); federica.fanton@unito.it (F.F.); paola.brusa@unito.it (P.B.)
2 Aid Progress Pharmacist Agreement Non-Profit Association, Via Pietro Giuria 9, 10125 Turin, Italy; gaetano.dlascio@gmail.com
3 Pharmacy Service, Foyer Saint Camille Hospital, 48 Rue Eben Ezer Marin 12, Route Nationale # 1, Varreux, Croix-des-Bouquets, Port-au-Prince HT6110, Haiti; leditson@gmail.com
* Correspondence: francesca.baratta@unito.it; Tel.: +39-0116706665

Abstract

Background/Objectives. The paediatric population is a heterogenous group that is known to be a therapeutic orphan despite the recent incentives to promote the development of children's formulations. Especially in low and middle-income countries, there is still a worldwide shortfall for the treatment and prevention of a variety of paediatric conditions. In this context, we developed a formulation specifically intended to administer metronidazole to paediatric patients using basic and low-cost excipients and with a simple set-up method. **Methods**. Various mixtures of excipients were prepared to obtain a suitable metronidazole liquid formulation at a concentration of 250 mg/5 mL. The best formula was tested for its quality and stability, assessing the uniformity of content, the pH, and the dispersion quality. We evaluated the stability of the preparation for 180 days at room temperature (25 +/− 2 °C), in a thermostatic oven (40 +/− 2 °C), and in a fridge (4 +/− 2 °C). **Results.** The tests performed gave excellent results. No variation greater than 10% was detected in the metronidazole concentration or in pH values after 180 days regardless of the temperature conditions during storage. Moreover, the microscope analysis confirmed the absence of significant differences over time. **Conclusions.** The results were consistent in different environmental conditions, ensuring the possibility of using the formulation even in those tropical countries where is not always possible to guarantee the conservation of medicines in controlled conditions. Moreover, the simple composition and easy preparation procedure make it possible to produce the suspension in any context, ensuring the quality of the finished product.

Keywords: metronidazole suspension; paediatric formulae; compounding; pharmacy; developing countries

1. Introduction

The paediatric population is a heterogenous group, from new-born to adolescent, that may be affected by the same pathologies as adults and, consequently, require treatment with the same active molecules. However, these are often commercially unavailable in formulations that contain paediatric dosages. In addition, there is a lack of data that specify the efficacy and tolerability amongst children for industrial products approved for adult use [1,2]. The paucity of child-friendly formulations means that in the field of paediatric therapy, the practice of using off-label prescriptions is widespread, with the risk of administering non-optimal dosages, inefficacious therapies, or increasing the risk of adverse reactions [3,4]. Moreover, the excipients contained in these products may also be unsuitable for children, even in small quantities [5].

In recent years, there have been a number of initiatives worldwide that have attempted to foster and improve the development of paediatric medicines [4]. Although these initiatives have resulted in an increase in the number of paediatric medicines available, providing new directions for the use of approved medicines in the paediatric field [6,7], little attention has been given to improving the situation for older or off-patent medicines in formulations and dosages suitable for the paediatric population. The active ingredients in question account for most of the medicines listed as essential for children by the World Health Organisation (WHO), but only a third of the oral preparations are commercially available in formulations appropriate for children in the age group between one and five years old [8,9]. Despite regulatory incentives, there is still a worldwide shortfall for the treatment and prevention of a variety of conditions, especially in low- and middle-income countries [10].

Considering all the issues above regarding the availability of paediatric medicines, the prescription of extemporaneous preparations becomes a necessity and, thus, a common activity among paediatricians [5].

Oral liquid formulations are generally recommended for children: these are easily swallowed, and facilitate, in younger children, the adjustment of the dosage according to the body weight of the patient. However, there are also some disadvantages: the dosage and volume of the medicine may be limited by the solubility of the substance to be administered. Moreover, ensuring the stability of the formulation may require buffers, antioxidants, or preservatives [11,12]. Another factor, which must not be overlooked, is the palatability of the formulation. In the 1964 film *Mary Poppins* by Walt Disney, Mary sings "Just a spoonful of sugar makes the medicine go down." Nobody could have imagined that this idea would be the subject of extensive research in the following decades to understand how the "sugar" helps to mask the bitter taste of medicines [13,14].

It is a fact that many active ingredients indeed have a bitter taste and this represents a potential hurdle to adherence among the paediatric population. Taste is of primary importance to children in deciding whether a food is acceptable or not; hence, this aspect must also be taken into consideration when developing medicines for the paediatric population: the sensory system matures gradually after birth and the responses of children to certain tastes differ greatly from those of an adult. Among these differences is the preference for sweet foods and a greater rejection of bitter tastes. Experimental studies have indicated that this preference for sweet tastes is a consequence of the basic biology of children [15–17].

Metronidazole is a synthetic nitroimidazole antibiotic with a particularly unpleasant taste. In developing countries (DCs), according to the WHO's list of essential medicines for children [8], metronidazole is prevalently employed for the treatment of amoebic dysentery and giardiasis, infections that are associated with a high infant mortality and morbidity rate in DCs, as these are the cause of approximately 2.5 million deaths every year and have long-term effects on growth and cognitive function. Oral forms of metronidazole are commercially available but generally not in DCs, particularly in rural areas.

The *A.P.P.A.*® Project [18–21] is an international health cooperation project whose main aim is to open galenic laboratories for the compounding of personalised medicines in DCs. The project was established at the University of Turin more than twenty years ago in collaboration with the non-profit association named Aid Progress Pharmacist Agreement. In the areas where the *A.P.P.A.*® project is active—currently Angola, Cameroun, Chad, Haiti, and Madagascar—the availability of medicines designed specifically for paediatric use is extremely scarce, and, in any case, the few available products are likely to be counterfeited.

Therefore, it is of fundamental importance to enable the local health organisations to prepare their own medicines for the treatment of their patients, whether paediatric or adult, with high-quality, safe, and efficacious components.

In 2024, there was an outbreak of parasitic intestinal dysentery in the Haitian population (>30%) [22,23]. In this context, the aim of the present study was to develop an oral liquid metronidazole paediatric formulation using basic and economical excipients and employing a simple preparation procedure. Our goal is to obtain a formulation that is easy to prepare in the laboratories of the Haitian hospitals involved in the *A.P.P.A.*® Project and, more generally, in community pharmacies in low-income countries and that does not require temperature-controlled storage that make it difficult to store in a patient's home.

2. Materials and Methods

2.1. Selection of Excipients

Various mixtures of excipients were prepared to obtain a suitable formulation: the principal criterion was its organoleptic properties. In order to make the formulation accessible even in low-income countries, the cost of raw materials was also taken into consideration. For the same reason, only raw materials whose storage instructions did not entail the need for temperature-controlled storage of the finished medicinal product were considered.

Due to the poor solubility of metronidazole in solvents, such as water, that are suitable for administration to paediatric patients, it was decided to develop a suspension. Thereafter, various combinations of sweeteners and flavours were prepared to make the formulation palatable.

In particular, the following ingredients were considered as sweeteners: erythritol, glucose, maltodextrin, sodium saccharin, sorbitol solution 70%, sucrose, sucrose syrup, and xylitol. Water-soluble flavours were also used: banana, lemon, orange, and strawberry. Solubilisers (ethanol, glycerol, propylene glycol, polysorbate 80), suspending agents (microcrystalline cellulose, sodium carboxymethyl cellulose), preservatives (sodium benzoate, sodium methyl p-hydroxybenzoate), and pH regulators (citric acid monohydrate, sodium citrate) were also tested.

The various compositions prepared to identify the most suitable formulation are reported in Table 1. The detailed quantity of each raw material is available as Supplementary Material.

The raw materials complied with the relevant monograph of the *European Pharmacopoeia* and were all purchased from a pharmaceutical supplier company (Farmalabor s.r.l, Canosa di Puglia, Bari, Italy).

2.2. Suspension Preparation

The best formula as regards organoleptic properties was prepared with metronidazole at a concentration of 250 mg/5 mL. The preparation procedure is as follows: weigh out the hydrophilic components (sodium methyl p-hydroxybenzoate, sodium saccharin, orange flavour, erythritol, and maltodextrin), add each component to purified water and mix until completely dissolution (mixture A). Mix metronidazole, sodium carboxymethylcellulose, and microcrystalline cellulose according to the progressive dilution procedure (mixture B). Add mixture A to mixture B and mix until the powders are completely suspended. All suspensions were prepared manually.

Table 1. Excipient mixtures tested for metronidazole suspension.

Ingredients	1	2	3	4	5	6	7	8	9	10	11	12	13	14	15	16	17	18	19	20	21	22	23	24	25	26	27	28	29	30	31	32	33
Banana flavour (water-soluble)			×					×																									
Citric acid monohydrate																															×		×
Purified water	×	×	×	×	×	×	×	×	×	×	×	×	×	×	×	×	×	×	×	×	×	×	×	×	×	×	×	×	×	×	×	×	×
Erythritol									×	×	×						×		×	×			×		×	×		×		×	×		
Ethanol																																	×
Glucose																					×	×	×	×		×							
Glycerol																					×	×	×	×		×							
Lemon flavour (water-soluble)	×				×		×		×	×		×		×		×	×	×	×	×	×	×	×	×		×			×			×	×
Maltodextrin	×					×						×	×					×	×					×	×	×	×	×		×	×		
Microcrystalline cellulose	×	×	×	×	×	×	×	×	×	×	×	×	×	×	×	×	×	×	×	×	×	×	×	×	×	×	×	×	×	×	×	×	
Orange flavour (water-soluble)				×		×					×										×	×	×	×	×	×	×	×	×	×	×	×	
Propylene glycol																					×	×	×	×		×							
Sodium benzoate																											×	×	×	×	×		
Sodium carboxymethyl cellulose	×	×	×	×	×	×	×	×	×	×	×	×	×	×	×	×	×	×	×	×	×	×	×	×	×	×	×	×	×	×	×	×	
Sodium citrate																															×		×
Sodium methyl p-hydroxybenzoate	×	×	×	×	×	×	×	×	×	×	×	×	×	×	×	×	×	×	×	×	×	×	×	×	×	×						×	
Sodium saccharin												×	×	×	×	×	×	×	×	×	×	×	×	×	×	×	×	×	×	×	×		×
Sorbitol solution 70%																					×	×	×	×		×							
Strawberry flavour (water-soluble)		×											×		×																		
Sucrose					×																×												
Sucrose syrup	×	×	×	×	×	×	×	×	×	×	×	×	×	×	×	×	×	×	×	×									×			×	×
Polysorbate 80																					×	×	×	×		×	×		×	×	×		
Xylitol						×	×	×		×	×			×	×	×	×	×		×		×							×				

2.3. Suspension Quantitative Analysis

The evaluation of the uniformity of metronidazole content was carried out using a standard procedure designed in accordance with the directives set out in the *European Pharmacopeia* [24].

In particular, the quantity of metronidazole in the studied formulation batches was assessed by a high-performance liquid chromatography (HPLC) method. The instrument used was a YL9300 liquid chromatograph, Younglin Instruments Co., Anyang-si, Republic of Korea. It was equipped with an ultraviolet (UV) detector set at 230 nm. The column was the Agilent XDB-C18, 4.60 × 250 mm, 5 µm. The mobile phase was prepared as a mixture of methanol (20%) and water (80%). The flow rate was 1 mL/minute, the elution time was 6 min. The injection volume was 20 µL. The calibration curve of metronidazole was drawn using metronidazole analytical standard in methanol solution at concentrations between 0.020 and 0.330 mg/mL. The samples to be analysed were appropriately diluted with methanol to obtain a concentration within the range of the calibration curve. In particular, 980 µL of methanol was added to 20 µL of the suspension to be quantified. The sample was then vortexed (Velp Scientific ZX3 vortexer) for one minute and then filtered (Teknokroma nylon syringe filters 0.45 µm 13 mm ⌀ pk/100). The supernatant was appropriately diluted and analysed.

The concentration of metronidazole in the suspension samples was also evaluated by spectrophotometric assay between 190 and 600 nm. The instrument used was a V-730 UV-Visible Spectrophotometer, Jasko Inc., Tokyo, Japan. The calibration curve was made using metronidazole analytical standard in methanol ranging from 0.01 to 0.04 mg/mL. The samples to be analysed were appropriately diluted with methanol to obtain a concentration within the range of the calibration curve. In particular, 150 µL of each suspension lot to be analysed was added to 1 mL of methanol. The sample was then vortexed (Velp Scientific ZX3 vortex machine, Usmate Velate, Italy) for one minute and then centrifuged for 6 min at 6000 revolutions per minute (Beckman Coulter Microfuge 18, Cat model, Krefeld, Germany). The supernatant was then appropriately diluted and scanned. [25].

All chemicals were analytical grade (Merck KGaA, Darmstadt, Germany). Quantification experiments were performed at room temperature (15–25 °C).

2.4. Evaluation of Suspension Stability

The stability test for the metronidazole suspensions was conducted on nine lots (three production batches) of the selected formulation. Each lot was analysed after preparation to define the initial conditions and then subdivided into three samples: the first was stored at room temperature (25 +/− 2 °C), the second was stored in a thermostatic oven (40 +/− 2 °C), and the third was stored in a fridge (4 +/− 2 °C). Studies were conducted in conditions of relative humidity between 50 and 70%. The samples were analysed immediately after preparation and then every 30 days in each storage condition for a total period of six months. All of the samples were assessed for uniformity of content as described in Section 2.3, pH value (Hanna HI 9321 pH meter AC/DC input 110 V, Hanna Instruments Italia, Villafranca Padovana, Italy), and dispersion homogeneity.

In particular, the visual quality over time of the dispersion was assessed by an optical microscope (LEICA DM 2500 microscope, Leica Microsystems GmbH, Wetzlar, Germany) connected to a digital camera (630 magnification).

Moreover, it was also verified that each sample, even in case of phase separation as prescribed by the *European Pharmacopoeia* [24], could be redispersed by simple manual shaking.

Tests were repeated in triplicate. For each parameter, the mean of the results obtained and the standard deviation (SD) were calculated. The values were accepted for SD < 2%. All samples were stored away from light.

3. Results

To prepare a metronidazole suspension with a concentration of 250 mg/5 mL with organoleptic properties suitable for administering to paediatric patients, various formulations were prepared with the combinations of ingredients reported in Section 2.1. The formulation with the best organoleptic properties was sample no. 25, with the excipient combination reported in Table 2.

Table 2. Suspension composition for 100 mL.

Ingredients	Amount (g)
Metronidazole	5.00
Orange flavour (water-soluble)	4.72
Sodium carboxymethyl cellulose	1.00
Microcrystalline cellulose	5.00
Erythritol	9.40
Maltodextrin	9.40
Sodium methyl p-hydroxybenzoate	0.10
Sodium saccharin	0.19
Purified water	95.60

The selected formula was then tested for uniformity of content as described in Section 2.3 and for stability as described in Section 2.4.

The results obtained from the analysis of uniformity of content show that the concentration of metronidazole in each lot corresponds with the expected value. Both the chromatography and the spectrophotometric analyses reveal that, regardless of the temperature conditions during storage, the variation in concentration of metronidazole is less than 10% across all the lots.

The averages of the obtained results in the initial conditions and after 180 days are reported in Table 3 and in Table 4 for the analysis carried out using HPLC and spectrophotometry, respectively. The complete results are available as Supplementary Material.

Table 3. HPLC results.

		T0		T 180					
				Room Temperature		Thermostatic Oven		Fridge	
		Mean Area Values	Average	Mean Area Values	Δ % Compared to Average Value at T0	Mean Area Values	Δ % Compared to Average Value at T0	Mean Area Values	Δ % Compared to Average Value at T0
Batches	A	2429	2378	2343	−1.5%	2286	−3.8%	2535	6.6%
	B	2411		2387	0.4%	2264	−4.8%	2240	−5.8%
	C	2293		2189	−7.9%	2396	0.8%	2270	−4.5%

T0: initial conditions; T180: 180 days of storage.

Table 5 reports the average of the detected pH values: it is evident that no sample over time has undergone a significant change (<10%) in pH values.

The microscope analysis (Figure 1) confirms the absence of any substantial difference in the tested suspensions, either in the initial conditions and throughout the period of the tests. The average diameter of the suspended particles was found to be less than 300 nm during the entire test period for all the tested samples. For all the tested suspensions, the separation phase was evident approximately one month on average after the date of preparation in any of the applied storage conditions. However, as indicated by the *Pharmacopoeia*, it was possible to manually redisperse the solid phase.

Table 4. Spectrophotometric results.

		T0		T 180					
				Room Temperature		Thermostatic Oven		Fridge	
		Mean Absorbance Values	Average	Mean Absorbance Values	Δ % Compared to Average Value at T0	Mean Absorbance Values	Δ % Compared to Average Value at T0	Mean Absorbance Values	Δ % Compared to Average Value at T0
Batches	A	2.2171	2.2076	2.2744	3.02%	2.1736	−1.54%	2.2590	2.33%
	B	2.2449		2.3669	7.21%	2.2552	2.15%	2.0151	−8.72%
	C	2.1609		2.2994	4.16%	2.3295	5.52%	2.0817	−5.70%

T0: initial conditions; T180: 180 days of storage.

Table 5. pH values.

		T0		T 180					
				Room Temperature		Thermostatic Oven		Fridge	
		Mean pH Value	Average	Mean pH Value	Δ % Compared to Average Value at T0	Mean pH Value	Δ % Compared to Average Value at T0	Mean pH Value	Δ % Compared to Average Value at T0
Batches	A	8.41	8.35	7.88	−5.59%	8.36	0.16%	8.29	−0.68%
	B	8.16		7.83	−6.19%	8.30	−0.56%	8.70	4.23%
	C	8.47		7.96	−4.63%	8.26	−1.04%	7.80	−6.55%

T0: initial conditions; T180: 180 days of storage.

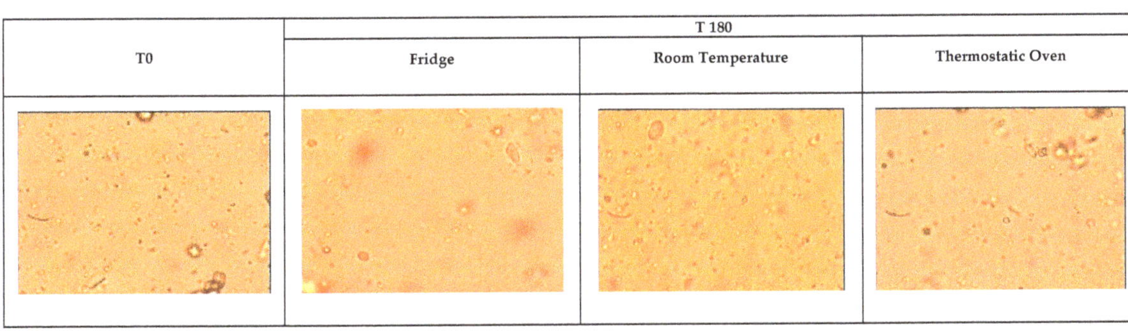

Figure 1. Microscope examination. T0: initial conditions; T180: 180 days of storage.

4. Discussion

The development of suitable paediatric formulations is certainly an issue of particular importance, in terms of both the scarcity of specific formulations for this age group and of liquid formulations.

Metronidazole may be administered intravenously, orally, or topically. For oral administration, it is commercially available in tablet, capsule, or suspension forms. In regards to suspensions, industrial medicines with concentrations of metronidazole or metronidazole benzoate ranging from 200 to 500 mg/5 mL are commercialised in some countries of the world. The administered dosage usually ranges between 35 and 50 mg/kg/day [26]. These preparations must be stored between 20 °C and 25 °C (brief exposure to 15 °C to 30 °C are usually permitted) [27–29]. The bitter metallic taste of metronidazole in its free base form in some commercial preparations has been masked by using the ester form, metronidazole benzoate, which has a blander taste. However, there are some questions over the bioavailability of the ester form that is, in any case, not widely available on the market as a raw material [13,30].

There are several factors that influence the choice of the antibiotic to be prescribed by a medical doctor, but the taste is not usually, or correctly, considered among these [31]. It is, therefore, fundamental to be able to treat the paediatric population with metronidazole in a suitable formulation.

In light of the above points, the study aimed to develop a pleasant-tasting oral liquid formulation for paediatric use in which the composition and preparation procedures are specifically designed for disadvantaged areas. Indeed, the suspension preparation method was designed to be very simple so as to be easily replicated in a compounding laboratory of any hospital or community pharmacy, even in DCs.

A variety of sweeteners and flavours were evaluated to identify the most suitable combination that was able to mask the taste of the metronidazole. The selection process for the formulation took into account their acceptable daily intake (ADI) and their potential side-effects [32–34]. The optimum sweetener system was identified in a combination of maltodextrin, erythritol, and sodium saccharin. Sodium saccharin, which for a long time had an ADI of 5 mg/kg/day in the general population, or 2.5 mg/kg/day in the paediatric population according to the literature, was recently revised in terms of its safety for food use. This revision led to a substantial increase in the safe daily dose to 9 mg/kg/day for the European Food Safety Authority (EFSA) in food [35,36]. This process confirmed the safe use of this sweetener in the developed formulation: the maximum dose foreseen for therapies with metronidazole totals a daily intake of 1.9 mg/kg/day of sodium saccharin, already consistent with the more restrictive indications above reported.

Polyalcohols such as erythritol are generally considered safe and are classified by the Food and Drug Administration (FDA) as generally recognised as safe (GRAS) [37]. In addition, children are not usually as sensitive as adults to the gastrointestinal effects of erythritol as adults [38]. In 2023, the EFSA established an ADI of 0.5 g/kg/day for erythritol as a safeguard against its immediate laxative effects, but also any adverse long-term effects secondary to diarrhoea, such as electrolyte imbalance [39] This ADI value is five times higher than the maximum dose of erythritol, which it is possible to assume in our suspension. Maltodextrin, which the FDA considers as a GRAS component [37], has no ADI for the ESFA, and, in general, any product for children containing maltodextrin is considered safe [40]. Orange flavour was added to the sweetening system as this is generally well accepted by the paediatric population.

Regarding the microbiological stability of the formulation, a key factor especially for DCs, it is important to underline that, according to the European Medicines Agency (EMA), the use of preservatives is deemed appropriate in multi-dose formulations but for many preservatives, only limited data are available regarding the maximum safe dose for children. The addition of such components would, therefore, be limited to the lowest quantity possible [41]. Parabens, a class of compounds including sodium nipagin (sodium methyl p-hydroxybenzoate) used in the formulation, are considered the safest class of compounds for paediatric use [35]. Parabens are usually used in concentrations ranging from 0.01% to 0.2% and the recommended maximum daily dose is 10 mg/kg/day [42]. This concentration is significantly higher than the one used in our study.

For oral liquid medicines, the EMA recommends that the administered volume should not more than 5 mL in children less than 5 years of age [41]. This indication considers the fact that lower volumes can generally be administered more easily and are more tolerable for children; hence, the developed formula adheres to this recommendation.

Once the composition of the formulation had been defined, it was fundamental to assess its stability. Therefore, tests were carried out in different environmental conditions: the tests performed at room temperature were applied to define the stability in the storage conditions generally foreseen for medicinal products. Stability tests performed at higher temperatures had two purposes: first, to reduce the duration of the analysis time, considering that one month's storage in these conditions is the equivalent of four months storage in standard conditions [20]; secondly, the applied temperatures help to predict stability in environments, such as those of DCs, where it is often impossible to ensure storage at temperatures below 25 °C. Finally, the tests carried out on samples stored in a fridge verify the stability of the product in these conditions if essential.

Regarding the quantification of metronidazole to evaluate the uniformity of content as well as the stability of the formulation, two analytical techniques were employed: chromatography and spectrophotometry. The scientific literature does not usually consider spectrophotometry as a quantitative method for active ingredients [25]. However, and in light of the fact that the *European Pharmacopoeia* does not prescribe a specific analytical method to quantify the concentration of active ingredients in a medicine (the *European Pharmacopoeia* states that "a suitable method" must be used) [24], we have also applied spectrophotometry as a quantitative method. The reasoning behind this choice is the need to develop a quantification method that can be performed using low-cost, easy-to-use instrumentation. The end is to ensure that the method, once its efficacy has been assured, can be used even in disadvantaged areas. In this light, the results obtained from the present study are certainly positive, because the data obtained from HPLC and spectrophotometry are substantially analogous.

5. Conclusions

The low availability of commercially oral paediatric formulations based on metronidazole inevitably means that many times, the therapy for this group must be prepared as a galenic formulation. Hence, we chose to focus our research on the development of a suspension with simple ingredients to make the preparation method feasible in any context using the equipment commonly available in any local or hospital galenic laboratory, but, at the same time, able to assure the quality of the finished product. Therefore, it was not only important but necessary to develop standard operating procedures that rely on low-cost instrumentation to assess on-site both the quality and the stability of the suspension.

Supplementary Materials: The following supporting information can be downloaded at: https://www.mdpi.com/article/10.3390/pharmaceutics17060787/s1.

Author Contributions: F.B. performed the conceptualization of the work. F.B., C.Z., F.F. and E.L. performed the investigation. F.B., G.D.L. and E.L. took care of the data and wrote the manuscript. F.B., C.Z. and F.F. performed the analytical data acquisition. P.B. and G.D.L. supervised the project. All authors discussed the results and contributed to the final manuscript. All authors have read and agreed to the published version of the manuscript.

Funding: The study was supported by the fund "Fondi Ricerca Locale" of the University of Turin provided by the Ministry of Education, Universities and Research (MIUR).

Institutional Review Board Statement: Not applicable.

Informed Consent Statement: Not applicable.

Data Availability Statement: Data is contained within the article.

Acknowledgments: The authors would like to thank Tom O Byrne for the linguistic revision of the text.

Conflicts of Interest: The authors declare that they have no known competing financial interests or personal relationships that could have appeared to influence the work reported in this paper.

Abbreviations

A.P.P.A.®	Aid Progress Pharmacist Agreement
ADI	Acceptable Daily Intake
DCs	Developing Countries
EFSA	European Food Safety Authority
FDA	Food and Drug Administration
GRAS	Generally Recognised As Safe
HPLC	High-Performance Liquid Chromatography
SD	Standard Deviation
T0	Initial conditions
T180	180 days of storage
UV	Ultraviolet
WHO	World Health Organisation

References

1. Lopalco, A.; Denora, N. Paediatric Formulation: Design and Development. *Int. J. Mol. Sci.* **2020**, *21*, 7118. [CrossRef]
2. US Government Accountability Office. Pediatric Drug Research: Studies Conducted Under Best Pharmaceuticals for Children Act: Report to Congressional Committees. 2007. Available online: https://www.gao.gov/assets/gao-07-557.pdf (accessed on 1 April 2025).
3. Milne, C.P.; Bruss, J.B. The economics of pediatric formulation development for off-patent drugs. *Clin. Ther.* **2008**, *30*, 2133–2145. [CrossRef]
4. Fadda, H.M.; Weiler, H.; Carvalho, M.; Lee, Y.Z.; Dassouki, H.; AbuBlan, R.; Iurian, S.; Hamid, A.; Şeremet, G.; Li, Z.; et al. Pediatric oral extemporaneous preparations and practices: International Pharmaceutical Federation (FIP) global study. *Eur. J. Pharm. Biopharm.* **2024**, *204*, 114483. [CrossRef]
5. Yuliani, S.H.; Putri, D.C.A.; Virginia, D.M.; Gani, M.R.; Riswanto, F.D.O. Prevalence, Risk, and Challenges of Extemporaneous Preparation for Pediatric Patients in Developing Nations: A Review. *Pharmaceutics* **2023**, *15*, 840. [CrossRef] [PubMed]
6. Commission to the European Parliament and Council. State of Paediatric Medicines in the EU: 10 Years of the EU Pediatric Regulation. 2017. Available online: https://eur-lex.europa.eu/legal-content/EN/TXT/?uri=CELEX:32006R1901 (accessed on 1 April 2025).
7. US Food and Drug Administration. Pediatric Labelling Changes. 2024. Available online: https://www.fda.gov/science-research/pediatrics/pediatric-labeling-changes (accessed on 1 April 2025).
8. World Health Organization. WHO Model List of Essential Medicines for Children—9th List. 2023. Available online: https://www.who.int/publications/i/item/WHO-MHP-HPS-EML-2023.03 (accessed on 1 April 2025).
9. Orubu, E.S.F.; Duncan, J.; Tuleu, C.; Turner, M.A.; Nunn, A. WHO essential medicines for children 2011–2019: Age-appropriateness of enteral formulations. *Arch. Dis. Child.* **2022**, *107*, 317–322. [CrossRef] [PubMed]
10. Walsh, J.; Masini, T.; Huttner, B.D.; Moja, L.; Penazzato, M.; Cappello, B. Assessing the Appropriateness of Formulations on the WHO Model List of Essential Medicines for Children: Development of a Paediatric Quality Target Product Profile Tool. *Pharmaceutics* **2022**, *14*, 473. [CrossRef]
11. Nunn, T.; Williams, J. Formulation of medicines for children. *Br. J. Clin. Pharmacol.* **2005**, *59*, 674–676. [CrossRef] [PubMed]
12. Baratta, F.; Zingarelli, C.; Felismè, F.; Lamy, E.; Cajuste, R.; Saint-Jean, P.H.; Ambreck, E.; Di Lascio, G.; Brusa, P. Spironolactone suspension for paediatric use: Formulation, quality and stability. *Pharm. Pract.* **2024**, *22*, 2987. [CrossRef]
13. McElhiney, L.F. Case Report: The Quest for a Palatable Compounded Metronidazole (Base) Suspension. *Int. J. Pharm. Compd.* **2021**, *25*, 24–28.
14. Mennella, J.A.; Reed, D.R.; Mathew, P.S.; Roberts, K.M.; Mansfield, C.J. "A spoonful of sugar helps the medicine go down": Bitter masking by sucrose among children and adults. *Chem. Senses* **2015**, *40*, 17–25. [CrossRef]
15. Mennella, J.A.; Bobowski, N.K. The sweetness and bitterness of childhood: Insights from basic research on taste preferences. *Physiol. Behav.* **2015**, *152 Pt B*, 502–507. [CrossRef]
16. Mennella, J.A.; Pepino, M.Y.; Reed, D.R. Genetic and environmental determinants of bitter perception and sweet preferences. *Pediatrics* **2005**, *115*, e216-22. [CrossRef] [PubMed]
17. Lipchock, S.V.; Reed, D.R.; Mennella, J.A. Relationship between bitter-taste receptor genotype and solid medication formulation usage among young children: A retrospective analysis. *Clin. Ther.* **2012**, *34*, 728–733. [CrossRef] [PubMed] [PubMed Central]

18. Baratta, F.; Germano, A.; Di Lascio, G.; Petieau, R.; Brusa, P. Establishment of galenic laboratories in developing countries to produce high quality medicines: Results of Aid Progress Pharmacist Agreement (A.P.P.A.®) Project. *Croat. Med. J.* **2014**, *55*, 662–668. [CrossRef]
19. Baratta, F.; Di Lascio, G.; Tarditi, F.; Petieau, R.; Brusa, P. Galenic formulations to fight the phenomenon of counterfeiting in developing Countries. *J. Drug Deliv. Sci. Technol.* **2016**, *32*, 313–315. [CrossRef]
20. Baratta, F.; Germano, A.; Brusa, P. Diffusion of counterfeit drugs in developing countries and stability of galenics stored for months under different conditions of temperature and relative humidity. *Croat. Med. J.* **2012**, *53*, 173–184. [CrossRef]
21. A.P.P.A.®. Non-Profit Association Website. Available online: https://www.progettoappa.it/ (accessed on 1 April 2025).
22. Moss, D.M.; Priest, J.W.; Hamlin, K.; Derado, G.; Herbein, J.; Petri, W.A., Jr.; Lammie, P.J. Longitudinal evaluation of enteric protozoa in Haitian children by stool exam and multiplex serologic assay. *Am. J. Trop. Med. Hyg.* **2014**, *90*, 653–660. [CrossRef]
23. Michel, D.; Raymond, L.; Apply, A.; Daphenide St Louis, D.; Balthazard-Accou, K.; Millien, M.F.; Emmanuel, E. Contribution to the Diagnostic Study of Intestinal Parasitosis, Haiti. *Eur. Sci. J.* **2021**, *17*, 64. [CrossRef]
24. European Directorate for the Quality of Medicines and HealthCare. *European Pharmacopoeia*, 11th ed.; Council of Europe: Geneva, Switzerland, 2023.
25. Moffat, A.C.; Osselton, D.M.; Widdop, B. *Clarke's Analysis of Drugs and Poisons*, 4th ed.; Pharmaceutical Press: London, UK, 2011.
26. Haque, R.; Mondal, D.; Duggal, P.; Kabir, M.; Roy, S.; Farr, B.M.; Sack, R.B.; Petri, W.A., Jr. Entamoeba histolytica infection in children and protection from subsequent amebiasis. *Infect. Immun.* **2006**, *74*, 904–909. [CrossRef] [PubMed] [PubMed Central]
27. US Food and Drug Administration. Drugs@FDA: FDA-Approved Drugs. Available online: https://www.accessdata.fda.gov/scripts/cder/daf/index.cfm?event=overview.process&ApplNo=216755 (accessed on 30 May 2025).
28. Drugs.com. Likmez: Package Insert/Prescribing Info. Available online: https://www.drugs.com/pro/likmez.html#s-34089-3 (accessed on 30 May 2025).
29. Medicines.ie. Flagyl-S 200mg/5mL Oral Suspension Information. 2024. Available online: https://www.medicines.ie/medicines/flagyl-s-200mg-5ml-oral-suspension-32159/patient-info (accessed on 30 May 2025).
30. Jarouche, M.; Ibrahim, M.; Pearson, J.; Low, M.; Rowe, J. Stability of Metronidazole Free-Base Oral Suspensions Formulated with United States Pharmacopeia-Grade Metronidazole Powder and Commercial Metronidazole Tablets. *Int. J. Pharm. Compd.* **2020**, *24*, 77–82. [PubMed]
31. Ausmed Education. Why Children's Medication Should Be Palatable. A Spoonful of Sugar—The Importance of Palatability in Children's Medication. Available online: https://www.ausmed.com/learn/articles/palatability-in-childrens-medication (accessed on 1 April 2025).
32. US Food and Drug Administration. Guidance for Industry and Other Stakeholders: Redbook 2000 Toxicological Principles for the Safety Assessment of Food Ingredients. Available online: https://www.fda.gov/regulatory-information/search-fda-guidance-documents/guidance-industry-and-other-stakeholders-redbook-2000 (accessed on 1 April 2025).
33. EFSA (European Food Safety Authority). Sweeteners. 2025. Available online: https://www.efsa.europa.eu/it/topics/topic/sweeteners (accessed on 1 April 2025).
34. Sylvetsky, A.; Rother, K.I.; Brown, R. Artificial sweetener use among children: Epidemiology, recommendations, metabolic outcomes, and future directions. *Pediatr. Clin. N. Am.* **2011**, *58*, 1467–1480. [CrossRef] [PubMed]
35. Rouaz, K.; Chiclana-Rodríguez, B.; Nardi-Ricart, A.; Suñé-Pou, M.; Mercadé-Frutos, D.; Suñé-Negre, J.M.; Pérez-Lozano, P.; García-Montoya, E. Excipients in the Paediatric Population: A Review. *Pharmaceutics* **2021**, *13*, 387. [CrossRef] [PubMed]
36. EFSA Panel on Food Additives and Flavourings (FAF); Castle, L.; Andreassen, M.; Aquilina, G.; Bastos, M.L.; Boon, P.; Fallico, B.; FitzGerald, R.; Frutos Fernandez, M.J.; Grasl-Kraupp, B.; et al. Re-evaluation of saccharin and its sodium, potassium and calcium salts (E 954) as food additives. *EFSA J.* **2024**, *22*, e9044. [CrossRef] [PubMed] [PubMed Central]
37. US Food and Drug Administration. GRAS Substances (SCOGS) Database. Available online: https://www.fda.gov/food/generally-recognized-safe-gras/gras-substances-scogs-database (accessed on 1 April 2025).
38. Jacqz-Aigrain, E.; Kassai, B.; Cornu, C.; Cazaubiel, J.M.; Housez, B.; Cazaubiel, M.; Prével, J.M.; Bell, M.; Boileau, A.; De Cock, P. Gastrointestinal tolerance of erythritol-containing beverage in young children: A double-blind, randomised controlled trial. *Eur. J. Clin. Nutr.* **2015**, *69*, 746–751. [CrossRef] [PubMed]
39. EFSA Panel on Food Additives and Flavourings (FAF); Younes, M.; Aquilina, G.; Castle, L.; Degen, G.; Engel, K.H.; Fowler, P.J.; Frutos Fernandez, M.J.; Fürst, P.; Gundert-Remy, U.; et al. Re-evaluation of erythritol (E 968) as a food additive. *EFSA J.* **2023**, *21*, e8430. [CrossRef]
40. Arnold, A.R.; Chassaing, B. Maltodextrin, Modern Stressor of the Intestinal Environment. *Cell. Mol. Gastroenterol. Hepatol.* **2019**, *7*, 475–476. [CrossRef]

41. European Medicines Agency. Guideline on Pharmaceutical Development of Medicines for Paediatric Use. 2013. Available online: www.ema.europa.eu/en/documents/scientific-guideline/guideline-pharmaceutical-development-medicines-paediatric-use_en.pdf (accessed on 1 April 2025).
42. European Medicines Agency. Reflection Paper on the Use of Methyl- and Propylparaben as Excipients in Human Medicinal Products for Oral Use. 2015. Available online: https://www.ema.europa.eu/en/documents/scientific-guideline/reflection-paper-use-methyl-propylparaben-excipients-human-medicinal-products-oral-use_en.pdf (accessed on 1 April 2025).

pharmaceutics

Article

Toward the Optimal Choice of Gelled Vehicles for Oral Drug Administration in Dysphagic Patients

Serena Logrippo [1,2], Roberta Ganzetti [3], Matteo Sestili [4], Diego Romano Perinelli [5], Marco Cespi [5,*] and Giulia Bonacucina [5]

1 Hospital Pharmacy, Santa Maria della Stella Hospital, USL Umbria 2, 05018 Orvieto, Italy
2 Hospital Pharmacy, Engles Profili Hospital, AST Ancona, 60044 Fabriano, Italy
3 Hospital Pharmacy, Carlo Urbani Hospital, AST Ancona, 60035 Jesi, Italy
4 Territorial Pharmaceutical Service, AST Ancona, 60035 Jesi, Italy
5 School of Pharmacy, University of Camerino, CHIP Building via Madonna delle Carceri, 62032 Camerino, Italy; diego.perinelli@unicam.it (D.R.P.); giulia.bonacucina@unicam.it (G.B.)
* Correspondence: marco.cespi@unicam.it

Abstract

Background/Objectives: Thickened waters are commonly used for dysphagic patients to ensure hydration, facilitate safer swallowing, and administer oral therapies, yet their impact on drug dissolution remains unclear. This study aims to investigate how thickening agents, viscosity, and solid oral dosage form (SODF) formulations influence drug release in gelled vehicles. **Methods**: Twelve commercially available thickened waters, including both ready-to-use products and powders for extemporaneous preparation, were used to disperse crushed sodium pravastatin tablets. The resulting preparations were evaluated for their rheological properties and dissolution performance. **Results**: Thickened water products vary in consistency, with starch-based thickeners providing more consistent results than gum-based ones. Pravastatin release profiles closely matched the original tablets with starch thickeners, while gum-based thickeners showed greater variability, primarily influenced by viscosity. **Conclusions**: These findings emphasize the importance of selecting the appropriate thickening agent for controlling drug release in thickened water products, highlighting the need to balance patient compliance with the potential impact on drug release during product development.

Keywords: thickened beverages; pravastatin sodium; swallowing difficulties; complex viscosity; rheological moduli; drug dissolution

1. Introduction

Thickened waters (also referred to as gelled waters or, more generally, thickened beverages) are water or other liquids (sometimes juices) that were modified by the addition of thickening agents to achieve a specific viscosity. From a regulatory perspective, thickened waters may be classified as food for special medical purposes (FSMPs) under EU Regulation No. 609/2013 [1], provided they are intended to meet the specific nutritional requirements of patients with impaired capacity to consume ordinary foodstuffs.

The modification of beverage consistency makes liquids easier and safer to swallow for individuals with swallowing difficulties, such as those suffering from dysphagia, who often struggle with certain consistencies, particularly solid foods and thin liquids [2,3]. For these individuals, thickened waters help ensure proper hydration while reducing the risk of aspiration and choking by providing a controlled consistency [4,5]. Several associations involved in the management, therapy, and support of dysphagic patients provided recommendations on using liquids with appropriate viscosity or consistency to reduce the risk of aspiration pneumonia [6]. Currently, the proper consistency of thickened waters is ensured by adherence to the NDD (National Dysphagia Diet) guidelines established by the American Dietetic Association and the National Dysphagia Diet Task Force [7], or to the IDDSI (International Dysphagia Diet Standardisation Initiative) recommendations, developed by an international multidisciplinary group (IDDSI Committee) supported by numerous International Reference Groups [8]. The market currently offers various thickened waters available in two forms: ready-to-use thickened liquids (RU_TL) and formulated powders designed for the extemporaneous preparation of thickened liquids (EP_TL). In both cases, the desired consistency is achieved through the use of thickening agents, which are polysaccharides belonging to the group of modified starches or gums. Among the starches, pregelatinized starches are commonly used for preparing thickened beverages, typically derived from corn starch, although alternatives, such as those sourced from potatoes, are also commercially available. On the other hand, the most commonly used gums include xanthan gum, guar gum, and other gum-like polysaccharides, such as carrageenan and pectin. In gum-based products, these agents are typically used in combination to achieve optimal consistency and functionality [9,10]. The use of liquids with appropriate consistency is the most suitable approach for dysphagic patients, except for those unable to swallow or in cases where oral nutrition does not ensure proper hydration. In such situations, an enteral nutrition strategy, such as administration via a nasogastric tube or percutaneous endoscopic gastrostomy, is required [11].

Thickened waters are used not only for hydration but also for administering the oral therapies when alternative dosage forms suitable for dysphagic, such as suppositories or transdermal patches, are not commercially available. A common practice in dysphagic patients is to crush tablets or open capsules, then disperse or dissolve their contents in modified-consistency beverages [10,12]. This practice can modify drug bioavailability by influencing the drug release process, due both to the manipulation of the solid oral dosage form (SODF) and the interaction of the dispersed powder with the thickened vehicle. While the effects of manipulating the SODF were extensively studied in the literature [12–15], the latter aspect requires further investigation and clarification. Currently, there are few studies focusing on this aspect. Manrique et al. reported a reduction in the release rate of several drugs when crushed tablets were dispersed in gum-based and starch-gum-based vehicles, hypothesizing that the effect was due to the consistency and/or structure of the carrier vehicles [16,17]. Similar findings was reported by Ilgaz et al., which demonstrated that the gelling vehicles significantly influences the drug's dissolution rate, especially in thickened samples prepared with xanthan gum [18]. These studies highlight that the gelled vehicles affect the dissolution rate of the drugs. However, several aspects remain to be clarified. First, although all the studies suggest a relationship between the reduction in dissolution rate and viscosity, this correlation has never been conclusively proven. Additionally, the number of commercial thickened waters analyzed was limited, despite the wide variety of products available on the market. These include both ready-to-use thickened liquids (RU_TL), which may come in a single consistency or in multiple consistency grades, and formulated powders designed for the extemporaneous preparation of thickened liquids (EP_TL). Moreover, most commercial products are gum-based, containing thickening agents such as guar gum, xanthan gum, carrageenan, and pectin, typically used in blends. However, starch-based products are also available. The effect of the type of thickening agent (gum-based or starch-based) remains unclear, although some authors suggest that starch-based products have a lesser impact on the drug release rate. Finally, it remains to be clarified whether the reduction in the drug release rate is exclusively due to the gelled vehicles or if it can also be partially attributed to the amount of SODF added or their formulation (the presence of specific excipients).

This study aims to address existing knowledge gaps by clarifying how thickening agents (gum-based vs. starch-based), viscosity, and SODF formulation (including excipients) influence drug dissolution in gelled vehicles. To achieve this aim, four ready-to-use thickened liquids (one available in three different consistencies) and two formulated powders for extemporaneous preparation of thickened liquids (gum- and starch-based) were selected, for a total of twelve different gelled vehicles. Tablets of sodium pravastatin (PraNa) were chosen as the model drug, given their frequent use among the elderly population, who are most likely to experience swallowing difficulties or disorders. The selection was also motivated by the drug's high water solubility and its availability as immediate-release tablets. Additionally, the availability of several equivalent medicinal products allows testing across different formulations, including both coated and uncoated tablets.

2. Materials and Methods

2.1. Materials

Uncoated 20 mg pravastatin sodium tablets from two different manufacturers (Pravastatina Pensa, Pensa Pharma S.p.A., Milano, Italy and Pravastatina ratiopharm, Teva Italia s.r.l., Milano, Italy) and coated 20 mg pravastatin sodium tablets (Pravastatina EG, EG S.p.A., Milano, Italy) were purchased from a local pharmacy. Pravastatin sodium powder was kindly provided by Teva Pharmaceutical Industries Ltd. (Debrecen, Hungary) through Angelini Pharma s.p.a. (Rome, Italy).

Thickened water sweet fruit taste, Gelly'Gel sweetened, and Hydra'Fruit grade 1, 2 and 3 (Nutrisens Medical, Chaponost, France), as well as Resource bevanda gelificata (Nestlé Italiana S.p.A., Assago, Italy), were all ready-to-use thickened liquids (RU_TL). Resource ThickenUp Clear and Resource ThickenUp (Nestlé Italiana S.p.A., Italy) were formulated powders for preparing thickened liquids (extemporaneous preparation of thickened liquids EP_TL). Both the RU_TL and EP_TL were purchased from a local pharmacy.

Table 1 provides a schematic summary of all the ready-to-use gelled waters and formulated powders used in this study, including their thickening agents, available grades, and abbreviations used in the manuscript.

Table 1. General information and abbreviations of all thickened water products used in manuscript.

Product Type	Product Name	Manufacturer	Thickening Agents	Grades Available	Abbreviation
Ready-to-use thickened liquids (RU_TL)	**Thickened water sweet fruit taste**	Nutrisens	Guar gum, pectin xanthan gum and calcium lactate	1	ThW
	Gelly'Gel sweetened	Nutrisens	Carrageenan and xanthan gum	1	JeG
	Hydra'Fruit *	Nutrisens	Xanthan gum, guar gum and pectin	3 *	HyF_G1 HyF_G2 HyF_G3
	Resource bevanda gelificata	Nestlè	Carrageenan, xanthan gum and guar gum	1	Res

Table 1. *Cont.*

Product Type	Product Name	Manufacturer	Thickening Agents	Grades Available	Abbreviation
Powders for the preparation of extemporaneous thickened liquids (EP_TL)	**Resource ThickenUp**	Nestlè	Corn starch	All **	ThUp_Ne ThUp_Ho ThUp_Pu
	Resource ThickenUp Clear	Nestlè	Maltodextrin, xanthan gum	All **	ThUpCle_Ne ThUpCle_Ho ThUpCle_Pu

* The Hydra'Fruit products are labelled and described in the brochure as having consistencies classified as grade 1 (semiliquid), grade 2 (creamy), and grade 3 (semisolid). However, the meaning of these classifications is unclear, as they do not precisely align with the standard definitions proposed by the National Dysphagia Diet (NDD classification) or the International Dysphagia Diet Standardisation Initiative (IDDSI levels). ** Since the product is available in powder form, all consistencies can be achieved by adjusting the amount of powder used. The prepared consistencies recommended by the manufacturer align with the DDS classification, specifically nectar (Ne), honey (Ho), and pudding (Pu).

Through the manuscript, pravastatin sodium is abbreviated as PraNa.

2.2. Preparation of Thickened Water with Formulated Powders

The extemporaneous preparation of thickened liquids was carried out according to the manufacturers' instructions. A specified amount of powder (varying by product and the desired consistency grade) was dispersed in a defined volume of water to achieve three different consistencies for each product, nectar (Ne), honey (Ho), and pudding (Pu), as classified by the NDD system [7]. The exact quantities of powder and water used in the preparations are detailed in Table 2.

Table 2. The concentrations of ThUp and ThUpCle used for the preparation of the different grades according to the label information (following the NDD classification).

Consistency Grades	ThUpCle		ThUp	
	g/100 mL	% *w/w*	g/100 mL	% *w/w*
Nectar	1.2	1.2	4.5	4.3
Honey	2.4	2.3	6.8	6.3
Pudding	3.6	3.5	9.0	8.3

2.3. Weight and Content Uniformity for PraNa Tablets

All the PraNa tablets were characterized in terms of weight and PraNa content. The weight of the tablets was determined using a three-decimal digit balance on a sample of 10 tablets.

The content uniformity was evaluated using a UV-Vis spectrophotometric (UV-1800, Shimadzu, Kyoto, Japan) method. A calibration curve was prepared by dissolving PraNa powder in water to create standard solutions in the range of 5–25 μg/mL, with absorbance measured at 238 nm (R^2 = 0.999). Preliminary trials were conducted to assess whether specific tablet excipients, such as iron oxide, sodium stearyl fumarate, or PVP, interfered with PraNa quantification at the selected wavelength.

The quantification of PraNa in the tablets was performed by dispersing each tablet in 900 mL of water. After two hours of mechanical stirring, the absorbance was measured, and the PraNa content was determined using the calibration curve. The test was conducted on five tablets for each type of PraNa tablet.

2.4. Preparation of Thickened Water Containing PraNa Tablets

Pensa PraNa tablet (weighing 0.149 ± 0.003 g) was selected to be dispersed in 5 g of thickened water, resulting in a total quantity of 5.15 g. This amount is suitable for administration using a teaspoon and represents the single dose to be administered (S_D).

All batches were prepared by pulverizing the tablets in a mortar with a pestle and then dispersing the powder into RU_TL and EP_TL under manual agitation for 5 min. Each batch consisted of 5 tablets and 25 g of thickened water.

2.5. Content Uniformity for Thickened Water Containing PraNa Tablets

The content uniformity of the gelled samples prepared with Pensa tablets was evaluated similarly to that of the tablets (Section 2.3) by dispersing an S_D in 900 mL of water and analyzing the PraNa content after two hours of mechanical stirring. The quantification of PraNa was performed as described for the tablets, except for samples containing the preservative potassium sorbate, which interferes with UV-based determination. In such cases, a dual-wavelength spectrophotometric method was used, measuring absorbance at 238 nm and 259 nm. This method was previously applied for PraNa quantification in the presence of parabens [19].

2.6. Rheological Analysis

The rheological analyses were performed using a stress-controlled rotational rheometer (Kinexus lab+, Malvern, UK) using a C40/4 cone-plate geometry on RU_TL and EP_TL, both with and without the presence of dispersed Pensa PraNa tablets at 25 and 37 °C. All samples were subjected to small amplitude oscillation tests.

Stress sweep analysis was conducted by applying a stress from 0.05 to 100 Pa at a frequency of 1 Hz. The linear viscoelastic region (LVR) limit was determined as the stress value at which the complex modulus (G^*) deviated by 10% from the plateau value [20].

A frequency sweep test was then performed by increasing the oscillation frequency from 0.01 to 1 Hz while maintaining a constant stress within the LVR (1 Pa).

All the samples were analyzed in triplicate.

2.7. Dissolution Studies of Thickened Water Containing PraNa Tablets

The dissolution studies were carried out in thickened waters prepared with Pensa PraNa tablets using a dissolution apparatus II (AT7 Smart, Sotax, Aesch, Switzerland) with 900 mL of deionized water as the dissolution medium, maintained at 37 °C. The paddle rotation speed was set to 50 rpm. A specific amount (the S-D) of thickened water containing the dissolved PraNa tablets was introduced into the bottom of the dissolution vessel using a modified syringe with a cut tip. Samples were withdrawn at 0, 5, 15, 30, 60, 90, and 120 min. If the PraNa dissolution was incomplete at 120 min, the test was extended up to 480 min. Considering that the solubility of PraNa is higher than 10 mg/mL [21], all dissolution tests are conducted under sink conditions.

The PraNa quantification was performed as described in Section 2.3, or in Section 2.5 for samples containing potassium sorbate [19].

Additional studies were conducted only on selected RU_TL and EP_TL samples prepared using double or half the amount of Pensa PraNa tablets or prepared with PraNa tablets from other brands (PraNa Ratiopharm and EG tablets). In these additional studies, the weight of a single dose was adjusted based on the weight of the tablets used to prepare the loaded gel, ensuring it contained a PraNa dosage equivalent to 40 mg (2 Pensa tablets), 10 mg (half a Pensa tablet), or 20 mg (Ratiopharm and EG tablets).

3. Results and Discussion

3.1. Content Uniformity of Tablets and Thickened Water

The tablets used in this study had a weight of approximately 150 mg (Pravastatina Pensa). Across all tablet batches, the maximum percentage deviation of a single unit from the average weight was 2.5%, well below the European Pharmacopoeia (Ph. Eur.) limit of 7.5%, confirming that all these commercial products comply with Ph. Eur. standards [22]. The average amount of PraNa in the tablets ranged from 20.1 to 21.4 mg, compared to the nominal dose of 20 mg. In all cases, the PraNa content was compliant with Ph. Eur. requirements [23].

The thickened waters loaded with Pensa PraNa tablets were analyzed in terms of PraNa concentration and of PraNa amount administered using a single dose (S-D) (Table 3). Across the different preparations, the PraNa concentration ranged from 3.51 to 4.34 mg/g, while the amount of PraNa administered with an S-D (5.15 g) ranged from 18.5 to 22.3 mg. In all cases, variability within each prepared thickened water was low, with the highest coefficient of variation being approximately 6% with an average value of 2.7% (for the PraNa tablets it was equal to 2.6%). The standard deviation in the PraNa amount between tablets and gelled beverages was comparable for the majority of the samples. Additionally, the maximum percentage deviation in PraNa administered between tablets and all gelled products was 13%, while the average deviation, calculated as absolute values, was 6.3%. These results suggest that thickened water loaded with tablets is a viable alternative method for tablet administration, ensuring consistent quality independent by the jellified system used.

Table 3. Pravastatin sodium concentration and amount administered in single dose (5.15 g) of thickened water prepared with Pensa PraNa tablets.

Product Type	Product Name	PraNa Concentration (mg/g)	PraNa Amount in the Single Dose (mg)
Ready-to-use thickened liquids (RU_TL)	ThW	4.34 ± 0.06	22.3 ± 0.3
	JeG	4.25 ± 0.15	21.9 ± 0.8
	HyF_G1	3.93 ± 0.10	20.2 ± 0.8
	HyF_G2	3.71 ± 0.09	19.1 ± 0.5
	HyF_G3	3.75 ± 0.11	19.3 ± 0.6
	Res	4.05 ± 0.25	20.8 ± 1.3
Powders for the preparation of extemporaneous thickened liquids (EP_TL)	ThUp_Ne	3.59 ± 0.09	18.5 ± 0.5
	ThUp_Ho	3.77 ± 0.09	19.4 ± 0.5
	ThUp_Pu	3.51 ± 0.11	18.1 ± 0.6
	ThUpCle_Ne	3.96 ± 0.03	20.4 ± 0.2
	ThUpCle_Ho	3.79 ± 0.07	19.5 ± 0.4
	ThUpCle_Pu	3.99 ± 0.10	20.6 ± 0.5

3.2. Rheological Behaviour

All the jellified vehicles, both with and without dispersed PraNa tablets, were compared in terms of rheological behaviour at 25 °C and 37 °C.

Initially, the samples were subjected to oscillation stress sweep analysis to identify the linear viscoelastic region (LVR), defined as the range of stress values within which the measured moduli remain independent of the applied stress. The samples exhibited typical stress sweep test profiles, with a constant complex modulus up to the LVR limit. The LVR limit values ranged from approximately 1.2–1.5 Pa for HyF grade 1 at both temperatures, to around 20–30 Pa for ThUp grade 3. Following this analysis, a stress value of 1 Pa was selected to perform the frequency sweep tests of all the samples.

The results of the frequency analysis (moduli vs. frequency) are reported in Figure 1 (data of viscosity are reported in Figure S1 of the Supplementary Materials). Comparing the traces with the typical viscoelastic spectrum [24] reveals that most samples align with the rubbery plateau at lower frequencies and the transition region at higher frequencies, reflecting the expected behaviour within these zones. At lower frequencies, the samples exhibit a behaviour characteristic of a strong gel, with G' exceeding G'' and both moduli remaining nearly independent of frequency. As the frequency increases beyond certain thresholds (ranging from 10 to 30 Hz, depending on the sample), both moduli increase, and G'' surpasses G', indicating a transition toward rubbery, solid-like behaviour. The only exception to this behaviour is observed in grade 1 of HyF. In this case, at frequencies below 1 Hz, the material exhibits a behaviour typical of the terminal region of the viscoelastic spectrum where the moduli are low, with G'' exceeding G', and both are highly frequency-dependent. This behaviour is characteristic of weak gels, with a crossover point, where the moduli invert, occurring around 1 Hz. A similar behaviour is partially observed for grade 2 of the same product, but only in tests conducted at 37 °C.

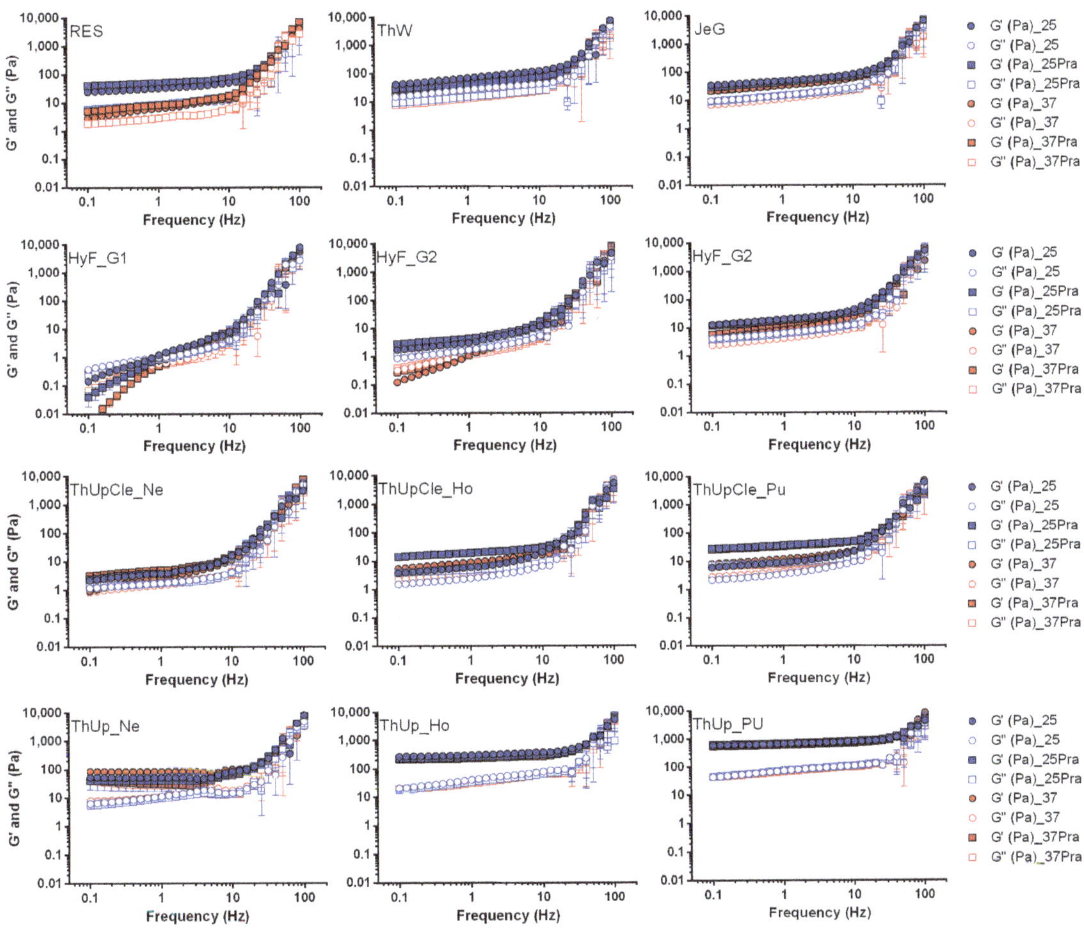

Figure 1. Frequency sweep tests for all jellified vehicles with and without pravastatin sodium at temperature of 25 and 37 °C. Thickened waters containing pravastatin were prepared with Pensa PraNa tablets.

Considering the absolute values of the moduli in the lower frequency region (characteristic of a gel under normal conditions of use), the samples can be divided into three distinct groups. Res, ThW, JeG, grades Ho and Pu of ThUpCle, ThUp_Ne, and grade 3 of HyF are characterized by moduli in the range of 3–40 Pa and complex viscosity between 3 and 10 Pa·sec. In contrast, HyF grades 1 and 2, as well as ThickenUp_Ne, have moduli lower than 3 Pa and complex viscosity below 1 Pa·sec. On the other hand, the higher grades of ThUp (Ho and Pu) show moduli higher than 20–30 Pa (with G' reaching values well above 100 Pa) and complex viscosity greater than 40 Pa·sec. Among all the samples, only the Resource sample showed a certain temperature dependency, while the presence of PraNa tablets did not significantly affect the rheology results. Clearly, the classification based on the frequency results is not absolute, and most samples exhibit their own specific behaviour. However, it is evident that HyF at the lowest grades stands out markedly from all other products due to its lower consistency, while the highest grades of ThickenUp are distinguished by their highest consistency.

3.3. *Dissolution Studies*

3.3.1. Effect of Gelled Vehicle

The Pensa tablets, as well as the gelled vehicles containing the Pensa tablets, were analyzed in terms of dissolution performance to evaluate potential effects related to the composition or consistency of the gels.

Comparing the dissolution rates of tablets and gels is not straightforward, and no official guidelines exist for this specific comparison. However, in this case, since the tablets are designed for immediate-release, the gels could be considered almost equivalent if they achieve a comparable immediate-release. For this reason, it was decided to classify the release from a gelled vehicle as immediate if at least 75% of PraNa is released within the first 15 min, based on one of the acceptance criteria suggested by EMA in the Reflection paper on the dissolution specification for generic solid oral immediate-release products with systemic action [25]. This criterion is not intended as a measure of bioequivalence but rather as a tool to identify gelled vehicles that significantly alter the drug's release kinetics.

The dissolution profiles of all gelled products are shown in Figure 2. Significant variability among the gelled vehicles is immediately apparent. The vehicles thickened with ThUp exhibited almost uniform results in terms of PraNa release, delivering the drug with immediate-release kinetics (lower right panel of Figure 2) despite having very different consistencies. In contrast, the other vehicles available in different grades (ThUpCle and HF) displayed markedly different PraNa release patterns depending on their consistency levels. Only those with lower consistencies achieved immediate-release profiles comparable to the original tablets. Finally, the three vehicles RU_TL Res, ThW, and JeG demonstrated distinctly different release behaviours, with only Res ensuring immediate-release. This highlights a contrasting situation: for ThUp-based products, consistency does not play a role (even though ThUp Pu has the highest consistency among all the gels tested), whereas for the other vehicles, the release profiles appear to depend on the gel's composition (thickening agents) and/or its consistency.

These results can be explained by considering the thickening agents used in the different products. ThUp is the only product containing starch as a gelling agent and is specifically based on corn starch (although the label indicates corn starch, according to Methacanon et al. [9], it is a modified corn starch). In contrast, all the other products consist of blends of gums (guar gum and xanthan gum) or gum-like thickeners (pectin and carrageenan). Starch-based gels are reported to have low thickening power and a low gelling tendency. Moreover, their products often exhibit a grainy or pulpy texture and an opaque appearance. On the other hand, gum- and gum-like-thickened products generally possess higher viscosity (depending on the type and grade of the gum), with a smoother, slippery, or slimy mouthfeel and a transparent appearance [9].

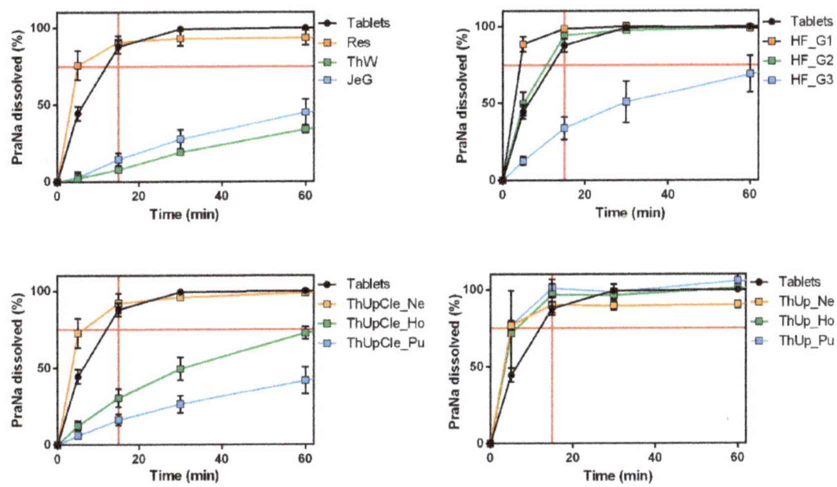

Figure 2. The PraNa release profiles for the tablets (Pensa) and all the jellified vehicles. The red lines on the x and y axes indicate a time of 15 min and a release of 75%, respectively.

A slowing drug-release effect for gum-based vehicles has been reported since the 1980s by Sarisuta and Parrott [26], although their studies did not aim to evaluate the potential for administering tablets using a gelled vehicle. Manrique et al. reported a reduction in the release rate of several drugs when crushed tablets were dispersed in gum-based vehicles [16,17]. The only study comparing starch- and gum-based formulations is that of Ilgaz et al., which demonstrated that the gelling vehicle significantly influences the drug's dissolution rate, especially in thickened samples prepared with xanthan gum [11]. The findings of Ilgaz et al. partially align with those of this study. Specifically, the authors reported that the starch-based thickener exhibited a lower reduction in drug release compared to gum, although the effect depended on the drug's solubility. Notably, starch did not influence drug release kinetics when the drug had low solubility. It is important to highlight that Ilgaz et al. used crushed tablets as a control instead of whole tablets, which could strongly affect the comparison (the dissolution rate of a powder is undoubtedly higher than that of whole tablets). However, to clarify whether the specific release profiles observed for ThUp are exclusively due to the starch-based thickener, further experiments were conducted using Pensa PraNa tablets and another commercially available starch-based thickener, Gel M (in this case, the thickener is a modified potato starch). The results of the dissolution study, reported in Figure S2 in the Supplementary Materials, confirm that the use of starch-based thickeners does not remarkably alter the dissolution profiles of dispersed tablets.

Concerning the gum-based vehicles, it is difficult to determine from the literature whether the differing release profiles observed in the present study are attributable to the specific thickening agents used or the viscosity of the samples. For this reason, a correlation analysis between the complex viscosity (measured at 1 Hz) of each gum-based vehicle and the amount of drug released at 15 min was performed. The results, reported in Figure 3, show a strong and statistically significant correlation based on Pearson correlation analysis, indicating a linear trend in the data. However, when the correlation was assessed using Spearman's correlation (based on the monotonic relationship between the two variables), the correlation coefficient was 1, indicating a perfect correlation. These results clearly indicate that, for the gum-based vehicles, the release profiles depend on the gel consistency, almost independently of the specific thickeners used.

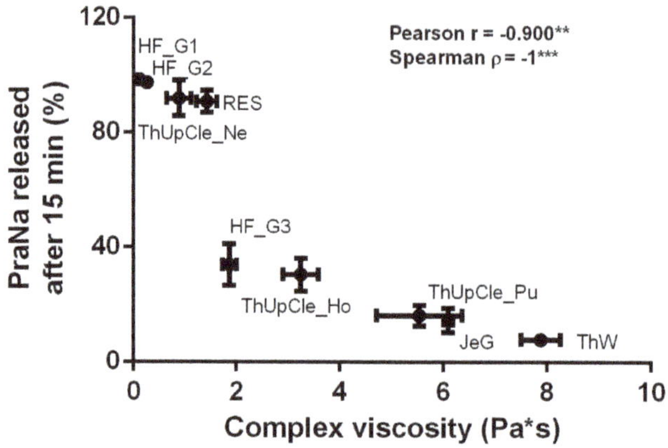

Figure 3. The correlation between the complex viscosity (measured at 1 Hz) of each gum-based vehicle and the amount of PraNa released at 15 min. The asterisks on the Pearson and Spearman coefficients indicate *p*-values between 0.01 and 0.001 (**) or lower than 0.001 (***).

3.3.2. Effect of PraNa Dose

The use of the gelled vehicles for PraNa administration could be applied not only for the standard dose of 20 mg (a single tablet) but also for personalized dosing. In the case of tablets, a personalized dose can be achieved by administering multiple tablets or using a portion of a single tablet. To verify any effects caused by increasing the amount of powder dispersed or dissolved in the vehicles, PraNa-loaded thickened water was prepared using either two Pensa PraNa tablets or half a tablet, simulating doses of 40 mg and 10 mg, respectively (10, 20, and 40 mg are all doses of PraNa usually administered [27]). Three different grades of a starch-based product (ThUp) and a gum-based product (HyF) were selected as vehicles The homogeneity data for PraNa in these gelled vehicles are reported in Table S1 in the Supplementary Materials. The dissolution results are reported in Figure 4. As evident, doubling or halving the dose yields almost identical results, indicating that dose personalization does not significantly affect the release kinetics.

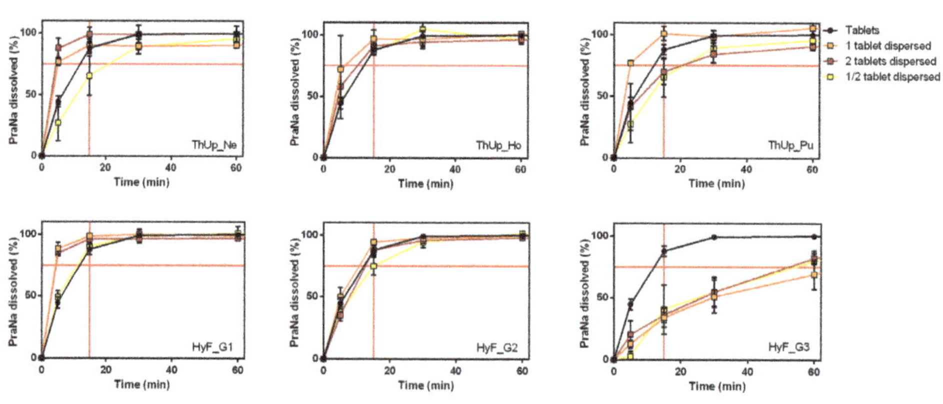

Figure 4. Effect of addition of 2 two tablets or half tablets on PraNa release from three different grades of ThUp (**upper panel graphs**) and HyF (**lower panel graphs**).

3.3.3. Effect of PraNa Formulation

PraNa is a drug with an expired patent, and several equivalent alternatives (generic medicinal products) are available on the market. All these generic products differ exclusively in terms of excipients. ThUp and HyF gelled waters at three different grades were used to test the effect of different formulations dispersed in the vehicle, comparing two medicinal product equivalents to Pensa PraNa tablets: PraNa Ratiopharm and PraNa EG. PraNa Ratiopharm consists of uncoated tablets, like the Pensa version, although its formulation is more complex due to the presence of additional diluents/binders and two superdisintegrants (crosspovidone and croscarmellose sodium). On the other hand, PraNa EG has a composition similar to PraNa ratiopharm but is formulated as coated tablets (water-soluble coating with hypromellose). The homogeneity data for PraNa in these gelled vehicles are reported in Table S1 in the Supplementary Materials.

The release profiles of Pensa PraNa, Ratiopharm PraNa, and EG PraNa tablets, as reported in Figure S3 of the Supplementary Materials, reveal that all three medicinal products exhibit nearly identical dissolution behaviour. When the Ratiopharm and EG PraNa tablets were incorporated into the three grades of ThUp and HyF gels, the dissolution profiles (Figure 5) were almost identical to those obtained with the PraNa tablets. This clearly indicates that the release kinetics are primarily determined by the composition and viscosity of the vehicle, while the effect of the formulation itself is practically negligible.

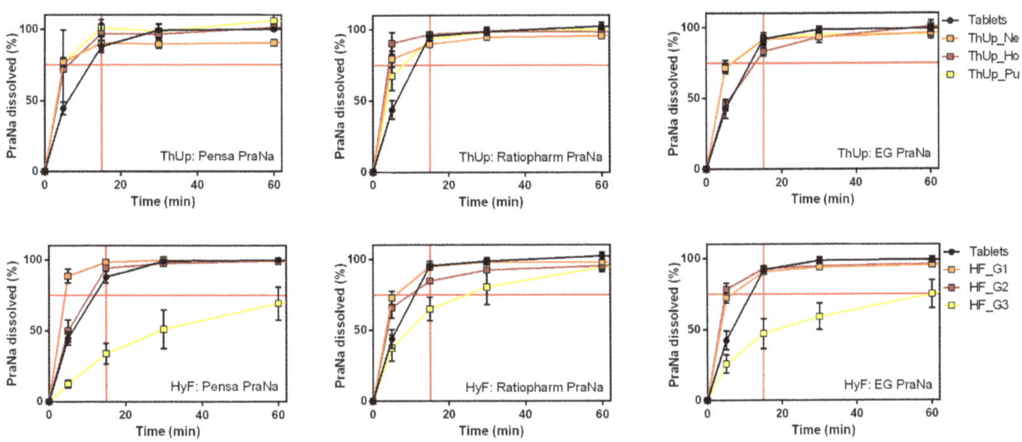

Figure 5. The effect of different tablet formulations on PraNa release from three grades of ThUp (**upper panel**) and HyF (**lower panel**). The graphs on the right show PraNa release from gelled water prepared with Pensa tablets, the middle graphs show release from gelled water prepared with Ratiopharm tablets, and the graphs on the left show release from gelled water prepared with EG tablets.

4. Conclusions

Thickened water products that are commercially available exhibit a wide range of consistencies, and in many cases, there is no perfect match between different brands or even between different products from the same brand. Among the tested products, those thickened with starch-based additives demonstrated higher consistency compared to those prepared with gum-based gelling agents. The in vitro release profiles varied significantly among the analyzed products. The main differences were attributed to the type of thickening agent used. Specifically, in the presence of starch-based thickeners, all gelled water samples exhibited nearly identical pravastatin release kinetics, closely resembling the immediate-release profiles of the original tablets. Conversely, the thickened waters prepared with gum-based gelling agents showed substantial variability in pravastatin release profiles, which were strongly correlated with their viscosity values. Changes in the amount of crushed tablets added or variations in tablet formulations did not significantly alter pravastatin release kinetics, indicating that the type and/or viscosity of the thickened water primarily governs drug release.

The results of this study demonstrated that starch-based gelled waters have the least impact on drug release. From this perspective, they represent the best option for administering solid oral dosage forms manufactured as immediate-release tablets. On the other hand, it is well-known that gum-based products are usually preferred by patients due to their better mouthfeel and transparent appearance. Therefore, developing products that combine both types of thickening agents in optimal proportions could offer acceptable drug release while maintaining good patient compliance.

It is important to emphasize that the results obtained in this study are specifically valid for drugs with high solubility, such as sodium pravastatin (a BCS Class III drug). The release behaviour observed in thickened water formulations may not be directly applicable to drugs with lower solubility, such as those in BCS Classes II and IV. These drugs often exhibit different solubility and release profiles due to their distinct physicochemical properties, which can significantly alter their interaction with the jelled vehicle. Consequently, caution should be exercised in generalizing these findings to drugs with limited solubility, as their behaviour in similar formulations could differ substantially. Future studies focusing on these drug classes are necessary to fully understand the effects of thickened water on their release dynamics.

Supplementary Materials: The following supporting information can be downloaded at: https://www.mdpi.com/article/10.3390/pharmaceutics17020251/s1, Figure S1. Complex viscosity of jellified vehicles (Panel A: RU_TL; Panel B: EP_TL) with and without Pravastatin sodium at 25 °C and 37 °C. The complex viscosity is presented as power-law viscosity, determined by analyzing the complex viscosity vs. frequency curves using a standard power-law model. The thickened water containing Pravastatin was prepared using Pensa PraNa tablets; Figure S2. PraNa release profiles from the tablets (Pensa) and jellified vehicles prepared with the powders for the preparation of extemporaneous thickened liquids Gel M (Nutrisens Medical, France). The red lines on the x and y axes indicate a time of 15 min and a release of 75%, respectively; Figure S3. PraNa release profiles from the tablets of the three different generic medicinal products The red lines on the x and y axes indicate a time of 15 min and a release of 75%, respectively; Table S1. Pravastatin sodium concentration and amount administered in a single dose of thickened water (Hydra'Fruit and Resource ThickenUp at all grades), prepared with two tablets or half a tablet of Pensa PraNa, or with a single tablet of PraNa Ratiopharm or PraNa EG.

Author Contributions: Conceptualization, R.G. and M.S.; methodology, D.R.P. and M.C.; investigation, S.L.; data curation, M.C.; writing—original draft preparation, S.L. and D.R.P.; writing—review and editing, M.C. and G.B.; visualization, D.R.P. and M.S.; supervision, M.C. and G.B.; project administration, G.B. and R.G. All authors have read and agreed to the published version of the manuscript.

Funding: This research received no external funding.

Institutional Review Board Statement: Not applicable.

Informed Consent Statement: Not applicable.

Data Availability Statement: The original contributions presented in this study are included in the article/Supplementary Material. Further inquiries can be directed to the corresponding author.

Acknowledgments: The authors thank Teva Pharmaceutical Industries Ltd. (Debrecen, Hungary) for the donation of sodium pravastatin, and Angelini Pharma s.p.a. (Roma, Italy), who allowed the material to be delivered at RG.

Conflicts of Interest: The authors declare no conflicts of interest.

References

1. European Parliament; Council of The European Union. *Regulation (EU) No 609/2013 on Food Intended for Infants and Young Children, Food for Special Medical Purposes, and Total Diet Replacement for Weight Control*; European Parliament: Strasbourg, France; Council of The European Union: Brussels, Belgium, 2013.
2. Carrau, R.L.; Murry, T.; Howell, R.J. *Comprehensive Management of Swallowing Disorders*; Plural Publishing: San Diego, CA, USA, 2016; ISBN 1944883258.
3. Saitoh, E.; Shibata, S.; Matsuo, K.; Baba, M.; Fujii, W.; Palmer, J.B. Chewing and food consistency: Effects on bolus transport and swallow initiation. *Dysphagia* **2007**, *22*, 100–107. [CrossRef] [PubMed]
4. Newman, R.; Vilardell, N.; Clavé, P.; Speyer, R. Effect of Bolus Viscosity on the Safety and Efficacy of Swallowing and the Kinematics of the Swallow Response in Patients with Oropharyngeal Dysphagia: White Paper by the European Society for Swallowing Disorders (ESSD). *Dysphagia* **2016**, *31*, 232–249. [CrossRef]
5. Steele, C.M.; Alsanei, W.A.; Ayanikalath, S.; Barbon, C.E.A.; Chen, J.; Cichero, J.A.Y.; Coutts, K.; Dantas, R.O.; Duivestein, J.; Giosa, L.; et al. The influence of food texture and liquid consistency modification on swallowing physiology and function: A systematic review. *Dysphagia* **2015**, *30*, 2–26. [CrossRef] [PubMed]
6. Cichero, J.A.Y. *How and Why Thickened Liquids Improve Swallowing Safety and Swallowing Efficiency*; Clinical Nutrition; Nestlé Nutrition Institute: Vevey, Switzerland, 2021.
7. National Dysphagia Diet Task Force. *National Dysphagia Diet: Standardization for Optimal Care*; American Dietetic Association: Chicago, IL, USA, 2002; ISBN 0880913150.
8. Cichero, J.A.Y.; Lam, P.; Steele, C.M.; Hanson, B.; Chen, J.; Dantas, R.O.; Duivestein, J.; Kayashita, J.; Lecko, C.; Murray, J.; et al. Development of International Terminology and Definitions for Texture-Modified Foods and Thickened Fluids Used in Dysphagia Management: The IDDSI Framework. *Dysphagia* **2017**, *32*, 293–314. [CrossRef] [PubMed]
9. Methacanon, P.; Gamonpilas, C.; Kongjaroen, A.; Buathongjan, C. Food polysaccharides and roles of rheology and tribology in rational design of thickened liquids for oropharyngeal dysphagia: A review. *Compr. Rev. Food Sci. Food Saf.* **2021**, *20*, 4101–4119. [CrossRef]
10. Cichero, J.A.Y. Thickening agents used for dysphagia management: Effect on bioavailability of water, medication and feelings of satiety. *Nutr. J.* **2013**, *12*, 54. [CrossRef]
11. Sura, L.; Madhavan, A.; Carnaby, G.; Crary, M.A. Dysphagia in the elderly: Management and nutritional considerations. *Clin. Interv. Aging* **2012**, *7*, 287–298. [CrossRef] [PubMed]
12. Logrippo, S.; Ricci, G.; Sestili, M.; Cespi, M.; Ferrara, L.; Palmieri, G.F.; Ganzetti, R.; Bonacucina, G.; Blasi, P. Oral drug therapy in elderly with dysphagia: Between a rock and a hard place! *Clin. Interv. Aging* **2017**, *12*, 241–251. [CrossRef] [PubMed]
13. Verrue, C.; Mehuys, E.; Boussery, K.; Remon, J.-P.; Petrovic, M. Tablet-splitting: A common yet not so innocent practice. *J. Adv. Nurs.* **2011**, *67*, 26–32. [CrossRef] [PubMed]
14. James, A. The legal and clinical implications of crushing tablet medication. *Nurs. Times* **2004**, *100*, 28–29. [PubMed]
15. Richey, R.H.; Hughes, C.; Craig, J.V.; Shah, U.U.; Ford, J.L.; Barker, C.E.; Peak, M.; Nunn, A.J.; Turner, M.A. A systematic review of the use of dosage form manipulation to obtain required doses to inform use of manipulation in paediatric practice. *Int. J. Pharm.* **2017**, *518*, 155–166. [CrossRef] [PubMed]
16. Manrique, Y.J.; Lee, D.J.; Islam, F.; Nissen, L.M.; Cichero, J.A.Y.; Stokes, J.R.; Steadman, K.J. Crushed tablets: Does the administration of food vehicles and thickened fluids to aid medication swallowing alter drug release? *J. Pharm. Pharm. Sci.* **2014**, *17*, 207–219. [CrossRef] [PubMed]
17. Manrique, Y.J.; Sparkes, A.M.; Cichero, J.A.Y.; Stokes, J.R.; Nissen, L.M.; Steadman, K.J. Oral medication delivery in impaired swallowing: Thickening liquid medications for safe swallowing alters dissolution characteristics. *Drug Dev. Ind. Pharm.* **2016**, *42*, 1537–1544. [CrossRef]
18. Ilgaz, F.; Timur, S.S.; Eylem, C.C.; Nemutlu, E.; Erdem, Ç.E.; Eroğlu, H.; Gökmen-Özel, H. Do Thickening Agents Used in Dysphagia Diet Affect Drug Bioavailability? *Eur. J. Pharm. Sci.* **2022**, *174*, 106197. [CrossRef] [PubMed]
19. Logrippo, S.; Ganzetti, R.; Sestili, M.; Perinelli, D.R.; Cespi, M.; Bonacucina, G. Enteral Delivery of Pravastatin Sodium Tablets: Effect of Compounding into a Liquid Form and Co-Administration of Enteral Nutrition. *Pharmacy* **2024**, *12*, 32. [CrossRef] [PubMed]
20. Agirre-Olabide, I.; Berasategui, J.; Elejabarrieta, M.J.; Bou-Ali, M.M. Characterization of the linear viscoelastic region of magnetorheological elastomers. *J. Intell. Mater. Syst. Struct.* **2014**, *25*, 2074–2081. [CrossRef]
21. Merck KGaA. Pravastatin Sodium Salt Hydrate. Available online: https://www.sigmaaldrich.com/IT/it/product/sigma/p4498?srsltid=AfmBOoqdgxLV799Q2aQ3vphB0J8mx_XTGpGXmhvne4dOzW9RVKf4mk9C&icid=sharepdp-clipboard-copy-productdetailpage (accessed on 28 November 2024).

22. European Pharmacopoeia Commission. Uniformity of mass of single-dose preparations. In *EUROPEAN PHARMACOPOEIA*, 10th ed.; European Pharmacopoeia Commission: Strasbourg, France, 2020; p. 335.
23. European Pharmacopoeia Commission. Uniformity of content of single-dose preparations. In *EUROPEAN PHARMACOPOEIA*, 10th ed.; European Pharmacopoeia Commission: Strasbourg, France, 2020; p. 336.
24. Barnes, H.A. Linear viscoelasticity and time effects. In *A Handbook of Elementary Rheology*; University of Wales, Institute of Non-Newtonian Fluid Mechanics: Aberystwyth, UK, 2000.
25. European Medicines Agency. *Reflection Paper on the Dissolution Specification for Generic Solid Oral Immediate Release Products with Systemic Action*; EMA/CHMP/CVMP/QWP/336031/2017; European Medicines Agency: London, UK, 2017.
26. Sarisuta, N.; Parrott, E.L. Relationship of dissolution rate to viscosity of polymeric solutions. *J. Pharm. Sci.* **1982**, *71*, 1375–1380. [CrossRef] [PubMed]
27. Sidhu, G.; Sapra, A. *Pravastatin*; StatPearls: Tampa, FL, USA; Available online: https://www.ncbi.nlm.nih.gov/books/NBK551621/ (accessed on 20 November 2024).

pharmaceutics MDPI

Article

Integrating Analytical Procedures in Routine Practices of Centralized Antiblastic Compounding Units for Valorization of Residual Compounded Drugs

Rita Patrizia Aquino [1], Giovanni Falcone [1], Paola Russo [1,*], Fabrizio Dal Piaz [2], Giulia Auriemma [1], Ferdinando Maria de Francesco [3], Stefania Cascone [3], Eduardo Nava [3] and Pasquale Del Gaudio [1]

1 Department of Pharmacy, University of Salerno, 84084 Fisciano, Italy; aquinorp@unisa.it (R.P.A.); gifalcone@unisa.it (G.F.); gauriemma@unisa.it (G.A.); pdelgaudio@unisa.it (P.D.G.)
2 Department of Medicine, Surgery and Dentistry, University of Salerno, 84084 Fisciano, Italy; fdalpiaz@unisa.it
3 Pharmaceutical Department, Local Health Authority Naples 3 South, 80059 Torre Del Greco, Italy; fm.defrancesco@aslnapoli3sud.it (F.M.d.F.); s.cascone@aslnapoli3sud.it (S.C.); e.nava@aslnapoli3sud.it (E.N.)
* Correspondence: paorusso@unisa.it; Tel.: +39-089-96-9256

Abstract

Background/Objectives: Although extemporaneous formulations of anticancer drug products for personalized therapy are produced according to Good Hospital Pharmacy Manufacturing Practice, the lack of knowledge about drug stability under clinical conditions limits the second-time use of these highly costly medications in clinical practice. Therefore, the residual compounded drugs are considered waste and a cost item that negatively affects the healthcare system. In the context of the ever-increasing interest of the health system in applying practices in line with personalized medicine and spending review policies, this research aimed to demonstrate the feasibility of incorporating analytical techniques into daily routine practice. Specifically, the present research focused on fast stability analysis of Active Pharmaceutical Ingredients (APIs) in antiblastic residual compounded drugs with the purpose of demonstrating their potentialities as a resource for possible second-time use. Methods: Two different subsets of drug products were analyzed, i.e., medicines containing small molecules and medicines containing monoclonal antibodies. In relation to their different physicochemical properties, two analytical approaches were optimized and involved in the stability investigation: HPLC-DAD for small molecules and a combined approach of LC-MS/MS with size exclusion chromatography for monoclonal antibodies analysis. Results: Results underlined that the stability data, as available in the summary of product characteristics related to each medicine, do not completely describe the physicochemical shelf-life of anticancer compounded drugs. Conclusions: In fact, for all tested products, our results suggested a longer shelf-life in comparison to the datasheet, giving hospital pharmacists the possibility to extend the clinical use of compounded drugs, improving the cost–benefit of anticancer personalized therapy.

Keywords: personalized medicine; anticancer medicines; hospital compounded drugs; physicochemical stability investigation

1. Introduction

The implementation of personalized medicine has the potential to improve patients' quality of life and life expectancy while reducing financial and time costs [1]. Although personalized medicine offers significant potential for improving therapeutic outcomes, its integration into resource-limited healthcare systems poses significant challenges [2]. Optimizing the allocation of healthcare resources is essential to ensure effective and efficient service delivery [3]. Hospitals and other healthcare providers constantly work to ensure the best possible care for the patient while navigating a challenging business and economic landscape [4]. The challenges of balancing the quality and cost of patient care are even more relevant to the adoption of personalized medicine in medical subsets such as chemotherapy [5,6]. In fact, the ongoing development of targeted therapies and a multidisciplinary approach to new treatment modalities have contributed to improved outcomes for cancer patients [7,8], but also treatment costs (USD 30,790 of the eight-week treatment regimens providing Bevacizumab or Cetuximab compared to USD 63 for the same period of 5-fluorouracil, leucovorin, and oxaliplatin regimens). This trend underscores the need to adopt new policies aimed at improving cost-effectiveness, cost–utility, and cost–benefit [9,10]. In the context of personalized therapy, customized and prescription-based compounded drugs are prepared in hospital pharmacies, mixing individual ingredients in personalized doses and dosage forms to meet patient-specific needs. Therefore, a wide range of anticancer drugs need to be manipulated, i.e., reconstructed or diluted, by the hospital pharmacist before administration, transforming the raw medicines into extemporaneous pharmacy or magistral preparations. Compounding activity requires that regulatory aspects be considered, i.e., dose accuracy, sterility assurance, and stability under clinical conditions [11]. In many European countries, the reconstitution and preparation of anticancer drugs are carried out in centralized compounding units in a controlled and validated environment by expert personnel to ensure standardization. In fact, centralized manufacturing of anticancer medicine responds to specific regulatory and procedural guidelines that have been developed over the years in consultation with regulatory authorities. Centralized compounding is an effective strategy for ensuring product quality, workers' and patients' safety, and reducing the risk of environmental contamination while rationalizing pharmaceutical expenditure [12]. However, if dosage accuracy and sterility requirements can be considered guaranteed by the adoption of Good Hospital Pharmacy Manufacturing Practice (GHPMP) (GMP) for the quality assurance of the preparation in hospital pharmacies [13], with periodically verified procedures and operative personnel in the routine of centralized units, the stability of the compounded drugs under clinical conditions remains an issue that limits the possible second-time use of residual compounded drugs in clinical practice. In fact, depending on the prescribed dosage for specific patient clinical needs and the amount of Active Pharmaceutical Ingredient (API) available in the packaging of the medicinal product, after reconstitution and dilution, a certain fraction of the medicinal product persists from compounding activity [14]. However, the lack of stability data for compounded drugs forces pharmacists to consider residual compounded drugs as waste, which has a negative impact on the hospital's bottom line. In fact, the stability data provided by the pharmaceutical industry in the summary of product characteristics (SmPCs) for each medicine are mostly related to the physicochemical stability of the raw drug product and the methods described in the pharmacopeias or ICH guidelines [15] do not fit the conditions of clinical practice [16]. The possibility of extending the validity of expensive medicine would be extremely helpful in providing hospital pharmacists with stability information on different drugs, as required for the proper management of a central compounding unit [17,18]. The availability of a longer period of use of the compounded drugs, which does not compromise the stability and safety of the drug, would facilitate the organization of centralized antiblastic units and would be economically advantageous, allowing the use of residual compounded drugs for subsequent preparations [19–21].

Considering this background, the present research, carried out in collaboration with the UFA Laboratory (Unità Farmaci Antiblastici-Centralized Antiblastic Drug Unit) of the

Gragnano Hospital managed by the ASL Na3 Local Health Authority Naples 3 South, aimed to demonstrate the feasibility of incorporating analytical techniques into the daily routine practice of a hospital centralized compounding unit. The study focused on the optimization of rapid methods to assess the physicochemical stability of each compounded API in a 21-day investigation. Six anticancer medicines were used as models, i.e., ALIMTA®, ABRAXANE®, and JEVTANA® as role models of small molecule drugs and HERCEPTIN®, AVASTIN®, and ERBITUX® containing monoclonal antibodies. HPLC-DAD protocol was established for small molecule analysis, and a combined approach of LC-MS/MS with SEC (size exclusion chromatography) was used for monoclonal antibodies assessment.

2. Materials and Methods

2.1. Materials

All medicinal products were provided by the Health Authority Naples 3 South (ASL NA3Sud), Italy. According to their SmPCs, quali-quantitative and dilution data are listed below:

- ALIMTA® 100 mg powder for concentrate for solution for infusion (Eli Lilly and Company, Indianapolis, IN, USA) (ALI). API: Pemetrexed disodium (Pemetrexed) at a final concentration of 25 mg/mL; other excipients: mannitol, hydrochloric acid, and sodium hydroxide [22];
- ABRAXANE® (ABR) 5 mg/mL powder for dispersion for infusion (Bristol Myers Squibb, New York, NY, USA). API: Paclitaxel formulated as albumin-bound nanoparticles (Nab-Paclitaxel) at a final concentration of 5 mg/mL; other excipients: human albumin solution (containing sodium caprylate and N-acetyl-L-tryptophan) [23];
- JEVTANA® (JEV) 60 mg concentrate and solvent for solution for infusion (Sanofi, Gentilly, France). API: Cabazitaxel at a final concentration of 10 mg/mL; other excipients: Polysorbate 80, citric acid, ethanol 96%, and water for injection [24];
- HERCEPTIN® (HER) 150 mg powder for concentrate for solution for infusion (Roche Products Limited, Grenzach-Wyhlen, Germany). API: Trastuzumab, a humanized IgG1 monoclonal antibody produced by mammalian (Chinese hamster ovary) cell suspension culture and purified by affinity and ion exchange chromatography, including specific viral inactivation and removal procedures at a final concentration of 21 mg/mL; other excipients: recombinant human hyaluronidase (rHuPH20), L-histidine, L-histidine hydrochloride monohydrate, α,α-trehalose dihydrate, L-methionine, Polysorbate 20, and water for injections [25];
- AVASTIN® (AVA) 25 mg/mL concentrate for solution for infusion (Genetech Inc., San Francisco, CA, USA). API: Bevacizumab, a recombinant humanized monoclonal antibody produced by DNA technology in Chinese hamster ovary cells, at a final concentration of 25 mg/mL; other excipients: trehalose dihydrate, sodium phosphate, Polysorbate 20, and water for injections [26];
- ERBITUX® (ERBI) 5 mg/mL solution for infusion (Merck, Readington, NJ, USA). API: Cetuximab, chimeric monoclonal IgG1 antibody produced in a mammalian cell line (Sp2/0) by recombinant DNA technology, at a final concentration of 5 mg/mL; other excipients: sodium chloride, Glycine, Polysorbate 80, citric acid monohydrate, sodium hydroxide, and water for injections [27].

Solvents (acetonitrile, acetic acid, phosphate-buffered saline—PBS) and materials for chromatographic analyses (polyacrylamide gels, trypsin) were purchased from Sigma-Aldrich (St. Louis, MO, USA) and ultra-pure solvents for LC/MS analysis from Romil (Cambridge, UK).

2.2. Methods

2.2.1. Residual Compounded Drugs: Shelf-Life Evaluation

All samples were prepared following the standardized protocols in use at the UFA Laboratory of the Gragnano Hospital:

ALI: The diluent, 4.2 mL of sodium chloride solution 9 mg/mL (0.9%) for injections, is injected into the Pemetrexed powder (100 mg) and gently stirred until complete powder dissolution with a final concentration of 25 mg/mL. The use of other solvents for reconstitution is avoided. The diluent is added slowly along the internal walls of the bottle, facilitating the dissolution of the powder with slow movements (at least 15 min) without shaking to avoid foam formation.

ABR: 20 mL of diluent solution is withdrawn with a syringe and injected through the spike very slowly into the API powder (100 mg of Nab-Paclitaxel) but along the internal walls of the bottle. The addition of the diluent is carried out in a time not shorter than 1 min. Once the syringe is disconnected from the spike, the latter is left inserted in the bottle for at least 7 min, slowly bringing it to a horizontal position and shaking. After the indicated time, the bottle is rotated with slow movements to avoid foaming, obtaining homogeneous dispersion (concentration 5 mg/mL) with a milky appearance and without visible precipitates.

JEV, the solvent, is quantitatively removed from the solvent bottle with a syringe and injected into the bottle containing Cabazitaxel (60 mg). Once the syringe and needle are removed, mixing is facilitated with slow, rotating movements of the vial without shaking to avoid foaming. Then, the solution (concentration of 10 mg/mL) is left to rest for at least 5 min until the solution appears clear, homogeneous, and with a light-yellow color.

HER: Trastuzumab (150 mg) was reconstituted with 7 mL of water for injections. The use of other solvents for reconstitution is avoided. This results in 10.2 mL of single-dose solution containing 21 mg/mL of Trastuzumab. The diluent is added slowly along the internal walls of the bottle, allowing powder dissolution with slow circular movements without shaking to avoid foam formation.

For AVA and ERB, no reconstitution is needed since the drugs are already in solution.

2.2.2. Small Molecules Stability Assays

The chemical stability of each API (Cabazitaxel, Pemetrexed, and Paclitaxel) was performed by HPLC-DAD on Agilent Technologies HPLC, model LC 1220 Infinity, equipped with a DAD UV detector using an injection volume of 20 μL and setting the temperature at 25 °C. The main parameters of optimized methods are reported in Table 1.

Table 1. Optimized HPLC-DAD set-up for each small molecule: Pemetrexed, Paclitaxel, and Cabazitaxel.

	Pemetrexed	**Nab-Paclitaxel**	**Cabazitaxel**
Chromatographic column	Phenomenex Luna C8 4.6 × 250 mm, (5 μm)	Agilent SB C18 4.6 × 250 mm, (5 μm)	Agilent Zorbax Eclipse XDB-C18, 4.6 × 250 mm, (5 μm)
Mobile phase composition	Acetonitrile/Buffer [1] (1.3:8.7)	Acetonitrile/Water (4.0:6.0)	Acetonitrile/Water (8.0:2.0)
Flow rate (mL/min)	1.00	1.5	1.5
DAD detector wavelength (nm)	285	228	232

[1] Buffer was water added with acetic acid 0.1% *v*/*v*.

For each API, the calibration curve in a range of concentration between 10 and 500 μg/mL was constructed, plotting peak area vs. concentration with six concentrations (10, 50, 100, 200, 300, and 500 μg/mL). Statistical analyses were performed using

GraphPad Prism 10 software to evaluate the specificity, the calibration response, and the accuracy of optimized methods.

Dynamic Laser Scattering Analysis

The physical stability of Nab-Paclitaxel, formulated as albumin-bound nanoparticles, was investigated in terms of size distribution and surface potential of nanoparticles by Dynamic Laser Scattering using a Litesizer™ 500 Particle analyzer (Anton Paar, Graz, Austria). Data acquisition was performed through Kalliope™ software *v*.2.34.3. Analyses were conducted at 25 °C on Paclitaxel solution at 1 mg/mL (0.9 mg/mL of albumin) obtained by product dilution in 0.9% NaCl solution.

2.2.3. Monoclonal Antibodies Stability Assays

The physicochemical stability of monoclonal antibodies was carried out by exploiting a combined assay: SEC and LC-MS/MS peptide mapping.

LC-MS/MS Peptide Mapping

Each monoclonal antibody was purified by one-dimensional electrophoresis on polyacrylamide gels. The band containing the proteins of interest underwent reduction and carboxyamidomethylation of cysteine residues and digestion using trypsin as a proteolytic enzyme, according to the method described in Figure 1.

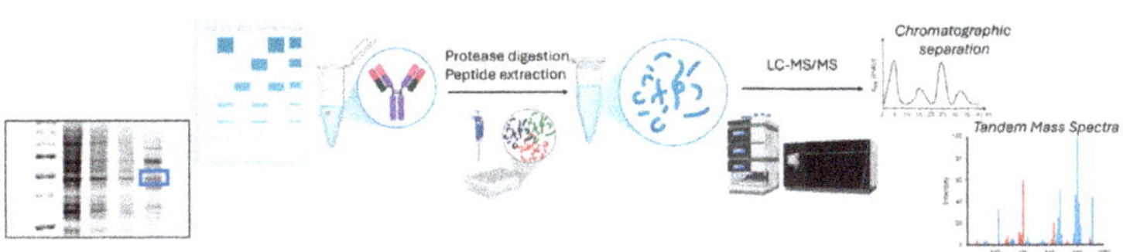

Figure 1. Protocol developed for protein peptide mapping.

The resulting peptide mixtures were analyzed using a system consisting of a nanoAquity (Waters, Milford, MA, USA) UPLC capillary chromatograph interfaced with a nanoSpray source mass spectrometer and equipped with an orbitrap-ion trap hybrid ion analyzer, Orbitrap XL (Thermo-Fisher, Carlsbad, CA, USA).

The data obtained were compared with those expected based on the amino acid sequence of the protein, thus revealing modifications of single amino acid residues or unexpected fragmentations of the polypeptide chain.

Size Exclusion Chromatography

For each monoclonal antibody, the hydrodynamic mobility, directly proportional to the conformation and the state of aggregation, was analyzed by molecular exclusion chromatography on a gel filtration column in Agilent Technologies HPLC, model LC 1220 Infinity. The column used was a Yarra3000 (300 × 4.6 mm; 3 µm), with a mobile phase consisting of phosphate-buffered saline (PBS) water solution and a flow rate of 0.5 mL/min. Before analysis, all samples were diluted from reconstructed concentration to a final concentration of 5 mg/mL, using an injection volume of 50 µL, and a spectrophotometric DAD detector settled at 280 nm to measure the absorption of the eluate.

2.2.4. Twenty-One Days Physicochemical Stability

Residual compounded drugs, both from medicine containing small molecules and antibodies, reconstructed as reported in Section 2.2.1, were subjected to a three-week stability study (21 days). Three batches of each drug product were used in the present study. Taking into account instructions about storage conditions of each drug product reported in SmPCs [22–27], batches were stored in a clean area inside a pharmaceutical-grade refrigerator according to DIN 13277:2022-05 [28] at 4 °C protected from light, each one closed within a sterile, sealed bag. For all compounded drugs, by convention, the day of powder reconstitution will be defined as Day 1. Samples diluted to 1 mg/mL on Day 1 were the controls for the stability study. The drug stability analyses were performed on days 1, 2, 3, 5, 8, 10, 15, 18, and finally 21. Each analysis was carried out in triplicate, and data were reported as average value ± standard deviation. Considering the very narrow therapeutic range of chemotherapy agents and the risks associated with the degradation products (DPs), the limit of acceptability of tested products was set at 5% of the reference values (i.e., drug products on Day 1).

2.2.5. Statistical Analysis

All statistical analyses were conducted using GraphPad Prism Software (v. 10.2). For methods validation, simple linear regression was carried out, choosing a confidence interval of 95% with a *p*-value of <0.05.

The one-way ANOVA (Analysis of Variance) test was applied to assess the significance of differences during stability studies (Tukey's test α 0.05, *p*-value < 0.05).

3. Results and Discussion

The growing interest of healthcare providers in applying resource recovery policies underlines the need to identify methods that allow them to fill the gap between available data in the SmPCs of medicine and data about compounded drugs in clinical practices [29]. Compliance with good manufacturing practices for the quality assurance of the preparation in hospital pharmacies (GHPMPs [13]), notably in the reconstitution of pharmaceutical products, is a mandatory requirement aimed at ensuring safety in terms of dosage and microbiological steadiness. Therefore, the main issue that limited the implementation of the secondary use of these drug products was the absence of universal guidelines that ensure the quality of analysis to evaluate the shelf-life of antiblastic compounded drugs [14]. To overcome this limitation, starting in the past decade, many research groups worked to establish baseline unifying procedures applied in the physicochemical evaluation of antiblastic post-compounding formulations. Considering the high relevance of standard procedures, to carry out the present investigation, we followed "Methodological guidelines for stability studies of hospital pharmaceutical preparations Part 1: liquid preparations" disclosed by SFPC (French Society of Clinical Pharmacy) and GERPAC (Evaluation and Research Group on Protection in Controlled Atmosphere) [30].

The preliminary step of the present study was the selection of drug products that could be considered candidates for a resource recovery policy. Two different subsets of antiblastic drug products were evaluated, i.e., medicinal products containing small molecules or monoclonal antibodies, selecting three different medicines for each group. In both cases, medicines were selected according to the annual financial report of ASL Na3, in the function of the worst rating in terms of balance between frequency of use and costs. Products containing small molecules, Cabazitaxel, Pemetrexed disodium, and Paclitaxel (i.e., JEV, ALI, and ABR, respectively), are almost indicated as second-line treatment, thus representing expensive products in comparison to their frequency of use. On the other hand, considering the high costs of all products in the monoclonal antibodies subset, the selection of Trastuzumab, Bevacizumab, and Cetuximab in the related patented products was almost driven by the frequency of use.

Looking at the purpose of introducing analytic control into routine practices, the choice of specific analytical techniques is the result of a balance between the quality of the achievable results, the cost of running the instrumentation, and the ease of use.

Thus, in the function of physicochemical differences between the two subsets, different analytical approaches were exploited to perform the stability study of the API in the residual compounded drugs: HPLC-DAD for small molecules and a combined approach of LC-MS/MS with SEC for monoclonal antibodies. Thus, results obtained from each drug product subset will be discussed separately.

3.1. Compounded Drug Products Containing Small Molecules

Usually, in a stability study performed for research purposes, the selection of the technique is driven by the physicochemical properties of the compounds to be determined. However, as also described in GERPAC guidelines, in hospital pharmacies, this selection is additionally dictated by what equipment is available and the costs connected to its routine use. For these reasons, HPLC is more recommended than other techniques, allowing the analysis of a very broad range of small molecules with different physicochemical properties and restrained running costs [30].

Starting from these premises, an HPLC-DAD method was selected and fine-tuned to provide an accurate response in a timely manner that fits with the practical needs of the hospital activities, performing serial analyses on several products using similar equipment and conditions (mobile phase, column system, and detector), in a short time.

Each drug product ALI, ABR, and JEV immediately after reconstruction was diluted to obtain a concentration of 1 mg/mL and used as a reference.

3.1.1. Methodological Approach to Define Small Molecules Chemical Stability Assays

In the U.S. Pharmacopeia 44th edition, there are specific monographies about Pemetrexed disodium and Paclitaxel; however, no info is available in the compendia for Cabazitaxel.

According to the USP method of Pemetrexed disodium [31], the following apparatus was used: C-8 reversed-phase column, DAD detector settled at 285 nm, mixture of acetonitrile and water buffer (i.e., water added with acetic acid 0.1% v/v to obtain a pH around 5.3) as mobile phase.

In detail, different ratios of the solvent mixture were evaluated from 1.0:9.0 to 2.5:7.5, varying also the flow rate from 0.8 to 1.2 mL/min, aiming to obtain API elution time of less than 10 min. The best results were obtained using a mobile phase in isocratic elution, consisting of 1.3 parts acetonitrile and 8.7 parts buffer, and a flow rate of 1.0 mL/min. In these conditions, the complete elution of the active ingredient from the column occurred in about 7 min.

A similar approach was exploited to find the optimal method set-up for the evaluation of Paclitaxel. According to the USP [31], the HPLC system was equipped with a C-18 reversed-phase column, and the DAD detector was settled at 228 nm. The mobile phase was an acetonitrile/water mixture in a ratio of 6.0:4.0. Testing different flow rates in a range between 1.0 and 1.5 mL/min and setting the final flow rate at 1.5 mL/min, a retention time of 10 min was obtained.

Differently from Pemetrexed and Paclitaxel, no information on quantitative assays of Cabazitaxel in official compendia is available, so two specific studies were considered the basement of the present study [32,33]. As a consequence, the following instrument configuration was settled: C-18 reversed-phase column, DAD detector (232 nm). Different mixtures of acetonitrile/water at a ratio between 9.0:1.0 and 1:1 v/v and a flow between 1.0 and 1.5 mL/min were evaluated, establishing as an optimal condition a mixture of 8.0:2.0 at 1.5 mL/min that allows us to obtain a very short retention time around 4 min.

The selectivity of each method was evaluated by the comparison of API and mobile phase chromatograms: no peak was detected at the retention time of each small molecule in the chromatograms of mobile phase blank. The calibration response was evaluated through linearity regression in a range of concentration from 10 to 500 μg/mL. Each linearity regression coefficient is listed as follows: Pemetrexed r^2 = 0.9975, Nab-Paclitaxel r^2 = 0.9998, and Cabazitaxel r^2 = 0.9991. Finally, the accuracy of each optimized method was evaluated by comparing the observed concentration with the theoretical concentration for all points of a calibration curve. In all cases, the statistical analysis highlighted non-significant differences between theoretical and observed concentrations ($p < 0.05$).

3.1.2. Chemical Stability Investigation of Compounded Drug Products Containing Small Molecules

The developed methods were used to analyze the chemical stability of each API in hospital drug residues daily compounded over three weeks. The evaluation was carried out starting from Day 1. Samples were diluted at a final concentration of 200 μg/mL, then several aliquots were picked up, and each one was analyzed at a different time (Table 2).

Table 2. Chemical stability data over 21 days of small molecules containing products: Cabazitaxel, Pemetrexed disodium, and Nab-Paclitaxel by HPLC analysis.

	Pemetrexed (% ± st. dev.)	**Nab-Paclitaxel (% ± st. dev.)**	**Cabazitaxel (% ± st. dev.)**
Day 1	100.00 ± 0.09	100 ± 0.31	100.00 ± 0.01
Day 2	100.00 ± 0.11	99.93 ± 0.47	100.00 ± 0.01
Day 3	99.97 ± 0.22	99.92 ± 0.53	99.80 ± 0.02
Day 4	99.72 ± 0.32	99.79 ± 0.92	99.22 ± 0.02
Day 5	99.34 ± 0.41	93.75 ± 1.02	99.10 ± 0.01
Day 8	98.94 ± 0.48	92.67 ± 2.51	98.90 ± 0.02
Day 10	97.96 ± 0.51	86.97 ± 2.55	97.95 ± 0.03
Day 12	97.70 ± 0.52	80.12 ± 2.75	97.50 ± 0.03
Day 15	97.58 ± 0.58	65.76 ± 3.53	97.20 ± 0.04
Day 18	95.00 ± 0.62	-	96.80 ± 0.03
Day 22	94.78 ± 0.63	-	94.60 ± 0.03

Results obtained from the stability studies of ALI shown in Table 2 evidenced a non-significant reduction in the Pemetrexed content up to 5 days of storage, less than 0.5% (99.72% recovery in API). After 5 days, a continuous reduction in drug content was observed: more than 1% after 8 days until it reached the 5% limit on the 21st day. SmPC of ALIMTA® reports the shelf-life of the reconstituted compounded drug as 24 h at refrigerated temperature (SmPC, Section 6.3 [22]), but our results highlighted that the chemical stability of Pemetrexed was ensured until three weeks after reconstitution if stored correctly at 4 °C.

Moving the attention to Nab-Paclitaxel (ABR), the HPLC-DAD investigation revealed a non-significant variation in API content up to 3 days of storage, followed by a minimum decrease on Day 4. On the other hand, from Day 5, it is possible to observe a relevant drop in the drug concentration from 5% in one day to a 35% drop after Day 15. To better highlight the mechanism behind this rapid down-drop of Nab-Paclitaxel concentration after Day 4, a Dynamic Laser Scattering study was performed to evaluate the physical stability. Nab-Paclitaxel particles on Day 1 showed a mean diameter of about 130 nm with a narrow size distribution (PDI < 0.1), while an apparent zeta potential of a −23 ± 3.1 mV was detected. This observation is in line with the presence of a partial negative charge on the particle surface due to interactions between the Paclitaxel and the albumin matrix in the nanoparticle structure. On Day 4, changes in both particle size and zeta potential were observed: particle size increased up to 85% until 220 nm diameter, PDI > 0.4, and the zeta potential moved to −22 ± 2.4 mV. Zeta potential reduced its absolute value over time until reaching a minimum value of −0.8 ± 2.4 mV after 15 days, suggesting a partial degradation of the Paclitaxel chains linked to the surface of the albumin nanoparticles. Considering that the shelf-life of ABR after the opening of reconstituted dispersion in the vial or of the infusion bag is 24 h at 2–8 °C in the original container and 24 h at 2–8 °C followed by 4 h at 25 °C, protected from light (as reported in Section 6.3 of its SmPC), the shelf-life of residual compounded drug comprehensive of nanoparticles stability until 3 days is still a very promising result.

Finally, the results of the Cabazitaxel (JEV) investigation indicated a very limited reduction in the API content over the first 8 days. Indeed, as shown in Table 2, Cabazitaxel content remains unchanged after 24 h of storage at 4 °C, and after 8 days of storage, it decreased by only 1.1%. Interestingly, the reduction in Cabazitaxel content has an almost linear relationship with time up to Day 15 (97.58% content). Although the in-use shelf-life of JEVTANA® after dilution is reported to be 1 h at ambient temperature and 24 h at 2–8 °C (as reported in Section 6.3 of its SmPC), our results about the chemical stability of Cabazitaxel open the possibility of using a residual compounded drug for a very long time (until 18 days); however, further studies are needed in order to make a conclusion.

3.2. Compounded Drug Products Containing Monoclonal Antibodies

In comparison to small molecules, protein drugs can undergo more complex degradation pathways related to both physical and/or chemical stress [34]. Moreover, the ability of a protein API, such as monoclonal antibodies, used in the therapeutic field to interact with its targets and partners is strictly associated with both the primary (amino acid sequence and any post-transcriptional modifications) and tertiary structures (conformation and intermolecular interactions). To evaluate whether the stability of these protein APIs is preserved even after any stress, it is necessary to verify that primary and tertiary structures are still retained [35]. In recent years, some research groups focused their attention on the development of methods to evaluate the stability of monoclonal antibody products after reconstruction [36]. For example, Vieillard et al. evaluated the stability of Cetuximab in opened vials exploiting a multiple techniques approach, i.e., SEC, DLS, derivative UV spectrophotometry, and fluorescence spectroscopy [37]. Carpanese et al. proposed an orthogonal assessment of the physicochemical, biological, and microbiological properties of ERBITUX® and VECTIBIX® in original opened glass vials [38]. They analyzed the tertiary structure changes in UV spectroscopy between 250 and 320 nm in second derivative mode, while changes in primary structure were evaluated by combining SDS_PAGE and SEC-HPLC. In both cases, an accurate evaluation of monoclonal antibody stability was performed. However, considering the final aim of the possible introduction of these investigations in daily routine practices of anticancer centralized units, the analytical techniques involved could not fit the daily routine. Thus, in accordance with the guidelines by GERPAC that suggested the possibility of using different analytical techniques as instruments for stability investigation, SEC and LC-MS/MS combined approaches were applied. In detail, SEC was exploited to evaluate the tertiary structure stability of monoclonal antibodies, while LC-MS/MS was used as a detection technique in a peptide mapping protocol settled to evaluate the stability of the primary structure. LC-MS/MS could be easier to introduce in routine practice for stability studies due to the high resolution of the process, as well as the shorter analysis times compared to ionic exchange chromatography, which is defined as the golden standard by GERPAC.

The studies carried out in this phase were conducted on residual compounded drugs Trastuzumab (HER), Bevacizumab (AVA), and Cetuximab (ERB).

3.2.1. Methodological Approach to Define Monoclonal Antibodies Stability Assays

To perform mAbs primary structure stability evaluation, it was necessary to optimize the peptide mapping approach. As well known, prolonged storage of proteins in aqueous solutions can also cause changes in their chemical structure; oxidation of methionine residues, deamination of glutamine residues, and hydrolysis of some peptide bonds (primarily those between asparagine and proline residues) are the most common events. The most effective analytical approach for the analysis and verification of the primary structure of a protein is the accurate measurement of its molecular weight coupled with the so-called peptide mapping. This technique is based on enzymatic digestion of the protein, aimed at generating peptide fragments that cover the entire sequence of the protein itself, and on their subsequent analysis using liquid chromatography techniques coupled with LC-MS/MS tandem mass spectrometry [39].

The method developed (Figure 1) involved the purification of each protein to be analyzed by one-dimensional electrophoresis on polyacrylamide gels, reduction and carboxyamidomethylation of cysteine residues, and digestion in gel, using trypsin as a proteolytic enzyme. The peptide mixtures generated were analyzed by a UPLC capillary chromatograph interfaced with a nanoSpray source mass spectrometer and equipped with an orbitrap-ion trap hybrid ion analyzer [40,41]. The comparison between the obtained data and those expected based on the amino acid sequence of the protein allowed us to highlight possible modifications of single amino acid residues or possible fragmentations of the polypeptide chains.

Preliminarily, full MS spectra of the three proteins were acquired. MS spectrum obtained from the Trastuzumab analysis showed the presence of a main species with a molecular weight—calculated from the average of three measurements—of 145,534 $\pm$ 4 g/mol (Trastuzumab theoretical weight 145,532 g/mol). The Bevacizumab spectrum showed a species with a molecular weight of 149,195 $\pm$ 4 g/mol (theoretical weight Bevacizumab 149,197 g/mol) and the Cetuximab a species with a molecular weight of 145,783 $\pm$ 5 g/mol (theoretical weight Cetuximab 145,782 g/mol). Subsequently, in-gel digestion coupled with a mass spectrometry approach was used to analyze samples containing Trastuzumab, Bevacizumab, or Cetuximab. The data obtained, processed manually and with the support of the Paws software, allowed us to confirm that this method was suitable to verify the amino acid sequence of the three proteins (Tables 3–5).

Table 3. Peptides identified after digestion of Trastuzumab with trypsin by LC/MS/MS analysis.

Light Chain		Heavy Chain	
Measured Molecular Weight (Da)	**Peptide Length**	**Measured Molecular Weight (Da)**	**Peptide Length**
1877.9	1–18	1881.1	1–19
691.4	19–24	1109.6	20–30
1989.5	25–42	1088.6	31–38
1771.9	46–61	829.5	44–50
4129.9	67–103	1083.5	51–59
1945.0	109–126	968.5	68–76
1739.9	127–142	1309.7	77–87
2134.9	150–169	1276.3	88–98
1501.6	170–183	2729.4	226–251
1817.5	191–207	834.4	252–295
		2081.2	259–277
		1676.8	278–291
		1188.5	296–304
		1806.9	305–320
		837.5	330–337
		1285.7	348–358
		1103.7	364–373
		2543.2	374–395
		1872.9	396–412
		2743.3	420–442
		787.5	443–450

Table 4. Peptides identified after digestion of Bevacizumab with trypsin by LC/MS/MS analysis.

Light Chain		Heavy Chain	
Measured Molecular Weight (Da)	**Peptide Length**	**Measured Molecular Weight (Da)**	**Peptide Length**
1877.9	1–18	1881.1	1–19
2743.3	19–42	2139.9	20–38
1761.9	46–61	2517.3	44–65
4602.4	62–103	1044.5	68–76
1945.0	109–126	1282.6	77–87
1739.9	127–142	1232.7	88–98
2134.9	150–169	3322.6	99–127
1501.6	170–183	1185.7	128–139
1817.5	191–207	1263.7	140–153
		2729.4	229–254
		834.4	255–261
		2081.2	262–280
		1676.8	281–294
		1188.5	299–307
		1806.9	308–323
		837.5	333–340
		1285.7	351–361
		1103.7	367–376
		2543.2	377–389
		1872.9	399–415
		2743.3	423–445

Table 5. Peptides identified after digestion of Cetuximab with trypsin by LC/MS/MS analysis.

Light Chain		Heavy Chain	
Measured Molecular Weight (Da)	**Peptide Length**	**Measured Molecular Weight (Da)**	**Peptide Length**
1923.2	1–18	3504.8	6–38
1787.9	25–39	2569.3	44–66
1265.4	50–61	754.4	76–81
4507.9	62–103	1848.8	82–97
1945.0	109–126	2904.4	98–123
1739.9	127–142	1185.6	124–135
2134.9	150–169	1263.6	136–149
1501.6	170–183	2729.4	229–254
1817.5	191–207	834.4	255–261
		2081.2	262–280
		1676.8	281–294
		1188.5	299–307
		1806.9	308–323
		837.5	333–340
		1285.7	351–361
		1103.7	367–376
		2543.2	377–389
		1872.9	399–415
		2743.3	423–445
		787.5	446–453

Results demonstrate that the obtained data allows the verification of the correctness of more than 80% of the amino acid sequence of the various proteins and is therefore suitable for the evaluation of the chemical stability of monoclonal antibodies and other proteins for therapeutic use.

Moving on to the investigation of tertiary protein structure, stability was investigated via SEC, applying an indirect quantization method. In detail, gel filtration chromatography equipped with UV-DAD detection was exploited to evaluate the hydrodynamic mobility, which was directly proportional to the conformation and the state of aggregation of the analyzed proteins. To optimize and verify this approach, for each mAbs, the exact retention time and the profile were determined on Day 1 and after 10 days of exposure to samples at stress conditions, i.e., light, not controlled humidity, and room temperature. Comparing obtained chromatograms, it was possible to observe no changes in both retention time and peak profile clearly attributable to the formation of oligomers of the analyzed monoclonal antibodies, confirming the accuracy of the present method to detect any changes to the tertiary structure.

3.2.2. Stability Investigation of Compounded Drug Products Containing Antibodies

We used the developed method to analyze the residual compounded HER, AVA, and ERB from compounding in Gragnano Hospital stored at 4 °C for three weeks.

For HER, the chemical and physical stability of the reconstituted solutions in water for injection under aseptic conditions is reported in its SmPC to be 48 h at 2–8 °C. Interestingly, after aseptic dilution in polyvinylchloride, polyethylene, or polypropylene bags containing sodium chloride 9 mg/mL (0.9%) solution for injection, physicochemical stability has been demonstrated at 24 h at temperatures not exceeding 30 °C and up to 30 days at 2–8 °C [17,42].

Regarding AVA, available data in its SMPC on physicochemical in-use stability of the diluted medicinal product is reported as 30 days at 2 °C to 8 °C plus an additional 48 h at 2 °C to 30 °C in sodium chloride 9 mg/mL (0.9%) solution for injection.

Considering the chemical and physical in-use stability of ERB, the expiration date is after 48 h at 25 °C.

Peptide mapping investigation of residual compounded drugs highlighted no changes in the primary sequence of the antibodies among data obtained during the time frame of the present stability study. In detail, LC-MS/MS analyses revealed that in all three cases, the average molecular weight did not vary significantly over the period analyzed (21 days, Table 6), demonstrating that no modification of the primary structure of the proteins occurred.

Table 6. Stability data expressed as average MW of Trastuzumab, Bevacizumab, and Cetuximab after LC-MS/MS analysis.

	Trastuzumab (Mw ± st. dev.)	**Bevacizumab (Mw ± st. dev.)**	**Cetuximab (Mw ± st. dev.)**
Day 1	145,534 ± 4	149,195 ± 4	145,783 ± 5
Day 2	145,533 ± 5	149,195 ± 4	145,786 ± 3
Day 3	145,534 ± 2	149,198 ± 3	145,784 ± 4
Day 4	145,536 ± 5	149,196 ± 5	145,784 ± 5
Day 5	145,532 ± 2	149,197 ± 3	145,784 ± 4
Day 8	145,535 ± 3	149,194 ± 6	145,787 ± 2
Day 10	145,538 ± 6	149,199 ± 8	145,783 ± 6
Day 12	145,530 ± 5	149,197 ± 2	145,782 ± 5
Day 15	145,534 ± 5	149,195 ± 3	145,782 ± 6
Day 18	145,535 ± 2	149,195 ± 7	145,784 ± 4
Day 22	145,531 ± 2	149,197 ± 4	145,783 ± 3

Finally, results obtained from gel filtration analysis demonstrated that for none of the three antibodies, it was possible to observe significant variations in the state of oligomerization during the entire investigation period. Retention time, intensity, and shape of the chromatographic peaks relating to each species do not show significant changes, suggesting the conformational stability of the antibodies during the three weeks of storage at 4 °C. This finding is very interesting considering the short half-life normally defined for compounded drug products containing antibodies, though depending on the product.

We have to consider that the short half-life indicated for this subset of antiblastic medicine is largely based on the possible biological risk and not on intrinsic physicochemical instability. However, results from the present research suggest that the selected monoclonal antibody-based compounded drugs have stability over time greater than that reported, and the residues can be safely used, providing that preservation in aseptic conditions can be guaranteed.

4. Conclusions

The ever-increasing adoption of personalized medicine approaches underlines the need for healthcare providers to optimize the balance between the quality of patient care and the financial aspects of the healthcare system. Resource recovery policy could be a valid pathway to meet this aim.

This policy became more relevant in application to the extemporaneous magistral formulation of antiblastic medicines characterized by high costs, high frequency of administration to different patients in different doses, and large waste production. In fact, the stability of antiblastic compounded drugs, frequently established to a few hours/days for microbiological needs, becomes a limiting factor to clinical practice, whereas the physicochemical stability of specific molecules may be much longer, and the content of API may remain steady in compounded formulations. However, the limit for a second use is still in the absence of universal guidelines that describe procedures to be applied for the evaluation of the stability of drug product residues, and, as a consequence, residual compounded drugs are considered waste.

The actual shelf-life of compounded drugs must be evaluated by analytical techniques, i.e., HPLC-DAD, or LC-MS/MS, with good sensitivity and capability of identification of target analyte and effective in protein analysis (LC–MS/MS). These techniques can be integrated into the routine practices of centralized compounding units to perform fast physicochemical stability assays of daily residual compounded drugs.

In this respect, results reported in the present paper, though at a preliminary stage, are very informative for the daily practice of hospitals and may offer a tool for the safe and efficient reduction of waste production and disposal and re-use of the preparations because the drug sensitivity to physicochemical factors during the preparation, managing, and storage phases seems to be limited for the studied API.

In fact, the present case study showed how several compounded drugs with different physicochemical characteristics are stable until three weeks post-compounding.

The re-use for other patients represents a potentially valuable resource to enhance cost-effectiveness in personalized anticancer therapy.

In particular, considering the possible shelf-life extension overall evidenced by this case study in relation to the annual financial report of ASL Na3, comprising medicines frequency of use and costs, it is possible to forecast an annual economic resource recovery for these medicines of about EUR 820,000, taking into account the total value recovered for potential medicine packages saved and the total value recovered for potential residual product secondary use. At this point, an optimization of the workflow and working time must be added, as well as a reduction in the costly operators' engagement.

These interesting results obtained integrating a centralization of drug administration with a proper re-use of residuals can be a valid foothold to the hospital pharmacist for a conscious decision to go beyond the expiration date reported in the SmPCs of a specific anticancer medicine and to obtain economically advantageous exploiting a potential extended use of the residues.

Other studies focusing on the clinical outcomes are necessary for an extended adoption in clinical practice in the near future, hoping for concrete support from regulatory agencies in the definition of standard guidelines.

Author Contributions: Conceptualization, R.P.A., P.R. and E.N.; methodology, P.D.G., G.F. and F.D.P.; formal analysis, P.D.G., F.D.P. and G.A.; resources, E.N. and S.C.; data curation, P.D.G., G.F. and F.D.P.; writing—original draft preparation, R.P.A., P.R. and F.M.d.F.; writing—review and editing, R.P.A., P.R. and F.M.d.F.; supervision, P.R.; funding acquisition, R.P.A. and P.R. All authors have read and agreed to the published version of the manuscript.

Funding: This research was funded by Local Health Authority Naples 3 South, within the following project: Supporto tecnico scientifico per l'implementazione delle attività previste dal progetto denominato implementazione UFA.—centralizzazione preparazione farmaci antiblastici—galenica oncologica.

Institutional Review Board Statement: Not applicable.

Informed Consent Statement: Not applicable.

Data Availability Statement: The original contributions presented in this study are included in the article. Further inquiries can be directed at the corresponding author.

Conflicts of Interest: The authors declare no conflicts of interest.

Abbreviations

API	Active Pharmaceutical Ingredient
ABR	Abraxane®
ALI	Alimta®
ASL Na3	Local Health Authority Naples 3 South
AVA	Avastin®
ERBI	Erbitux®
GERPAC	Evaluation and Research Group on Protection in Controlled Atmosphere
GHPMP	Good Hospital Pharmacy Manufacturing Practice
HER	Herceptin®
JEV	Jevtana®
MS	Mass spectroscopy
PBS	Phosphate-buffered saline
PDI	Polydispersity index
SDS_PAGE	Sodium Dodecyl Sulfate—PolyAcrylamide Gel Electrophoresis
SEC	Size exclusion chromatography
SFPC	French Society of Clinical Pharmacy
SmPCs	Summary of product characteristics
UFA	Unità Farmaci Antiblastici-Centralized Antiblastic Drug Unit
USP	United States Pharmacopeia

References

1. Mathur, S.; Sutton, J. Personalized medicine could transform healthcare (Review). *Biomed. Rep.* **2017**, *7*, 3–5. [CrossRef]
2. Chan, I.S.; Ginsburg, G.S. Personalized medicine: Progress and promise. *Annu. Rev. Genom. Hum. Genet.* **2011**, *12*, 217–244. [CrossRef]
3. Savchenko, E.; Bunimovich-Mendrazitsky, S. Investigation toward the economic feasibility of personalized medicine for healthcare service providers: The case of bladder cancer. *Front. Med.* **2024**, *11*, 1388685. [CrossRef] [PubMed]
4. Khashayar, V.; Jason, R.; Linda, S.F.; Samir, F. Optimizing physician staffing and resource allocation: Sine-wave variation in hourly trauma admission. *J. Trauma* **2007**, *62*, 610–614.
5. Arnedos, M.; Soria, J.-C.; Andre, F.; Tursz, T. Personalized treatments of cancer patients: A reality in daily practice, a costly dream or a shared vision of the future from the oncology community? *Cancer Treat. Rev.* **2014**, *40*, 1192–1198. [CrossRef] [PubMed]
6. Sewell, G.; Plumridge, R. Dose-banding of cytotoxic drugs: A new concept in cancer chemotherapy. *Am. J. Health-Syst. Pharm.* **2001**, *58*, 1760–1764.
7. Gonzalez-Angulo, A.M.; Hennessy, B.T.; Mills, G.B. Future of personalized medicine in oncology: A systems biology approach. *J. Clin. Oncol.* **2010**, *28*, 2777–2783. [CrossRef]
8. Buma, A.I.; Piet, B.; Ter Heine, R.; van den Heuvel, M.M. Integrating treatment cost reduction strategies and biomarker research to reduce costs and personalize expensive treatments: An example of a self-funding trial in non-small cell lung cancer. *Front. Pharmacol.* **2023**, *14*, 1274532. [CrossRef] [PubMed]
9. Massimiliano, B.; Raffaele Di, F. Editorial: The Real Impact of Target Therapy in Cancer Patients: Between Hope and Reality. *Curr. Cancer Drug Targets* **2018**, *18*, 402–404. [CrossRef]

10. Handorf, E.A.; McElligott, S.; Vachani, A.; Langer, C.J.; Bristol Demeter, M.; Armstrong, K.; Asch, D.A. Cost effectiveness of personalized therapy for first-line treatment of stage IV and recurrent incurable adenocarcinoma of the lung. *J. Oncol. Pract.* **2012**, *8*, 267–274. [CrossRef] [PubMed]
11. Bakshi, M.; Singh, S. Development of validated stability-indicating assay methods—Critical review. *J. Pharm. Biomed. Anal.* **2002**, *28*, 1011–1040. [CrossRef]
12. Adade, C.A.; Benabbes, M.; Belahcen, M.J.; Rahali, Y. Centralization impact and cost-saving study in a Moroccan hospital's centralized unit of chemotherapy preparation. *J. Oncol. Pharm. Pract.* **2020**, *26*, 1630–1636. [CrossRef] [PubMed]
13. Bouwman, Y.; Andersen, L.M. GMP and preparation in hospital pharmacies. *Eur. J. Hosp. Pharm. Sci. Pract.* **2012**, *19*, 469. [CrossRef]
14. Bardin, C.; Astier, A.; Vulto, A.; Sewell, G.; Vigneron, J.; Trittler, R.; Daouphars, M.; Paul, M.; Trojniak, M.; Pinguet, F. Guidelines for the practical stability studies of anticancer drugs: A European consensus conference. *Ann. Pharm. Françaises* **2011**, *69*, 221–231. [CrossRef] [PubMed]
15. International Conference of Harmonization (ICH). Guidelines for Stability. Available online: https://www.ich.org/page/quality-guidelines (accessed on 4 March 2024).
16. Rai, K.; Potphode, P.; Gupta, C.; Rao, N. Comparitive study between ICH guideline and anvisa guideline. *Int. J. Res. Pharm. Chem.* **2020**, *10*, 173–190. [CrossRef]
17. Astier, A. Practical stability studies: A powerful approach for reducing the cost of monoclonal antibodies. *Eur. J. Oncol. Pharm.* **2012**, *6*, 4–6.
18. Chiumente, M.; Rivano, M.; Severino, D.; Bertoli, S.; Gasbarro, A.R.; Santeramo, R.; Pasqualini, A.; Provasi, R.; Mengato, D.; Palozzo, A.C. Oncostability: Stability of reconstituted and diluted anticancer medicines for a possible extension of use. *Eur. J. Hosp. Pharm.* **2023**, *30*, e112. [CrossRef]
19. Fasola, G.; Aita, M.; Marini, L.; Follador, A.; Tosolini, M.; Mattioni, L.; Mansutti, M.; Piga, A.; Brusaferro, S.; Aprile, G. Drug waste minimisation and cost-containment in Medical Oncology: Two-year results of a feasibility study. *BMC Health Serv. Res.* **2008**, *8*, 70. [CrossRef] [PubMed]
20. Ioele, G.; Chieffallo, M.; Occhiuzzi, M.A.; De Luca, M.; Garofalo, A.; Ragno, G.; Grande, F. Anticancer Drugs: Recent Strategies to Improve Stability Profile, Pharmacokinetic and Pharmacodynamic Properties. *Molecules* **2022**, *27*, 5436. [CrossRef] [PubMed]
21. Vigneron, J.; Astier, A.; Trittler, R.; Hecq, J.D.; Daouphars, M.; Larsson, I.; Pourroy, B.; Pinguet, F. SFPO and ESOP recommendations for the practical stability of anticancer drugs: An update. *Ann. Pharm. Françaises* **2013**, *71*, 376–389. [CrossRef] [PubMed]
22. EMA. Summary of Product Characteristics (Alimta). Available online: https://www.ema.europa.eu/en/medicines/human/EPAR/alimta (accessed on 28 November 2024).
23. EMA. Summary of Product Characteristics (Abraxane). Available online: https://www.ema.europa.eu/en/medicines/human/EPAR/abraxane (accessed on 28 November 2024).
24. EMA, Summary of Product Characteristics (Jevtana). Available online: https://www.ema.europa.eu/en/medicines/human/EPAR/jevtana (accessed on 28 November 2024).
25. EMA. Summary of Product Characteristics (Herceptin). Available online: https://www.ema.europa.eu/en/medicines/human/EPAR/herceptin (accessed on 28 November 2024).
26. EMA. Summary of Product Characteristics (Avastin). Available online: https://www.ema.europa.eu/en/medicines/human/EPAR/avastin (accessed on 28 November 2024).
27. EMA. Summary of Product Characteristics (Erbitux). Available online: https://www.ema.europa.eu/en/medicines/human/EPAR/erbitux (accessed on 28 November 2024).
28. Deeb, T.; Brunotte, R.; Hubenia, O.; Leal-Marin, S.; Glasmacher, B. Advancements in Cryogenic Freezing Instrumentation for Cryopreservation. *Annu. Rev. Heat Transf.* **2024**, *27*, 2024053933. [CrossRef]
29. de Lemos, M.L.; Hamata, L. Stability issues of parenteral chemotherapy drugs. *J. Oncol. Pharm. Pract.* **2007**, *13*, 27–31. [CrossRef]
30. SFPC (French Society of Clinical Pharmacy); GERPAC (Evaluation and Research Group on Protection in Controlled Atmosphere). *Methodological Guidelines for Stability Studies of Hospital Pharmaceutical Preparations*; Print Conseil: Romagnat, France, 2013; Volume 1.
31. *United States Pharmacopeia 44, National Formulary 39*; U.S. Pharmacopeial Convention Inc.: Rockville, MD, USA, 2021.
32. Venkatesh, B.; Mathrusri Annapurna, M.; Pramadvara, K. Analytical stress degradation studies of cabazitaxel (a semi synthetic natural taxoid) using liquid chromatography. *Pharm. Methods* **2015**, *6*, 137. [CrossRef]
33. D'Huart, E.; Sacrez, M.; Vigneron, J.; Sobalak, N.; Demoré, B. Physicochemical stability of Cabazitaxel Zentiva® solution in vials after opening and diluted solutions in three infusion bags. *Pharm. Technol. Hosp. Pharm.* **2023**, *8*, 20220009. [CrossRef]
34. Manning, M.C.; Chou, D.K.; Murphy, B.M.; Payne, R.W.; Katayama, D.S. Stability of Protein Pharmaceuticals: An Update. *Pharm. Res.* **2010**, *27*, 544–575. [CrossRef] [PubMed]

35. Hawe, A.; Wiggenhorn, M.; van de Weert, M.; Garbe, J.H.O.; Mahler, H.-c.; Jiskoot, W. Forced Degradation of Therapeutic Proteins. *J. Pharm. Sci.* **2012**, *101*, 895–913. [CrossRef] [PubMed]
36. Kaur, H. Stability testing in monoclonal antibodies. *Crit. Rev. Biotechnol.* **2021**, *41*, 692–714. [CrossRef]
37. Vieillard, V.; Le Guyader, G.; Jallades, A.; Astier, A. Extended physicochemical stability of cetuximab in opened vials and infusion bags when stored at 4 °C and 25 °C. *J. Oncol. Pharm. Pract.* **2023**, *30*, 142–150. [CrossRef]
38. Carpanese, D.; Rossi, V.; Di Paolo, V.; Quintieri, L.; Penna, A.; Zuccolotto, G.; Sebellin, J.; Saran, C.; Pipitone, F.; Miolo, G.; et al. Prolonging the stability of cetuximab (Erbitux®) and panitumumab (Vectibix®): An orthogonal assessment of physicochemical, biological and microbiological properties of original opened glass vials and diluted saline preparations. *Int. J. Pharm.* **2024**, *649*, 123643. [CrossRef]
39. Aebersold, R.; Mann, M. Mass-spectrometric exploration of proteome structure and function. *Nature* **2016**, *537*, 347–355. [CrossRef] [PubMed]
40. Izzo, V.; Charlier, B.; Bloise, E.; Pingeon, M.; Romano, M.; Finelli, A.; Vietri, A.; Conti, V.; Manzo, V.; Alfieri, M.; et al. A UHPLC–MS/MS-based method for the simultaneous monitoring of eight antiblastic drugs in plasma and urine of exposed healthcare workers. *J. Pharm. Biomed. Anal.* **2018**, *154*, 245–251. [CrossRef] [PubMed]
41. Charlier, B.; Coglianese, A.; De Rosa, F.; Cozzolino, A.; Boccia, G.; Borrelli, A.; Capunzo, M.; Genovese, G.; De Caro, F.; Filippelli, A.; et al. A LC-MS/MS based methodology for the environmental monitoring of healthcare settings contaminated with antineoplastic agents. *J. Public Health Res.* **2023**, *12*, 22799036231160629. [CrossRef]
42. Nalenz, H.; Köpf, E.; Dietel, E. Prolonged In-use Stability of Reconstituted Herceptin in Commercial Intravenous Bags. *Int. J. Pharm. Compd.* **2018**, *22*, 417–423. [PubMed]

pharmaceutics

MDPI

Article

Evaluation of Five Ready-to-Use Bases for the Topical Administration of Propranolol Hydrochloride to Treat Infantile Hemangioma

Chiara Lacassia [1], Annalisa Cutrignelli [1], Flavia Maria la Forgia [2], Sergio Fontana [2], Antonio Lopalco [1,*], Nunzio Denora [1] and Angela Assunta Lopedota [1]

[1] Department of Pharmacy-Pharmaceutical Sciences, University of Bari Aldo Moro, 70125 Bari, Italy; chiara.lacassia@uniba.it (C.L.); annalisa.cutrignelli@uniba.it (A.C.); nunzio.denora@uniba.it (N.D.); angelaassunta.lopedota@uniba.it (A.A.L.)

[2] Centro Studi Ricerche "Dr. S. Fontana 1900–1982", Farmalabor s.r.l., 76012 Canosa di Puglia, Italy; f.laforgia@farmalabor.it (F.M.l.F.); s.fontana@farmalabor.it (S.F.)

* Correspondence: antonio.lopalco@uniba.it; Tel.: +39-0805442764

Abstract

Background/Objectives: Since 2008, following clinical studies conducted on children that revealed the ability of the β-adrenergic antagonist propranolol to inhibit capillary growth in infantile hemangiomas (IHs), its oral administration has become the first-line treatment for IHs. Although oral propranolol therapy at a dosage of 3 mg/kg/die is effective, it can cause systemic adverse reactions. This therapy is not necessarily applicable to all patients. Topical skin applications could help maintain a high drug concentration at local sites and also represent a characteristically easy method of administration for pediatric patients. Because no topical propranolol dosage forms are commercially available, such formulations may be prepared at hospitals and pharmacies. **Methods**: In the present study, we identified a simple method for preparing topical propranolol hydrochloride formulations at 1% *w/w* with five commercial ready-to-use bases and evaluated the pharmaceutical profiles. The physical stability of the extemporaneous formulations was predicted by performing an accelerated centrifuge test and assessed by visual inspection after one month storage at 25 °C. The chemical stability of the drug in the five formulations was assessed by using a high-performance liquid chromatography (HPLC) method. In vitro drug-release and permeability experiments were conducted through synthetic membranes and the outer pavilion of a pig's ear by utilizing Franz-type diffusion cells. **Results**: The results indicated that the release of the drug was significantly influenced by the internal structure and physicochemical properties of each base. **Conclusions**: Specifically, the formulations prepared with the hydrophilic bases could be easily prepared and yield satisfactory results, representing a potential effective therapy for IHs in pediatric patients.

Keywords: propranolol hydrochloride; formulation; topical; hemangioma; pediatric; compounding; off-label; repurposing; repositioning

1. Introduction

Infantile hemangiomas (IHs) are the most common childhood benign tumors [1], caused by uncontrolled proliferation from vascular endothelial cells. IHs appear soon after birth, forming skin spots that may be light in hue and covered with dilated small capillaries named telangiectasias. These tumors grow rapidly in size, intensity, color (red or bluish spots), and texture and tend to stabilize or regress in 7 to 8 years [2,3]. Often, IHs do not cause significant concern and only require careful monitoring of the skin lesion. However, in about 12% of cases, especially in multiple or segmental forms, complications can arise that may require specialist consultation and prompt treatment [4].

Until 2008, local or oral administration of corticosteroids, interferon-alpha, and vincristine was the first-line treatment of choice for IHs together with highly invasive therapy, such as surgical and laser interventions. In 2008 in France, the "off-label" therapeutic benefits of oral propranolol in the benign tumor IHs were randomly discovered in a clinical trial conducted on children with hypertrophic obstructive cardiomyopathy [5]. Since then, the oral administration of propranolol [6] has become the first-line treatment for IHs, showing its ability to block the tumor's growth phase and rapidly induce regression, leading to its repurposing for the treatment of various rare diseases [7,8].

Propranolol hydrochloride (PRP-HCl) (Figure 1) is a non-specific β1- and β2-adrenergic receptor (ADRB1-2) antagonist, prescribed for hypertension, irregular heart rate, essential tremor, and anxiety.

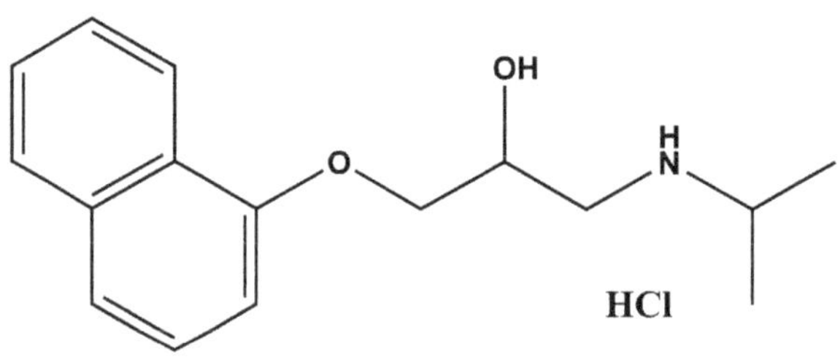

Figure 1. Chemical structure of propranolol hydrochloride (PRP-HCl).

However, oral administration of PRP-HCl for the treatment of IHs can cause several adverse effects, such as bradycardia, hypotension, and hypoglycemia [9]. Therefore, topical formulations of PRP-HCl are considered an appealing approach to selectively deliver the drug at the focal sites of the tumor and easily administer the therapy to pediatric patients [6]. Nowadays, there is no industrial topical medicine of PRP-HCl, so to provide appropriate therapy for IHs, the only alternative is to prepare extemporaneous formulations in a pharmacy or hospital.

Several studies have highlighted substantial variability in the formulations of topical propranolol, employing diverse pharmaceutical vehicles. For instance, Xu et al. prepared an ointment by combining crushed propranolol tablets with petroleum jelly [10], Kunzi-Rapp compounded a hydrophilic ointment in a hospital pharmacy [11], and Price et al. reported the development of a nano-propranolol hydrogel designed to enhance transdermal delivery [12].

The preparation of topical propranolol demonstrates a high degree of customization across studies, underscoring the adaptability of pharmaceutical compounding to meet specific therapeutic requirements. However, no universally recognized optimal dosage for topical propranolol in the treatment of IHs has been established. The concentrations employed in studies ranged from 0.5% to 5% *w/w*. Notably, Price et al.'s systematic review found no correlation between higher concentrations and improved efficacy [12], suggesting that lower concentrations may be equally effective while reducing the risk of local adverse effects. Although a single optimum dosage regimen remains elusive, the evidence suggests that a PRP-HCl concentration of 1% to 2% *w/w* appears effective [13,14].

In the galenic field, vehicle preparation is the longest and most delicate phase of setting up an extemporaneous formulation. A series of small-scale tests to fine-tune the most suitable vehicle for incorporating a given active are necessary, investing considerable time and raw materials. Pharmacists can expedite extemporaneous formulation by employing ready-to-use vehicles while upholding the highest quality standards [15,16]. The composition of the ready-to-use base, however, must be carefully evaluated as it can influence the stability of the active ingredient, its release properties, and its ability to permeate through the skin, determining the effectiveness of the therapy. Therefore, a systematic study on different ready-to-use bases could be useful to identify an appropriate vehicle for a topical drug to minimize the risk of errors during compounding, leading to safer and more effective treatments for patients.

This study aimed to rationalize the choice of a ready-to-use base able to vehicle PRP-HCl for the topical treatment of IHs. In earlier investigations, a preliminary assessment was conducted to evaluate the incorporation of various active pharmaceutical ingredients (APIs), including PRP-HCl [17,18], across a broader range of ready-to-use bases already on the worldwide market. This effort aimed to provide pharmacists with optimized bases and preparation protocols that ensure the requisite quality and safety standards for galenic products. Building on these findings, five ready-to-use bases were selected as vehicles for the preparation of 1% *w*/*w* PRP-HCl formulations. Their physical stability was evaluated in real time and accelerated by centrifugation studies at 25 °C. In vitro drug-release tests were performed using Franz diffusion cells equipped with a cuprophane membrane, while for the permeability tests, the skin of the inner pinna of a pig's ear was used. Data collected from these in vitro analyses were used to elaborate mathematical models to describe the drug-release phenomena with the best relevance. The high-performance liquid chromatography (HPLC) method demonstrated the drug's chemical stability in the five formulations.

2. Materials and Methods

PRP-HCl (Lot No. F2400149), Klimt (Lot No. W2204038), Caravaggio (Lot No. W2303637), Modigliani (Lot No. W2002165), Burri (Lot No. R1818671), and Warhol (Lot No. R1811917) were provided by Farmalabor s.r.l. (Canosa di Puglia, Italy). The characteristics and compositions of the five bases are reported in Table 1: as shown in their composition, the first four bases (Burri, Caravaggio, Klimt, and Modigliani) are oil-in-water creams, while the last one (Warhol) is a hydrophobic ointment, able to emulsify a small amount of water due to the presence of lanolin and the two surfactants cetyl and stearyl alcohol.

Methanol (Lot No. M1230S, Honeywell, Charlotte, NC, USA), Water for HPLC (Lot No. 2223457), NaH_2PO_4 (Lot No. BCBJ8797V, Sigma-Aldrich, Milan, Italy), hydrogen peroxide (H_2O_2, 35%, Lot No. 21.4722903.500, CHEMLAB Analytical), NaOH pellets for analysis (Lot No. B1543269 847, Merk, Milan, Italy), H_3PO_4 (>85%, Lot No. SZBC 1860V, Merk), and HCl (ACS reagent 37%, Lot No. 1320A, Honeywell Fluka™) were supplied by Levanchimica s.r.l. (Bari, Italy). The glass beakers, vials, graduated cylinders and pipettes, and volumetric flasks used were in borosilicate and supplied by Levanchimica s.r.l. (Bari, Italy).

Table 1. Characteristics and composition of ready-to-use bases.

Base	pH and Viscosity (cP)	Composition
Burri Cream base	3.5 ± 0.5; 4000–30,000	Aqua q.s. to 100%; Glyceryl stearate SE 8%; Cetyl Alcohol/Stearyl Alcohol 2%; Oryza sativa brain oil 5%; Ethylhexyl Palmitate 7%; Tocopheryl acetate 0.25%; Sodium Cetearyl sulfate 1.5%; Glycerin 2%; Benzyl alcohol 0.5%; Xanthan gum 0.3%; Lecithin 0.2; Tocopherol 0.2%; Ascorbyl Palmitate 0.1; Citric Acid 0.05%; Tartaric acid q.s. to the required pH.
Caravaggio Amphiphilic cream base	5.5 ± 0.5; 20,000–100,000	Aqua q.s. to 100%; Petrolatum 25.5%; Propylene Glycol 10%; Caprilyc/Capric Triglyceride 7.5%; PEG-40 stearate 7%; Cetearyl Alcohol 6%; GlycerylStearate 4%; Phenoxyethanol 0.5%; Sodium Benzoate 0.4%; Potassium Sorbate 0.3%; Citric Acid q.s. to the required pH.
Klimt Cetomacrogol cream base	5.5 ± 0.5; 4000–40,000	Aqua q.s. to 100%; Petrolatum 15%; Cetearyl Alcohol 50/50 7.2%; Paraffinum Liquidum 6%; Ceteareth-20 1.8%; Benzyl Alcohol 0.5%; Sodium Benzoate 0.4%; Potassium Sorbate 0.3%; Disodium EDTA 0.1%; Citric Acid q.s. to the required pH.

Table 1. *Cont.*

Base	pH and Viscosity (cP)	Composition
Modigliani Antioxidant cream base	5.5 ± 0.5; 20,000–100,000	Aqua q.s.to 100%; Petrolatum 25.5%; Propylene Glycol 10%; Caprilyc/Capric Triglyceride 7.5%; PEG-40 stearate 7%; Glyceryl Stearate 4%; Cetyl Alcohol 3%; Stearyl alcohol 3%; Phenoxyethanol 0.5%; Sodium Benzoate 0.4%; Sodium Metabisulfite 0.4%; Potassium Sorbate 0.3%; Disodium EDTA 0.1%; Citric Acid q.s. to pH.
Warhol Petrolatum-lanolin base	-	Petrolatum q.b. a 100%; Lanolin 5%; Cetyl alcohol 2.5%; Stearyl alcohol 2.5%.

2.1. Preparation of Topical PRP-HCl Formulations

The semisolid formulations were prepared as described in the procedures reported in the Good Preparation Practices guidelines [19,20] by solubilizing approximately 100 mg of PRP-HCl weighed on a balance in 200 μL of distilled water [17,18]. Then, the solution of the API was mixed (for 5 min) with 9.7 g of the selected base weighed on a balance in the same beaker with a glass stick until evenly dispersed and then put in a plastic pack (PP, 20 mL volume capacity, Farmalabor s.r.l.). The samples were prepared in triplicate, and the qualitative–quantitative compositions are shown in Table 2.

Table 2. Samples prepared and their qualitative–quantitative composition.

Sample	Base (g)	API (mg)	Solvent (μL)
Modigliani 1	9.745	100.01	200
Modigliani 2	9.777	100.20	200
Modigliani 3	9.721	100.39	200
Sample	**Base (g)**	**API (mg)**	**Solvent (μL)**
Caravaggio 1	9.746	100.84	200
Caravaggio 2	9.669	100.61	200
Caravaggio 3	9.676	101.18	200
Sample	**Base (g)**	**API (mg)**	**Solvent (μL)**
Burri 1	9.744	98.50	200
Burri 2	9.745	99.95	200
Burri 3	9.770	98.55	200
Sample	**Base (g)**	**API (mg)**	**Solvent (μL)**
Klimt 1	9.681	98.90	200
Klimt 2	9.696	98.29	200
Klimt 3	9.736	98.86	200
Sample	**Base (g)**	**API (mg)**	**Solvent (μL)**
Warhol 1	9.704	99.34	200
Warhol 2	9.776	99.40	200
Warhol 3	9.774	99.95	200

2.2. HPLC Method

Quantitative analysis of the samples was conducted by a Shimadzu HPLC Nexera series equipped with a photodiode array detector and an SIL-40C autosampler using the method described by Lopalco A. and coworkers [21]. The system was equipped with a hyperclone ODS C18 250 mm × 4.6 × 5 μm column thermostated at 35 °C. An isocratic elution at a flow rate of 1.0 mL/min was used, and the ultraviolet detection was carried out at 254 nm. Each sample injection had a 20 μL volume. The mobile phase was acetonitrile, methanol, and an aqueous solution of 0.01 M sodium phosphate dibasic adjusted to pH = 2.7 with phosphoric acid in a ratio of volumes 50:35:15 (% *v*/*v*).

A stock solution of 1 mg/mL PRP-HCl in a 30% (*v*/*v*) methanol/water mixture was used to create six different diluted solutions for the calibration curve and verify the linearity. The mean area of each sample, calculated on triplicate injections, was plotted against its concentration using the least squares regression method. The linearity range was demonstrated between 1.008 µg/mL and 100.8 µg/mL ($R^2 > 0.9999$). Each analysis lasted 8 min, and the drug peak retention time was about 5 min. The slope of the calibration curve and the standard deviation of the curve response (Sy) were used to calculate the lower limit of detection (LOD) and lower limit of quantification (LOQ) by using equation 1 and 2, respectively:

$$\text{LOD} = 3.3\frac{\text{Sy}}{\text{Slope}} \quad (1)$$

$$\text{LOQ} = 10\frac{\text{Sy}}{\text{Slope}} \quad (2)$$

LOD and LOQ were 0.18 µg/mL and 0.54 µg/mL, respectively.

2.3. Accelerated and Real-Tme Physical Stability Studies

An accelerated centrifuge test was conducted to assess the formulations' physical stability. The protocol was established starting from the evidence reported by Sopyan and coworkers [22], who reported that centrifuge tests could simulate the effect of gravity for a specific period. A total of 10 g of each sample was put in a 15 mL falcon tube and subjected to 5 centrifugation cycles of 30 min each in a ThermoScientific SL 16R centrifuge (Thermo Fisher Scientific, Rodano, Milan, Italy). The temperature and the speed were set at 25 °C and 3800 rpm, respectively. Under these conditions, one centrifugation cycle corresponded to the effect of gravity of approximately 1.2 months.

For the assessment of the real-time physical stability, each formulation was kept at 25 °C and 60% RH in a climatic chamber (Climacell; MMM Medcenter; Munich; Germany) for 30 days. The samples were observed, simulating a daily use condition, in terms of organoleptic characteristics (color and odor), pH values, and phase separation phenomena, which may serve as indicators of degradation processes or contamination over time.

2.4. Chemical Stability Study

The chemical stability of the API in the same samples subjected to real-time physical stability studies was investigated by HPLC analysis. Aliquots of 0.5 g of each formulation were taken and diluted in 10 mL of a 30% (*v*/*v*) methanol/water mixture, vortexed in a falcon tube, sonicated with an ultrasonic cleaner CP102 (FIOA International s.r.l., Arezzo, Italy) for two minutes, and finally centrifuged for 10 min at 25 °C and 13,000 rpm. After being separated, the supernatant was filtered with a PTFE 0.25 µm filter and diluted 10-fold with a 30% (*v*/*v*) methanol/water mixture before being analyzed by HPLC. By examining the chromatographic peaks and their areas in relation to the drug calibration curve, the concentration of PRP-HCl was determined.

2.5. In Vitro Release and Permeation Studies

Drug-release and permeation profiles were obtained by performing in vitro studies using Franz diffusion cells equipped with a cuprophane membrane and the skin of the inner pinna of a pig's ear, respectively. The membrane was first hydrated with the receptor solution to facilitate interaction with the formulation. The donor compartment was filled with 200 mg of each sample (corresponding to 2 mg of API), while a 0.1 M phosphate buffer solution at pH 7.4 was placed in the receiver compartment. The system was maintained at

37 °C throughout the experiment with a circulating water bath, and air bubbles between the solution and the membrane in the receptor compartment were properly eliminated. The 500 μL samples were withdrawn from the receiver compartment at predetermined times (0, 1, 2, 3, 4, 5, 6, 24 h), replaced with fresh receiver medium, and analyzed by using the HPLC method previously described. Sample collection up to 48 h was carried out in the case of releases through a synthetic membrane. The cumulative amount permeated through the membrane was calculated from the drug concentration in the receiving medium and plotted as a function of time. The amount of drug retained in the skin was determined by extraction from the tissue incubated overnight at 4 °C in 1 mL of acetonitrile. Data are the mean of three experiments, each one conducted in duplicate.

2.6. Mathematical Models and Kinetic Studies

Four mathematical models, i.e., zero-order, first-order, Higuchi–Connor, and Kosmeyer–Peppas, were used to investigate the PRP-HCl kinetic release from each formulation and rationalize the involved mechanisms. The experimental data, collected before reaching equilibrium, were processed as the cumulative amount of drug released over time using the four predefined equations. The correlation coefficient (R^2) for each mathematical model greater than 0.95 was taken into account and used as a first criterion to discard the models least suitable for describing the drug-release phenomenon. The mechanism of drug diffusion was evaluated considering the release exponent n calculated from the Kosmeyer–Peppas equation.

2.7. Statistical Analysis

Data are the mean of three experiments, each one conducted in duplicate. The relative values of the standard deviations (S.D.) were calculated using Microsoft Excel, and GraphPad Prism version 5.0 (San Diego, CA, USA) was used to fit the mathematical models in the release studies.

3. Results and Discussion

Currently, no commercial topical formulations of PRP-HCl are available for the treatment of IHs. To address this gap, this study aimed to evaluate five semisolid formulations prepared by using different ready-to-use bases as vehicles for the API. Ready-to-use bases in pharmaceutical compounding offer significant advantages over formulations from individual components, including greater efficiency, safety, and precision. These pre-formulated bases simplify preparation by ensuring ingredient stability and compatibility, allowing for pharmacists to focus on customizing therapies. They reduce errors, enhance stability by preventing degradation or incompatibility, and are compatible with a wide range of APIs, enabling tailored patient-specific medications without compromising formulation quality.

The five extemporaneous preparations were analyzed in terms of physical stability and in vitro drug-release and permeability profiles. The chemical stability of the drug within the formulations was also investigated, with the goal to propose a robust galenic alternative to effectively meet clinical needs.

3.1. Accelerated and Real-Time Physical Stability Studies

The parameters used in the accelerated assay, realized by a centrifugation procedure that typically exacerbates instability, simulated the effect of gravity on the sample for six months under storage conditions in order to predict phenomena such as phase separations or drug precipitation. Figure 2 shows the effect of different centrifugation cycles on each sample.

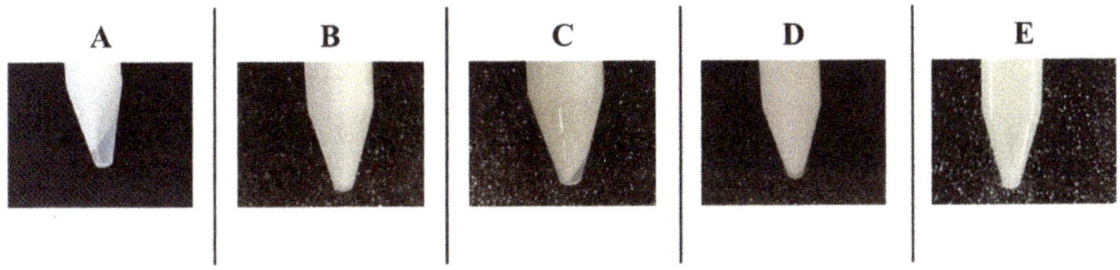

Figure 2. Representative images of 1% *w/w* PRP-HCl semisolid formulations in each ready-to-use base (Burri (**A**) at 4 cycles, Caravaggio (**B**) at 5 cycles, Klimt (**C**) at 4 cycles, Modigliani (**D**) at 5 cycles, Warhol (**E**) at 5 cycles) after the centrifugation test.

The lack of significant changes in the physical appearance of the creams prepared with the Caravaggio (B) and Modigliani (D) bases and the ointment prepared with the Warhol (E) base after five centrifugation cycles indicates the physical stability of these formulations up to 6 months (Figure 2). This result highlights strong excipient–drug interactions that balance well the overall formulation matrix, providing its structural integrity during the time. This is an important consideration for topical formulations, as physical stability is crucial for ensuring uniformity and consistency throughout the shelf-life of the product. In contrast, the creams prepared with the Burri (A) and Klimt (C) bases show an evident phase separation after four centrifugation cycles, highlighting a physical stability below 4 months. The different behavior observed among the formulations could be explained considering the composition and characteristics of the ready-to-use bases (Table 1). The Burri and Klimt bases are characterized by a lower viscosity (below 40,000 cPoise) compared to the Caravaggio and Modigliani bases (viscosity up to 100,000 cPoise). The viscosity of a dispersed system, such as a cream, influences its physical stability: as known from Stokes' law, the higher the viscosity the lower the speed with which phase separation phenomena (oil and water) occur. In regards to the formulation prepared with the Warhol base, its physical stability could be explained considering several aspects: it is a lipophilic ointment in a single phase constituted prevalently by petrolatum in which the quantity of water (200 µL) necessary to solubilize PRP-HCl is well dispersed for the presence of the excipient's lanolin, which has self-emulsifying properties, and the two surfactants cetyl and stearyl alcohol.

The real-time stability assay confirms the results observed with the accelerated test. All the formulations were stable after one month in a climatic chamber as described above. Furthermore, since the test was conducted by simulating in-use conditions of the products, the absence of variations in pH, odor, color, phase integrity, and microbiological contaminants observable by visual inspection may also indicate microbiological stability of the preparations. The lack of pH variations suggests that the formulations are well buffered and resilient to environmental factors that could otherwise cause acid–base shifts, affecting both the stability of the API and the overall product performance.

3.2. Chemical Stability Study

The chemical stability test represents a fundamental aspect of ensuring product quality and therapeutic efficacy. The chemical stability of PRP-HCl was demonstrated by HPLC at predefined time points (0, 15, 30 days) to quantitatively monitor the API in the formulations. Residual drug content values in the formulations stored at 25 °C are reported in Table 3. The results show that no drug degradation occurs after 30 days, since the HPLC chromatograms analyzed at each time did not highlight the presence of degradants. These findings show the suitability of the selected bases for maintaining the integrity of PRP-HCl in semisolid topical applications, providing a foundation for further in vitro investigations and clinical studies.

Table 3. Residual concentrations (%) of PRP-HCl and standard deviations (S.D.) in each sample stored at 25 °C for 30 days. Data are the mean of three experiments, each one conducted in duplicate.

Sample	PRP-HCl (%)		
	0	15 Days	30 Days
Modigliani	95.41 ± 3.81	95.06 ± 3.98	100.78 ± 2.58
Caravaggio	97.13 ± 1.22	96.96 ± 1.5	98.43 ± 5.41
Burri	99.37 ± 1.14	94.50 ± 6.6	99.64 ± 2.97
Klimt	96.62 ± 4.16	96.67 ± 1.5	97.13 ± 2.2
Warhol	88.74 ± 6.17	87.10 ± 4.12	90.74 ± 5.2

However, it is important to underline that, in the case of the formulation prepared with the ready-to-use Warhol base, the extracted quantity of API is always around 90%. These results can be explained by considering the nature of the base used, which is a single-phase lipophilic ointment. This type of vehicle probably has a high affinity towards the drug that is retained in the formulation and not completely extracted. In fact, PRP-HCl is a lipophilic molecule characterized by an octanol/water partition coefficient (Log P) equal to 2.81 [23]. This hypothesis will be further confirmed by the results obtained in the release studies with Franz cells.

3.3. *In Vitro Release and Permeation Studies*

Figure 3 illustrates the release profiles of PRP-HCl from creams formulated with the Caravaggio, Modigliani, and Klimt bases. The data obtained with the Burri and Warhol bases are not shown because it was not possible to quantify the drug in the receptor chamber due to its inadequate release from the formulations. As underlined previously in the chemical stability, the active ingredient has a Log P value that denotes its affinity towards the Warhol lipophilic base, resulting in a poor ability to pass into the aqueous receiving medium. Instead, in the case of the Burri base, the parameter limiting the drug release could be represented by its pH value (~3.5, see Table 1), lower than that of the other creams. Since the API is a hydrochloride salt, at that pH value, it is probably present in a dispersed form that is not able to cross the cuprophane membrane.

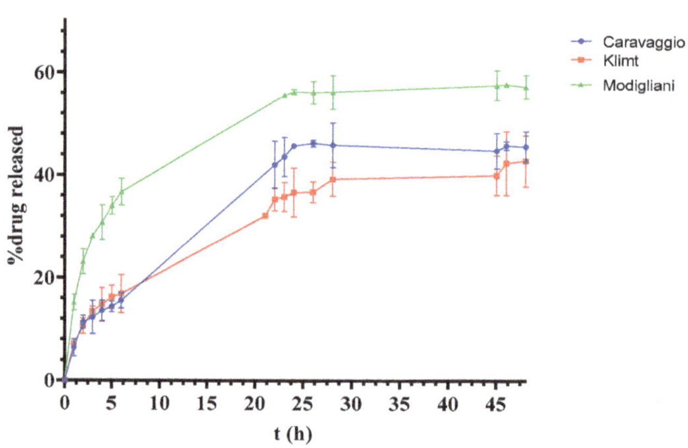

Figure 3. PRP-HCl release profile by Franz cell equipped with cuprophane membrane.

The Franz cell drug-release study revealed differences in the profiles among the other three tested formulations over 48 h. The Modigliani base exhibited the highest release percentage, with 57.61% ± 1.33 of PRP-HCl diffused through the membrane, followed by the Caravaggio base at 39.63% ± 1.73 and the Klimt base at 37.89% ± 2.84. These results suggest that the composition of the Modigliani base may enhance the solubilization or diffusion of PRP-HCl, potentially due to optimized interactions between the drug and the excipients. In details, as shown in Table 1, disodium EDTA, a well-known chelating agent, is present in the Modigliani base. EDTA can chelate metal ions, which are sometimes involved in the formation of insoluble salts or complexes with certain drugs. By binding these ions, EDTA could increase the solubility of the drug, enhancing its release from the formulation. In fact, the Caravaggio base, which has no EDTA in its composition, shows a lower drug-release value. On the other hand, the Klimt base, although containing EDTA, has a lower petrolatum content in its composition, partly replaced by liquid petrolatum (Table 1). Liquid petrolatum could likely create a real barrier on the hydrophilic cuprophane membrane, preventing the drug from crossing it.

Further investigation into the rheological properties and microstructural characteristics of these formulations may provide insights into the factors influencing release performance.

These findings emphasize the critical role of the base composition in determining the release kinetics of PRP-HCl and highlight the importance of tailoring formulation properties to achieve the desired therapeutic outcomes.

In contrast, the permeability study using the skin of the inner pinna of a pig's ear as the membrane demonstrated a markedly different trend in the percentage of PRP-HCl permeated over 24 h, specifically 13.75% ± 1.35, 17.68% ± 0.65, and 41.22% ± 0.35 for the Modigliani, Klimt, and Caravaggio bases, respectively (Figure 4). These findings suggest that, while the Modigliani base exhibited the highest release rate in the Franz cell studies with the cuprophane membrane, its permeation across a biological membrane was significantly lower compared to the Caravaggio base. This discrepancy may be attributed to the differing structural and chemical characteristics of the membranes. The cuprophane membrane, being synthetic and relatively inert, primarily reflects the release capacity of the formulation, whereas the pig's ear membrane, which better mimics human skin, provides a more physiologically relevant barrier, where factors such as lipid compatibility, excipient–drug interactions, and formulation viscosity could play a critical role in drug permeation.

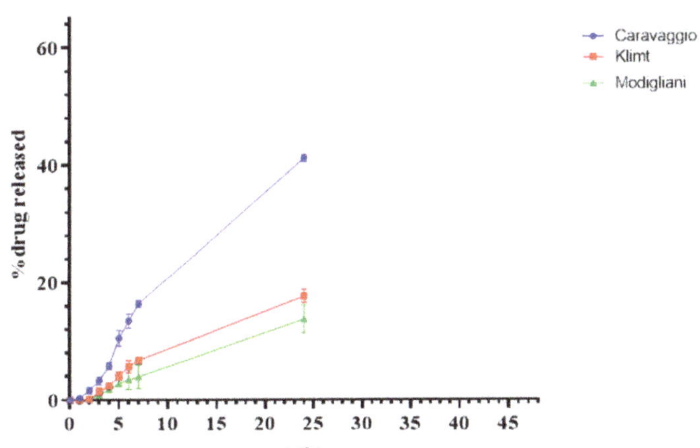

Figure 4. PRP-HCl release profile by Franz cell equipped with pig ear inner pavilion membrane.

It is important to underline that, in the permeability study, the intact skin of a pig's ear was used without separating the epidermis from the dermis. It is, therefore, a multilayer barrier with a lipophilic (stratum corneum) and hydrophilic (living epidermis and dermis) character in which the skin appendages are also present. Therefore, it is difficult to rationalize the result obtained by simply considering the compositions of the three ready-to-use bases. The superior permeation performance of the Caravaggio base (41.22%) across the pig's ear skin compared to the Modigliani (13.75%) and Klimt (17.68%) bases suggests that its composition may enhance drug partitioning into and diffusion through the lipid-rich environment of the biological membrane.

This highlights the importance of integrating both release and permeability studies when evaluating topical formulations. While synthetic membranes provide valuable insights into release profiles, biological membranes are essential for assessing real-world drug-delivery potential. Further characterization of the bases, including their lipid compatibility, partition coefficients, and interaction with skin components, will be necessary to fully elucidate the mechanisms driving these observed differences.

In addition to drug permeation, the amount of PRP-HCl accumulated in the pig's ear skin over 24 h was also evaluated, revealing values of 7.94% ± 0.3, 5.18% ± 0.23, and 4.45% ± 0.19 for the Modigliani, Caravaggio, and Klimt bases, respectively. These results are fully in agreement with the release and permeability data. In fact, the Modigliani base, which is the one that allows for a greater release of PRP-HCl, showed a lower permeability due to a lower ability to promote drug diffusion through the skin, guaranteeing a greater accumulation therein. This suggests that the Modigliani formulation may promote stronger interaction or binding of the drug to components of the biological membrane, such as lipids or proteins, leading to higher accumulation. Such retention could be advantageous for formulations designed for localized action, as it may prolong the presence of the drug at the site of application and potentially enhance therapeutic efficacy.

Conversely, the Caravaggio and Klimt bases exhibited lower drug accumulation in the skin, having higher drug permeation compared to the Modigliani base, favoring systemic absorption rather than localized retention. This behavior could decrease the therapeutic efficacy of the topical treatment, leading to the potential appearance of side effects. Furthermore, the possibility to have the lowest PRP-HCl permeated amounts seems interesting for a topical preparation intended to treat newborn patients. The limited drug permeation profile of the Modigliani base compared to that of the Caravaggio and Klimt creams evaluated on the pig ear inner pavilion membrane can be advantageous in such patients because their skin barrier is more permeable to xenobiotics in comparison to adults or children older than three-years old [13,14]. These observations underline the importance of balancing drug retention and permeation based on the therapeutic goals of the formulation. For conditions requiring localized drug delivery, such as in the treatment of IHs, cream formulations, like that obtained with the Modigliani ready-to-use base, may be preferable due to their enhanced accumulation within the dermis, where capillaries are localized.

3.4. Mathematical Models and Kinetic Studies

For the analysis of release profiles (Figure 3), in order to obtain valuable insights into the underlying mechanisms governing drug release from the different formulations [24], the most widespread kinetic models that best describe the release from semisolid systems are taken into consideration, i.e., the zero-order model, the first-order model, and the Higuchi–Connors model (Table 4). As described in Section 2.6, the correlation coefficient (R^2) for each mathematical model greater than 0.95 was taken into account and used as a first criterion to discard the models least suitable for describing the drug-release phenomenon. In a second moment, once the kinetic model that best fit the experimental data was identified, the mechanism of drug diffusion was evaluated considering the release exponent n calculated from the Kosmeyer–Peppas equation, as described in the literature [25].

This was further supported by the release exponent n, calculated by the Korsmeyer–Peppas equation, being less than 0.5, suggesting that the drug release follows a diffusion-controlled process, where the rate is primarily governed by the concentration gradient and the drug diffusion through the matrix of the base. The Higuchi–Connors model is commonly observed in systems where the drug is released from a homogeneous matrix, and its release is not significantly hindered by the base itself.

Table 4. Mathematical models of PRP-HCl release kinetics from the Modigliani, Klimt, and Caravaggio ready-to-use bases by Franz cell equipped with cuprophane membrane.

Mathematical Model		Modigliani	Klimt	Caravaggio
Zero Order	Equation	y = 2.0466x + 16.08	y = 1.2196x + 6.2199	y = 1.7843x + 6.1141
	R^2	0.8575	0.9425	0.9716
First Order	Equation	y = −0.0149x + 1.9304	y = −0.0067x + 1.9741	y = −0.0109x + 1.9785
	R^2	0.9432	0.9655	0.987
Higuchi—Connors	Equation	y = 12.178x + 3.5964	y = 6.9394x − 0.5024	y = 9.8998x − 3.1504
	R^2	0.9858	0.9907	0.9711
Kosmeyer–Peppas	Equation	y = 0.4419x + 1.193	y = 0.4978x + 0.8261	y = 0.5653x + 0.8607
	R^2	0.9829	0.9815	0.9612
	n	0.4419	0.4978	0.5653

In contrast, the Caravaggio base exhibited a different release profile, following first-order kinetics with an anomalous drug transport mechanism. The release exponent *n* for this formulation was greater than 0.5, indicating a non-Fickian or anomalous transport process (Table 4). This suggests that the release from the Caravaggio base may involve complex mechanisms, such as drug diffusion coupled with matrix relaxation or swelling, which could result in a release rate that is not solely dependent on the drug concentration gradient. The first-order behavior is often seen in systems where the drug release is controlled by both diffusion and the dissolution of the base, leading to a more sustained release over time.

These findings underscore the significant role that the vehicles, such as the ready-to-use bases, play in determining the release kinetics of the drug. The Modigliani and Klimt bases, which favor Fickian diffusion, may be more suitable for controlled-release systems, where a predictable and linear release is desired. On the other hand, the Caravaggio base, with its anomalous transport mechanism, could be advantageous for applications requiring more complex or sustained drug release, where the rate of release is not strictly linear.

Overall, this study highlights the importance of carefully selecting and optimizing formulation bases to tailor the release profile to meet specific therapeutic needs. Understanding the underlying release mechanisms, as revealed by the kinetic modelling, is crucial for designing more effective drug delivery systems that can achieve desired pharmacokinetic profiles.

4. Conclusions

Since 2008, propranolol has gained approval as the first-line treatment for IHs associated with risks of dysfunction and esthetic problems due to its high effectiveness. Following the success of oral treatment, topical formulations of the API have been explored, particularly for curing superficial IHs in pediatric patients who may be more prone to oral treatment side effects. In fact, topical skin applications could help maintain high drug concentrations at local or focal sites and also represent an easy method of administration to pediatric patients. Because no topical propranolol formulations are commercially available, such dosage forms may be prepared as extemporaneous formulations at hospitals and pharmacies. In the present study, we identified a simple method for preparing topical PRP-HCl formulations at 1% *w/w* with four hydrophilic creams and one lipophilic ointment commercially available. The five bases guaranteed physical stability of the dosage form and chemical stability of the API when the formulations were stored at 25 °C for one month. An in vitro drug-release screening showed that the Modigliani, Caravaggio, and Klimt hydrophilic creams could be identified as the most suitable candidates for the preparation of topical formulations. Further in vitro permeation studies highlighted the most critical formulative aspects for dermal delivery of PRP-HCl and allowed for the rational selection of the most appropriate cream. In particular, the Modigliani base ensured both higher drug release from the vehicle and higher drug concentration in the skin. Moreover, the in vitro results on full-thickness skin suggested a lower permeation pattern that could suggest lower systemic side effects induced by topical propranolol rather than oral treatment. The overall results discussed in this work may be, therefore, useful for physicians for driving the selection of a semisolid matrix according to the therapeutic needs of pediatric patients. Additionally, this systematic study allowed for the identification of an appropriate ready-to-use vehicle for a topical treatment of IHs in order to minimize the risk of errors that a pharmacist could make during compounding. By addressing critical aspects of safety, stability, and customization while reducing preparation time, these bases enable pharmacists to deliver high-quality, patient-specific medications with greater confidence and precision. Topical formulations of PRP-HCl for the treatment of IHs offer a safer and less toxic alternative to oral administration. By applying the drug directly to the affected area, the dose required is significantly lower, further decreasing the potential for systemic toxicity. However, it is essential to monitor the skin's response and the potential for local irritation or other mild side effects, although these are generally rare and less severe than the systemic effects associated with oral propranolol therapy.

Author Contributions: Conceptualization, A.L., A.C. and N.D.; methodology, A.L., A.A.L., A.C. and C.L.; software, A.C.; validation, A.A.L., A.C. and A.L.; formal analysis, A.L., A.A.L. and A.C.; investigation, C.L.; resources, A.A.L.; data curation, F.M.l.F. and S.F.; writing—original draft preparation, C.L.; writing—review and editing, A.L., A.C., A.A.L. and N.D.; visualization, A.L., A.A.L., A.C. and N.D.; supervision, A.L., A.C. and N.D.; project administration, A.L., F.M.l.F. and S.F.; funding acquisition, N.D. All authors have read and agreed to the published version of the manuscript.

Funding: This research received no external funding.

Institutional Review Board Statement: Not applicable.

Informed Consent Statement: Not applicable.

Data Availability Statement: Data are contained within the article.

Acknowledgments: The authors would like to acknowledge the University of Bari Aldo Moro and Centro Studi Ricerche "Dr. S. Fontana 1900-1982", Farmalabor s.r.l., Giuseppe Francesco Racaniello, Antonio Spennacchio, and Angelica Franchini for their precious help in HPLC analysis and graphic support in designing images and tables.

Conflicts of Interest: Authors Flavia Maria la Forgia and Sergio Fontana were employed by the Company Farmalabor s.r.l. The remaining authors declare that the research was conducted in the absence of any commercial or financial relationships that could be construed as potential conflicts of interest.

References

1. Hoeger, P.H.; Harper, J.I.; Baselga, E.; Bonnet, D.; Boon, L.M.; Atti, M.C.D.; El Hachem, M.; Oranje, A.P.; Rubin, A.T.; Weibel, L.; et al. Treatment of Infantile Haemangiomas: Recommendations of a European Expert Group. *Eur. J. Pediatr.* **2015**, *174*, 855–865. [CrossRef] [PubMed]
2. Léauté-Labrèze, C.; Harper, J.I.; Hoeger, P.H. Infantile Haemangioma. *Lancet* **2017**, *390*, 85–94. [CrossRef] [PubMed]
3. Holland, K.E.; Drolet, B.A. Infantile Hemangioma. *Pediatr. Clin. N. Am.* **2010**, *57*, 1069–1083. [CrossRef]

4. Rodríguez Bandera, A.I.; Sebaratnam, D.F.; Wargon, O.; Wong, L.C.F. Infantile Hemangioma. Part 1: Epidemiology, Pathogenesis, Clinical Presentation and Assessment. *J. Am. Acad. Dermatol.* **2021**, *85*, 1379–1392. [CrossRef]
5. Léauté-Labrèze, C.; de la Roque, E.D.; Hubiche, T.; Boralevi, F.; Thambo, J.-B.; Taïeb, A. Propranolol for Severe Hemangiomas of Infancy. *N. Engl. J. Med.* **2008**, *358*, 2649–2651. [CrossRef] [PubMed]
6. Chen, Z.-Y.; Wang, Q.-N.; Zhu, Y.-H.; Zhou, L.-Y.; Xu, T.; He, Z.-Y.; Yang, Y. Progress in the Treatment of Infantile Hemangioma. *Ann. Transl. Med.* **2019**, *7*, 692. [CrossRef] [PubMed]
7. Cuesta, A.M.; Gallardo-Vara, E.; Casado-Vela, J.; Recio-Poveda, L.; Botella, L.-M.; Albiñana, V. The Role of Propranolol as a Repurposed Drug in Rare Vascular Diseases. *Int. J. Mol. Sci.* **2022**, *23*, 4217. [CrossRef]
8. Wassef, M.; Blei, F.; Adams, D.; Alomari, A.; Baselga, E.; Berenstein, A.; Burrows, P.; Frieden, I.J.; Garzon, M.C.; Lopez-Gutierrez, J.-C.; et al. Vascular Anomalies Classification: Recommendations From the International Society for the Study of Vascular Anomalies. *Pediatrics* **2015**, *136*, e203–e214. [CrossRef] [PubMed]
9. Kwon, E.-K.M.; Joachim, S.; Siegel, D.H.; Drolet, B.A.; Holland, K. Retrospective Review of Adverse Effects From Propranolol in Infants. *JAMA Dermatol.* **2013**, *149*, 484. [CrossRef] [PubMed]
10. Xu, G.; Lv, R.; Zhao, Z.; Huo, R. Topical Propranolol for Treatment of Superficial Infantile Hemangiomas. *J. Am. Acad. Dermatol.* **2012**, *67*, 1210–1213. [CrossRef] [PubMed]
11. Kunzi-Rapp, K. Topical Propranolol Therapy for Infantile Hemangiomas. *Pediatr. Dermatol.* **2012**, *29*, 154–159. [CrossRef]
12. Price, A.; Rai, S.; Mcleod, R.W.J.; Birchall, J.C.; Elhassan, H.A. Topical Propranolol for Infantile Haemangiomas: A Systematic Review. *J. Eur. Acad. Dermatol. Venereol.* **2018**, *32*, 2083–2089. [CrossRef] [PubMed]
13. Piraccini, B.M.; Alessandrini, A.; Dika, E.; Starace, M.; Patrizi, A.; Neri, I. Topical Propranolol 1% Cream for Pyogenic Granulomas of the Nail: Open-label Study in 10 Patients. *J. Eur. Acad. Dermatol. Venereol.* **2016**, *30*, 901–902. [CrossRef] [PubMed]
14. Casiraghi, A.; Musazzi, U.M.; Rocco, P.; Franzè, S.; Minghetti, P. Topical Treatment of Infantile Haemangiomas: A Comparative Study on the Selection of a Semi-Solid Vehicle. *Ski. Pharmacol. Physiol.* **2016**, *29*, 210–219. [CrossRef]
15. Spennacchio, A.; Lopalco, A.; Racaniello, G.F.; Cutrignelli, A.; la Forgia, F.M.; Fontana, S.; Cristofori, F.; Francavilla, R.; Lopedota, A.A.; Denora, N. Mucoadhesive Budesonide Solution for the Treatment of Pediatric Eosinophilic Esophagitis. *Pharmaceuticals* **2024**, *17*, 550. [CrossRef] [PubMed]
16. Lacassia, C.; Spennacchio, A.; Lopedota, A.A.; Denora, N.; Lopalco, A.; Maria La Forgia, F.; Fontana, S. Physical-Chemical Stability of the Extemporaneous Paracetamol Oral Suspension in Puccini Base. *Int. J. Pharm. Compd.* **2024**, *28*, 146–150. [PubMed]
17. Lacassia, C.; Spennacchio, A.; Lopalco, A.; Lopedota, A.A.; la Forgia, F.; Fontana, S.; Franco, M.; Denora, N. Lipophilic Ready to Use Vehicles Compounded Topical Medications. *Int. J. Pharm. Compd.* **2024**, *28*, 146–150.
18. Spennacchio, A.; Lacassia, C.; Lopalco, A.; Lopedota, A.A.; la Forgia, F.; Fontana, S.; Franco, M.; Denora, N. Hydrophilic Ready-to-Use Vehicles and Compounded Topical Medications. *Int. J. Pharm. Compd.* **2024**, *28*, 138–145.
19. Procedure per Unguenti Secondo Le Norme Di Buona Preparazione. Available online: https://www.sifap.org/procedure-norme-di-buona-preparazione/procedure-unguenti (accessed on 30 December 2024).
20. Procedure per Creme Secondo Le Norme Di Buona Preparazione. Available online: https://www.sifap.org/procedure-norme-di-buona-preparazione/procedure-creme (accessed on 30 December 2024).
21. Lopalco, A.; Denora, N.; Laquintana, V.; Cutrignelli, A.; Franco, M.; Robota, M.; Hauschildt, N.; Mondelli, F.; Arduino, I.; Lopedota, A. Taste Masking of Propranolol Hydrochloride by Microbeads of EUDRAGIT® E PO Obtained with Prilling Technique for Paediatric Oral Administration. *Int. J. Pharm.* **2020**, *574*, 118922. [CrossRef]
22. Sopyan, I.; Gozali, D.; Tiassetiana, S. Formulation of Tomato Extracts (*Solanum lycopersicum* L.) as a Sunscreen Lotion. *Natl. J. Physiol. Pharm. Pharmacol.* **2017**, *8*, 453–458. [CrossRef]
23. SCHEDA DATI DI SICUREZZA PROPRANOLOLO CLORIDRATO. Available online: https://materie-prime.farmalabor.it/sds_completa/01907_it.pdf (accessed on 28 November 2012).
24. Racaniello, G.F.; Balenzano, G.; Arduino, I.; Iacobazzi, R.M.; Lopalco, A.; Lopedota, A.A.; Sigurdsson, H.H.; Denora, N. Chitosan and Anionic Solubility Enhancer Sulfobutylether-β-Cyclodextrin-Based Nanoparticles as Dexamethasone Ophthalmic Delivery System for Anti-Inflammatory Therapy. *Pharmaceutics* **2024**, *16*, 277. [CrossRef]
25. Bialik-Wąs, K.; Miastkowska, M.; Sapuła, P.; Sycz, A.; Pluta, K.; Malina, D.; Chwastowski, J. Kinetic Analysis of in Vitro Release Profiles of Salicylic Acid and Fluocinolone Acetonide from Dual Delivery Systems Composed of Polymeric Nanocarriers and a Hydrogel Matrix. *J. Drug Deliv. Sci. Technol.* **2024**, *92*, 105355. [CrossRef]

pharmaceutics

MDPI

Article

Development of an Adaptable Qualification Test Set for Personnel Involved in Visual Inspection Procedures of Parenteral Drug Products Manufactured Under Good Manufacturing Practice Conditions in Hospital Pharmacy Compounding Facilities

Tessa van den Born-Bondt [1,†], Harmen P. S. Huizinga [1,†], Koen R. Kappert [1,2], Hans H. Westra [1], Jacoba van Zanten [1], Herman J. Woerdenbag [2], Jacoba M. Maurer [1] and Bahez Gareb [1,*]

[1] Department of Clinical Pharmacy and Pharmacology, University Medical Center Groningen (UMCG), 9713 GZ Groningen, The Netherlands

[2] Department of Pharmaceutical Technology and Biopharmacy, Groningen Research Institute of Pharmacy (GRIP), University of Groningen, Antonius Deusinglaan 1, 9713 AV Groningen, The Netherlands

* Correspondence: b.gareb01@umcg.nl

† These authors contributed equally to this work.

Abstract

Objectives: Parenteral drug products manufactured under GMP conditions should be visually inspected for defects and particulate contamination by trained and qualified personnel. Although personnel qualification is required, no practical protocols or formal guidelines are available for the development of qualification test sets (QTSs) used for qualification procedures. The current practice is to either procure a standardized QTS from a commercial supplier or amass sufficient manufacturing rejects during visual inspection procedures to compile in-house QTSs. However, both strategies inherently possess disadvantages and limitations. The objective of this study was to develop a manufacturing protocol for an optimal and adaptable QTS for training and qualification procedures. **Methods:** We combined the results of a literature search, survey of five Dutch hospital pharmacy compounding facilities, semi-structured personnel interviews, and extensive pre-GMP formulation studies to develop an optimal and adaptable QTS manufacturing protocol. **Results:** The literature search did not identify a manufacturing protocol for an optimal and adaptable QTS, but did identify specifications and requirements for optimal QTSs. The survey among hospital pharmacy compounding facilities revealed considerable variability in the qualification procedures and used QTSs. Semi-structured personnel interviews and pre-GMP formulation studies demonstrated that defects encountered during routine productions could be realistically simulated with pharmaceutical-grade excipients. As a proof-of-concept, we manufactured two different QTSs under GMP conditions and assessed these for formal GMP training and qualification purposes, which were considered a significant improvement compared to using manufacturing rejects. **Conclusions:** To the best of our knowledge, this is the first study presenting these data and our adaptable protocol, which is provided in the Supplemental Materials, may aid compounding facilities in the standardization, training, and qualification of personnel involved in visual inspection procedures.

Keywords: good manufacturing practice (GMP); qualification; visual inspection; parenteral drugs; hospital pharmacy; pharmaceutical compounding; qualification test set; particulate matter

1. Introduction

Hospital pharmacy compounding facilities play an essential role in providing patients with extemporaneous preparations when no adequate pharmaceutical alternatives are commercially available. Moreover, hospitals with a GMP manufacturing license also play an essential role in providing clinicians and investigators with experimental medication intended for clinical trials (phase I/II). Small-scale productions, such as those for individual patients or clinical trial medication at limited costs, are often not facilitated by pharmaceutical companies. Additionally, hospital pharmacy compounding facilities usually have a wider range of products compared to a pharmaceutical company, including aseptically prepared, terminally sterilized, and non-sterile preparations. Taken together, these activities highlight the indispensable contribution of hospital pharmacies to innovation and personalized treatment of patients.

Parenteral preparations are sterile drug products that are either aseptically manufactured or terminally sterilized. All parenteral drug products manufactured under GMP conditions should be visually inspected by qualified personnel for possible particulate contamination [1]. Particulate contamination is defined as the presence of extrinsic and/or intrinsic particulate matter in the drug product [2]. Extrinsic particles are not part of the formulation, packaging, or assembly process. They include, for example, clothing fragments, fibers, and hair. Intrinsic particles are particles that can be attributed to the formulation, packaging, and assembly process, such as glass and rubber particles originating from the primary packaging material or precipitates due to instable active pharmaceutical ingredients or excipients [3]. Since the source and characteristics of these particles can vary, so do their size and visibility under standardized lighting conditions.

There is no single particle size defined as the smallest observable size by the human eye. The United States Pharmacopeia (USP) <1787> monograph considers particles larger than 100 μm to be visible [4]. However, under conditions of increased light intensity, particles smaller than 100 μm may be distinguished by the human eye [5].

The European Pharmacopoeia (Ph. Eur.) method 2.9.20 and USP monograph <1790> describe the visual inspection methods and acceptance criteria for parenteral drugs manufactured in the European Union (EU) and United States of America (USA), respectively [6,7]. In general, these methods require that the drug products are visually inspected in bright light against white and black backgrounds. Any observed defect to the primary container or the presence of particulate matter in the drug product should be rejected and discarded [8].

The EU GMP Annex 1 states that all manufacturing activities should be performed by trained and qualified personnel [1]. Guidelines describing the qualification of personnel involved in visual inspection procedures of parenteral drugs state that inspectors must demonstrate proficiency of removing defects from a seeded population of typical "in-house" defects. Before being trained and formally qualified, an operator should undergo a visual acuity test [1]. Subsequently, personnel are qualified using qualification test sets (QTSs) containing representative defects that are typically encountered during routine productions. To warrant the qualification status, personnel should be requalified with a predetermined and justified frequency, which is typically at least annually [8].

An optimal QTS should meet a number of requirements [8–10]. First, it should contain a subset of defect-free containers and a subset (10–20% of the total) of containers containing at least one defect. This ensures that personnel are not only qualified to detect the presence of any defects but also qualified to accept containers without defects. Second, the QTS should contain a representative number of units (batch size) to simulate a typical visual inspection procedure encountered during routine productions. Furthermore, the QTS units should ideally be identical to units manufactured during routine productions, i.e., similar primary packaging materials, fill volumes, and color/turbidity of solution. Third, the QTS should contain a wide range of representative defects (e.g., particles, fibers, and damages) to optimally qualify the personnel for the defects that can be encountered during routine productions. Finally, in view of practicality, the QTS should have a long shelf life (years) and should withstand repeated handling over time [9].

The units of the QTS may be sourced from actual manufacturing rejects encountered during routine productions. It is also possible to procure standardized QTSs from commercial suppliers [8]. However, both strategies inherently possess disadvantages. For instance, using manufacturing rejects may not yield a wide range of defects in a timely manner, especially if the compounding facility manufactures multiple drug product formulations (e.g., syringes, bags for intravenous infusion, containers, and ampoules) with different fill volumes in relatively small batch sizes (e.g., 100–200 units). Furthermore, commercially available QTSs are expensive, especially when multiple sets need to be procured to train personnel for qualification procedures of multiple drug product formulations. Moreover, such sets may lack representative units or defects typically encountered during routine productions. The high costs associated with commercially available QTSs are generally the result of the standardized particle size and count present in the containers. However, these features are not necessary nor required for the qualification of personnel since the qualification procedure is a qualitative (present/absent of defect) rather than a quantitative test (not tested for particle size and count).

As an alternative, QTSs may be manufactured by the compounding facility itself. This strategy is relatively easy, cheap, and adaptable and yields fully representative QTS units with the possibility to include colored, viscous, and opalescent solutions (if desired) in the same packaging materials as used during routine productions. Furthermore, the batch size of the manufactured QTS can be as large as needed, which ensures that the QTS simulates the circumstances of a visual inspection procedure during routine productions. In addition, each desired and representative defect can be introduced in any given frequency based on historic visual inspection or trend analysis data. These in-house manufactured QTSs are thus more representative for routine practice and provide a more reliable qualification procedure. Although such QTSs are more suitable for training and qualification procedures, methods and requirements to manufacture these test sets are lacking in the current literature.

The objective of this study was to develop a manufacturing protocol for an adaptable QTS that can be used for the qualification of personnel involved in visual inspection procedures of parenteral drug products manufactured under GMP conditions. First, a literature search was performed to investigate whether manufacturing protocols and requirements for a QTS are available. Second, a survey was conducted to assess the visual inspection qualification procedures and used QTSs in five Dutch hospital compounding pharmacies. Subsequently, personnel involved in visual inspection procedures were interviewed to gather data on typical and rarer defects encountered during routine visual inspection procedures and these defects characteristics. Based on these results, QTS requirements and formulation studies were conducted to develop a manufacturing protocol for an adaptable and in-house manufactured QTS ready for GMP tech transfer. As a proof-of-concept, two QTSs were manufactured under GMP conditions with the developed manufacturing protocol and were evaluated for feasibility and suitability for visual inspection qualification procedures under GMP conditions.

2. Materials and Methods

2.1. Study Design

This study was conducted in the compounding facility of the University Medical Center Groningen (UMCG), The Netherlands, which is a tertiary hospital with a GMP manufacturing license for parenteral drug products manufactured under EU GMP Annex 1 conditions. A wide range of parenteral drug products are manufactured in our compounding facility, including fluorescent-labelled monoclonal antibodies.

We used a mixed methods study design, combining the results of a literature search, survey of five Dutch hospital pharmacy compounding facilities (including our own facility), semi-structured interviews of qualified personnel involved visual inspection procedures of parenteral drugs, and pre-GMP formulation studies to manufacture two QTSs under GMP conditions with the developed manufacturing protocol (Figure 1).

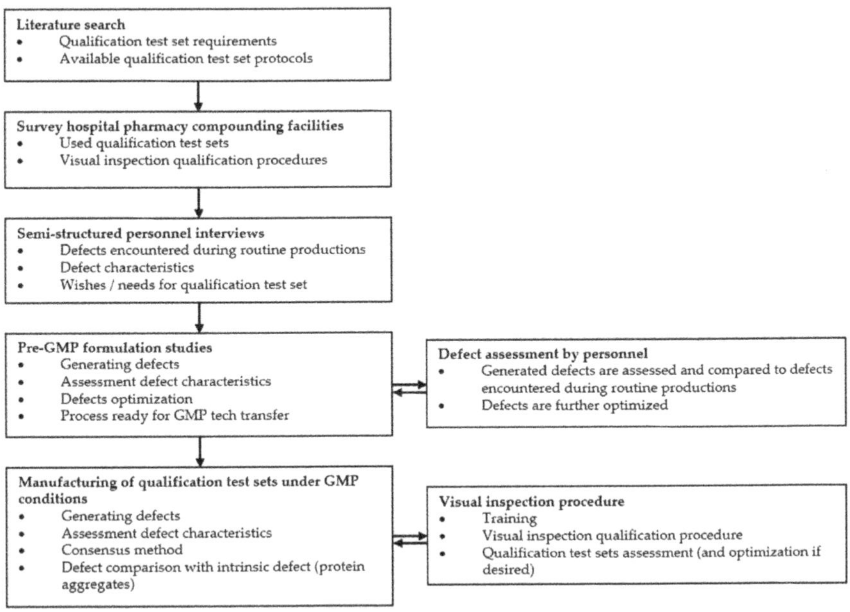

Figure 1. Study design and flow chart of the present study.

To show proof-of-concept, the present study focused on fluorescent-labeled monoclonal antibodies, in particular, bevacizumab-800CW [11]. This parenteral drug product is a clear, blue-greenish, aqueous solution with a protein concentration of 1 mg/mL and packaged in clear type I glass 10R vials (APG Europe, Uithoorn, The Netherlands) with a bromobutyl rubber stopper (Brocacef Supplies & Services, Maarssen, The Netherlands) and aluminum crimp with a plastic cap (Brocacef Supplies & Services, Maarssen, The Netherlands) with a fill volume of 5–6 mL and with a batch size of 100–200 units. Possible causes and sources of particulate contamination or defective containers were identified with a risk assessment using a Ishikawa diagram (Appendix A).

2.2. Literature Search

To investigate whether manufacturing protocols and requirements for a QTS are available in the literature, the PubMed, Embase, and Web of Science databases were searched.

The search term for the PubMed database was '(qualification[tiab] OR qualification set[tiab] OR test set[tiab] OR training set[tiab] OR challenge set[tiab]) AND (good manufacturing practices[tiab] OR GMP[tiab] OR visual inspection[tiab] OR parenteral[tiab] OR visible particles[tiab] OR particles[tiab] OR particulate matter[tiab])'.

The search term for the Embase database was '('qualification':ti,ab OR 'qualification set':ti,ab OR 'test set':ti,ab OR 'training set':ti,ab OR 'challenge set':ti,ab) AND ('good manufacturing practice':ti,ab OR 'GMP':ti,ab OR 'visual inspection':ti,ab OR 'parenteral':ti,ab OR 'visible particles':ti,ab OR 'particles':ti,ab OR 'particulate matter':ti,ab)'.

The search term for the Web of Science database was '(TI=(qualification) OR AB=(qualification) OR TI=(qualification set) OR AB=(qualification set) OR TI=(test set) OR AB=(test set) OR TI=(training set) OR AB=(training set) OR TI=(challenge set) OR AB=(challenge set)) AND (TI=(good manufacturing practices) OR AB=(good manufacturing practices) OR TI=(GMP) OR AB=(GMP) OR TI=(visual inspection) OR AB=(visual inspection) OR TI=(parenteral) OR AB=(parenteral) OR TI=(visible particles) OR AB=(visible particles) OR TI=(particulate matter) OR AB=(particulate matter))'.

The titles as well as abstracts of all articles were read to assess whether the articles described manufacturing protocols or requirements for QTSs. The reference list of articles describing QTS manufacturing protocols or requirements were also screened for potential relevant articles.

To investigate the requirements for a QTS intended for GMP qualification purposes, guidelines from the EU GMP (Annex 1), FDA, Parental Drug Association (PDA), USP, British Pharmacopoeia (BP), and Ph. Eur. were reviewed and summarized [1,6–8,10,12]. The obtained data were used for the development of the manufacturing protocol described in the present study and to warrant that the QTS complied with the relevant guidelines for manufacturing parenteral drug products.

2.3. Survey Hospital Pharmacy Compounding Facilities

To assess the current practices in GMP qualification of personnel involved in the visual inspection of parental drug products, a survey was distributed to six different hospital pharmacy compounding facilities in the Netherlands with a GMP manufacturing license to manufacture parenteral drug products (including the UMCG compounding facility). The survey was conducted via e-mail and aimed to assess the general qualification procedure, the used QTSs, and coding/decoding method of the test set. The survey questions of this survey are presented in Appendix B.

2.4. Semi-Structured Personnel Interviews

Semi-structured interviews were conducted with qualified personnel (four participants) involved in visual inspection procedures of parenteral drug products manufactured under GMP conditions by the UMCG. The interview questions were directed to identify which routine defects were typically encountered with what frequency, what typical defect characteristics (e.g., size, motion, ease of dispersion, sedimentation rate, and interaction with light in solution) were during visual inspection procedures according to Ph. Eur. 2.9.20, which defects were easy/difficult to spot, and what the specific wishes of the personnel were regarding the training and qualification procedures. Open-ended questions were used with additional probing questions when necessary to avoid researcher bias. The semi-structured interview questions are available in Appendix C.

2.5. Pre-GMP Formulation Studies

Pre-GMP formulation studies were conducted to assess the suitability of different pharmaceutical excipients and cleanroom materials for the QTS defects that were identified in the semi-structured interviews (see Section 2.4). Pre-GMP production was performed in a laminar airflow cabinet (LAF) with EU GMP grade A air situated in an unclassified area.

Ideally, excipients compatible with GMP conditions should be used, since the final production process must comply with GMP standards. Therefore, Ph. Eur. and GMP-grade materials, such as pharmaceutical excipients and sterile wipes, were chosen. Talc (VWR, Radnor, PA, USA), microcrystalline cellulose ((MCC), Pharmacel® 102, particle size distribution ×10: 40 μm; ×50: 90 μm; ×90: 180 μm, DFE Pharma, Goch, Germany), barium sulfate (Thermo Scientific, Waltham, MA, USA), magnesium stearate (Spruyt Hillen, Capelle aan den IJssel, The Netherlands), sodium carbonate (Merck, Darmstadt, Germany), and silicon dioxide (colloidal anhydrous silica) (Merck, Darmstadt, Germany) were selected to simulate particulate matter.

Talc particles were generated either from talc agglomerates directly deposited into the glass vials or by first depositing talc agglomerates onto the surface of water for injection (WFI), which remained afloat by the surface tension of the water. Subsequently, a small portion of the agglomerate was transferred into the sterile 10R vials (Ph. Eur. Type I glass, APG Europe, Uithoorn, The Netherlands). MCC particles were generated by first transferring a small amount of MCC into a glass beaker filled with WFI. A small portion of MMC particles was subsequently transferred into the glass vial with a spatula.

Glass shards were obtained by gently chipping the tip of a 150 mm Pasteur capillary pipette (Thermo Scientific, Waltham, MA, USA) with sterile tweezers. Rubber particles were generated by cutting a bromobutyl rubber stopper (Brocacef Supplies & Services, Maarssen, The Netherlands), which was part of the primary packaging, with a sterile surgical scalpel. Fibers were produced using either a paper towel (Tork, Zeist, The Netherlands) or a Sontara Micropure AP sterile cloth (IPS-Group A/S, Kvistgård, Denmark). Suitable fibers were then transferred into the containers containing WFI using sterile tweezers.

After the defects consisting of particulate matter were generated, the glass vials were filled with 5–6 mL WFI and sealed with a bromobutyl rubber stopper and aluminum crimp with a plastic cap. Furthermore, dents and chips were generated as defects in the aluminum crimp or plastic cap, respectively, by mechanical force applied to vials that did not contain particulate matter as a defect. All vials were coded with a number using a UV marker (Edding 8280, Ahrensburg, Germany). The mark could be made visible with a UV lamp (BASEY, BH-ZaklampUV, Nieuw Vennep, The Netherlands) (Figure 2).

A B

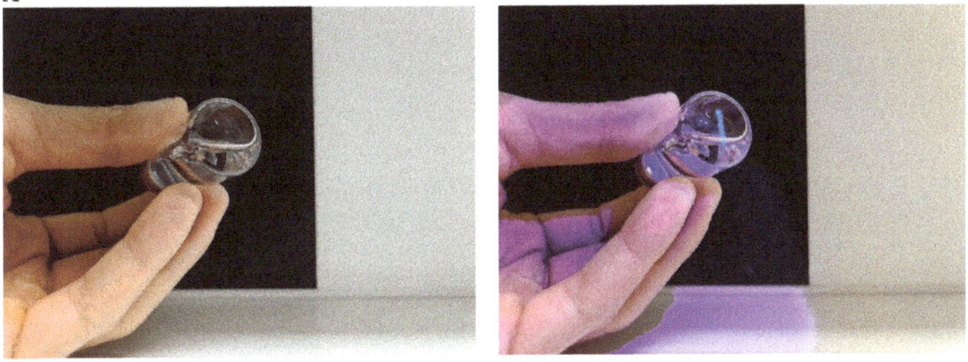

Figure 2. Coding and decoding of the QTS vials with a UV marker and UV lamp. (**A**) The test set vial code cannot be seen in visible light during visual inspection according to Ph. Eur. 2.9.20. (**B**) The code ("number 1") can be made visible with a UV lamp, which warrants a fully blinded qualification procedure of personnel.

The manufactured defects were assessed by qualified UMCG personnel involved in visual inspection procedures. The appearance as well as flow characteristics of particulate matter during visual inspection according to Ph. Eur. 2.9.20 (Apollo II Liquid Viewer,

Aldephi, United Kingdom) was assessed. In case the generated defects did not accurately simulate the defects encountered during routine GMP productions, defects were further formulated and optimized. This process was repeated until the generated defects accurately simulated the defects encountered during routine GMP productions and therefore was ready for tech transfer (Figure 1).

2.6. Manufacturing of Qualification Test Sets Under GMP Conditions

Two final GMP QTSs were manufactured according to a summary of the guidelines described in Section 2.2 and the procedures described in Section 2.5. The only difference between the pre-GMP and GMP QTSs was that the two GMP QTSs were manufactured under GMP conditions in a LAF cabinet with EU GMP-grade A air situated in an EU GMP-grade C cleanroom with a batch size of 100 units.

The first GMP QTS consisted of the primary container filled with 5–6 mL WFI with and without defects. The second GMP QTS consisted of the primary container filled with 5–6 mL WFI in which the fluorescent dye IRDye 800CW (LI-COR, Lincoln, NE, USA) was dissolved at a concentration of 10 μg/mL to mimic the color of the fluorescent-labelled monoclonal antibodies (e.g., bevacizumab-800CW [9]) that are routinely manufactured as clinical trial medication by the UMCG.

After the manufacturing process and batch release, the GMP QTSs were simultaneously visually inspected by two qualified persons according to Ph. Eur. 2.9.20 (Apollo II Liquid Viewer, Aldephi, UK). The objective of this inspection procedure was to confirm with the four-eye principle (i.e., consensus method) that the vials containing the defects were identified as such and to confirm that the vials that did not contain any defects were indeed identified as such.

2.7. Comparison Qualification Test Set Defects with Protein (Monoclonal Antibody) Aggregates

To assess whether the generated defects consisting of particulate matter simulated protein aggregates (intrinsic particles), GMP-produced bevacizumab-800CW vials were stored at 50 °C for 48 h in an oven (Salm & Kipp, Breukelen, The Netherlands). Subsequently, these vials were stored for an additional 7 days at room temperature (15–25 °C) to further stress the drug product. Bevacizumab-800CW manufactured by the UMCG under GMP conditions has a storage temperature of 2–8 °C with a shelf life of four years substantiated by in-house stability data presented in the product dossier. The high-temperature stress test induced protein aggregates, which is a common intrinsic particle encountered during routine production of parenteral protein drug products [13,14].

2.8. Evaluation of Qualification Test Sets for GMP Training and Qualification Purposes

The two GMP QTSs (Section 2.6) were implemented in the GMP training and qualification procedures with a change control strategy. GMP training and qualification procedures were conducted according to the in-house standard operating procedures of the UMCG. For the evaluation of the GMP QTSs and for comparison with the previous GMP training and qualification procedures using manufacturing rejects, four initial qualification and two requalification procedures were conducted with the in-house developed GMP QTSs. The experience of visual inspection personnel and the hospital pharmacist involved in the GMP training and qualification procedures were discussed and summarized. The focus of this discussion was whether the two developed GMP QTSs were a significant improvement and the factors attributing to this.

3. Results

3.1. Literature Search

On 28 December 2024, the searches yielded 320 (Pubmed), 634 (Embase), and 3631 (Web of Science) hits. The literature search did not reveal any publications from the databases describing an adaptable QTS manufacturing protocol for personnel qualification. However, two review articles [9,15] were identified that outlined certain considerations and specifications that contribute to defining an optimal QTS. Furthermore, one research article was identified that described a QTS manufacturing process [16].

The optimal QTS must meet a number of specifications (Table 1). First, the QTS must be stable (multiple years) and withstand repeated handling over time. Second, the number of QTS containers should ideally be representative of a routine visual inspection procedure to optimally train and qualify personnel. Third, the content of the QTS containers should be fully representative of the products encountered during routine productions since the physio-chemical characteristics of the content (e.g., viscosity, surface tension, turbidity, and colored solution) can have an impact on the motion of the content and the particulate matter. Fourth, the QTS should contain a wide range of defective containers that are representative of the defects encountered during routine production (e.g., small/large particles, fibers, glass shards, and mechanical damage), especially since these particulates interact differently with light and, therefore, the detection probability may differ. Fifth, the QTS should also contain defect-free containers, which aid in training personnel not to erroneously reject acceptable products, thereby maintaining inspection accuracy. Finally, the QTS should be adaptable and expandable with experience and based on visual inspection trend analysis data to further optimize personnel training and qualification.

Table 1. Specifications, requirements, and considerations for an optimal QTS for personnel training and qualification procedures.

Specification	Requirement and Consideration
Stability	Stable for years; withstand repeated handling over time
Number of containers	Fully representative of routine production; approximately 15–20% defective containers
Content containers	Fully representative of routine production; e.g., turbidity, viscosity, colored solutions, surface tension; physio-chemical characteristics may impact motion and light interaction of particulate matter
Primary packaging	Fully representative of routine production; e.g., colored glass, opaque, syringe, ampoules, vials; ease of dispersion of particulates in different containers may differ
Defects	Fully representative of routine production; particles, fibers, glass shards, mechanical damage; different particles interact differently with light; defects should be adaptable to manufacture less/more challenging containers for personnel training and qualification
Defect-free containers	Aids in training personnel not to erroneously reject acceptable products
Adaptability	Should expand based on experience and visual inspection trend analysis data; new defects may be introduced

Although the literature search did not reveal any publications describing an adaptable QTS manufacturing protocol, only one study was identified that described a QTS manufacturing process. This study used spherical cross-linked polystryrene divylbenzene beads with different diameters (40–180 µm) to manufacture a QTS. However, several limitations of this method were identified [16].

First, the authors noted that the beads were spherical and that the motion characteristics as well as light interaction of these beads did not always represent the wide range of defects that are encountered during routine productions. Furthermore, the beads could not always be readily dispersed, but either floated ('floaters') on the meniscus of the fluid or sticked to the sides of the containers. Consequently, personnel could not always identify these containers as defective units, which made training and qualification procedures challenging since it was not always evident whether personnel truly missed these defects or that the defects were simply not observable due these phenomena. These phenomena are likely the result of poor wettability and low surface energy of the beads [17]. Lastly, the proposed method was not adaptable and the QTS could not be expanded based on experience and visual inspection trend analysis data since the QTS only contained beads [16]. Taken together, we considered that this method did not comply with the specifications and requirements of an ideal and adaptable QTS for personnel training. Therefore, we continued with further research to develop an adaptable QTS protocol complying with the specifications listed in Table 1.

Common guidelines, including EU GMP Annex 1, FDA, PDA, USP, BP, and Ph. Eur. were reviewed and the information about QTSs was summarized [1,6–8,10,12]. According to all reviewed guidelines, 100% of the manufactured drug product batch must undergo visual inspection to ensure quality and safety. Defects found during these inspections should be categorized as critical, major, or minor [7,12]. Critical defects present a potential hazard capable of causing permanent injury and may compromise the integrity of the vial, rendering the product unsuitable for human use. Major defects, while not posing a risk of permanent injury, are likely to be noticeable to the user and may alter the usability of the drug product. Minor defects have no impact on user safety or product functionality but are typically of cosmetic nature [12].

To ensure operator competence, annual requalification is mandated according to the EU GMP Annex 1, including a visual acuity test [1,7]. Training requirements also specify that operators should be thoroughly trained in defect recognition, particularly in identifying particulate contamination [7,10]. The qualification procedure should be designed to reflect the actual production environment, incorporating relevant features such as container type, inspection duration, and batch size to accurately represent production conditions [7,9,10].

Additionally, a commercial QTS can be procured, or QTS units may be collected from manufacturing rejects encountered during routine productions. An in-house manufactured QTS is also permissible if needed to meet specific testing conditions [7].

Different methods are available for vial coding/decoding, including labeling, numbering, or using QR codes or UV markers, though each method has distinct limitations. For instance, QR codes require specialized scanning equipment, which can be costly and labor-intensive for decoding, while manual and observable numbering (e.g., using labels), although straightforward, may be subject to error if not updated regularly and do not provide fully blinded qualification procedures [7].

3.2. *Survey Hospital Pharmacy Compounding Facilities*

To evaluate existing procedures for personnel qualification involved in the visual inspection of parenteral drug products, we conducted a survey in which we contacted six hospital pharmacy compounding facilities in the Netherlands to gather insights into their practices. The survey involved the participation of five different hospital pharmacy compounding facilities besides the UMCG compounding facility. These included two tertiary and three secondary hospitals, all in possession of a GMP manufacturing license. The facilities produce various products that are visually inspected (e.g., ready-to-administer (RTA) syringes, bags for intravenous infusion, containers, and ampoules). All hospital pharmacy compounding facilities responded, and four (besides the UMCG) agreed to publish the synopsis of the observed methodologies, as detailed in Table 2. The results from the UMCG compounding facility describe the situation before development and implementation of the GMP QTSs.

It was observed that in-house developed QTSs were commonly used in the compounding facilities. However, there exists variability in the used excipients, manufacturing processes, and the QTS batch size across different facilities. Additionally, the acceptance criteria differ between the compounding facilities.

Table 2. Summary of results from the survey for hospital pharmacy compounding facilities in the Netherlands. Abbreviations: VAT: visual acuity testing. Opth.: ophthalmologist. QTS: qualification test set. MCC: microcrystalline cellulose. WFI: water for injection.

	UMCG	Hospital A	Hospital B	Hospital C	Hospital D
Level of healthcare	Tertiary care	Secondary care	Secondary care	Tertiary care	Secondary care
Personnel qualification	VAT via opht. and test set	VAT via opht. and test set	VAT via opht. and test set	VAT via opht. and test set	VAT via opht. and test set
Frequency of qualification	Annually	Annually	Annually	Annualy VAT, Once per two years test set	Annually
Development of QTS	Obtained from manufacturing rejects of routine productions	In-house developed Only particles	Commercial QTS	Obtained from manufacturing rejects of routine productions	In-house developed Only particles
Number of containers in the QTS	100	30	100	50	30
Composition of QTS	No distinction between types of particles	MCC	Glass, fibers, incorrect ampoule heads, volume variations	No distinction between types of particles	12.5 mg/L MCC and tap water
Acceptance criteria	Not more than 0 critical, 1 major, 5 minor defects should be missed. Incorrect rejection: ≤15%.	100% of all defects must be identified. Incorrect rejection: maximum of 2 syringes.	Three QTS's are visually inspected. ≥75% of all defects must be identified and ≥70% of defects must be identified per individual QTS. Incorrect rejection: ≤10%.	≥70% of all defects must be identified. Initial failure: repeat with double QTS, until the employee is proficient.	100% of all defects must be identified. Incorrect rejection: in WFI, 7 out of 9 is allowed.
Decoding of containers	Decoding table with visual numbers.	Decoding table with visual numbers. The numbers on the vials are replaced after qualification of 2–3 employees and when a new QTS is developed.	UV lamp.	Decoding table with visual numbers. A unique subset is used for each qualification. Employees are not informed which containers were rejected correctly.	UV lamp.

3.3. Semi-Structured Personnel Interviews

The semi-structured interview with GMP personnel revealed an overview of typical defects encountered during visual inspection of parenteral drug products. Among the visible particles encountered, fibers emerged as the most prevalent. Glass particles were found with lower frequency, and defects such as rubber particles from the stoppers were even rarer. Further, small particles such as aggregates or agglomerates were seldom detected.

Typical defect characteristics after gently swirling or inverting drug product containers were categorized on the basis of size (large or small), motion (fast, slow, or 'cloudy'), ease of dispersion (readily or difficult), sedimentation rate (fast or slow), and interaction with light (does or does not reflect light). The characteristics of small particulate matter were classified as small spheres that are easy to disperse with a fast, sometimes 'cloudy' motion and slow sedimentation rate that do not reflect light readily. Fiber characteristics were classified as easy to disperse thread-like particles that could either be large or small with a slow motion and sedimentation rate that do not reflect light readily. Rubber particle characteristics were classified as a relatively large pellet that is difficult to disperse with a slow motion and fast sedimentation rate that does not reflect light readily. Glass particle characteristics were classified as a relatively large particle (shard) that is difficult to disperse with a slow motion and fast sedimentation rate that reflects light readily.

To ensure an objective and fully blinded inspection procedure, personnel stated that the vials should ideally be coded with an invisible coding system, preventing inspectors from memorizing vial numbers. Additionally, the QTS should encompass a sufficient variety of defect types and vials with no defects to optimally train personnel for the range of defects typically encountered during routine GMP productions, next to rarer defects since these are more difficult to observe because these defects are not encountered frequently.

3.4. Pre-GMP Formulation Studies

Pre-GMP and formulation research evaluated a variety of defects to determine how these defects could be introduced under GMP conditions, focusing on pharmaceutical- and GMP-grade excipients to simulate representative defects. In different and subsequent sessions, the defects were improved based on the feedback provided by personnel, ensuring relevance and practical applicability.

The materials and defects selected during the pre-GMP formulations studies and their advantages and disadvantages are listed in Table 3. Glass and rubber were found suitable to simulate defects found during visual inspection procedures. Paper fibers were deemed unsuitable due to brittleness and instability in aqueous solution due to disintegration within several days. A paper pulp fiber can absorb 30% of its mass in water [18], aiding in the wetting of the fibers and subsequent disintegration in smaller, not readily observable particles. The fiber from a Sontara® Micropure AP cloth consists of a mixture of cellulose and polyester, making it more stable in an aqueous solution. Also, this material does not release other (undefined) particles that could contaminate the solution. Therefore, a fiber from this material was selected and found to be suitable for the QTS.

The introduction of talc and MCC particles as defects was challenging. On the one hand, larger talc particles (agglomerates) immediately disintegrated in the solution, yielding not readily observable particles. On the other hand, MCC agglomerates initially appeared to be stable, but also completely disintegrated within several days. These excipients proved to be useful to simulate small particles but could not be used to simulate larger particles for an extended period of time. Despite this, both talc and MCC provided realistic small-particle characteristics valued by personnel and, thus, were selected to be included in the final GMP QTS to simulate small particulate matter.

To overcome the limitations of talc and MCC, other materials were tested, namely barium sulfate, magnesium stearate, sodium carbonate, and silicon dioxide. Magnesium stearate was too hydrophobic and could not be optimally processed in aqueous solutions. The amount of sodium carbonate and silicon dioxide used during the experiments dissolved/disintegrated in water and yielded vials with defects that could not be readily detected. However, barium sulfate appeared to be suitable to simulate particulate matter in aqueous solution. Barium sulfate did not dissolve and had characteristics similar to protein aggregates in parental drug products, which has also been described elsewhere [5]. Furthermore, serial dilutions of barium sulfate suspensions could be produced to simulate high- and low-concentration aggregate solutions with varying degrees of difficulty to detect by the personnel, which was considered desired for training purposes.

Table 3. Defect types and materials used to simulate different intrinsic and extrinsic particles with their advantages and disadvantages.

Defect Materials	Simulates	Characteristics in Solution	Advantages	Disadvantages
Talc	Particulate mater (intrinsic, extrinsic)	• Small spheres • Easy to disperse • Slow sedimentation rate	• Available in pharmaceutical grade, compatible in cleanroom areas • Realistically simulates intrinsic and extrinsic particles	• Disintegrates in aqueous solution • Particle size may decrease over time
Microcrystalline cellulose (MCC)		• Small spheres • Easy to disperse • Slow sedimentation rate	• Available in pharmaceutical grade, compatible in cleanroom areas • Realistically simulates intrinsic and extrinsic particles	
Barium sulfate		• Small spheres • 'Cloudy' motion • Easy to disperse • Slow sedimentation rate	• Available in pharmaceutical grade, compatible in cleanroom areas • Insoluble in water • Serial dilution of known concentration can be produced to challenge personnel • Realistically simulates protein aggregates	None observed
Magnesium stearate		Large clumps	• Available in pharmaceutical grade, compatible in cleanroom areas	Too hydrophobic to properly process in aqueous solutions
Silicon dioxide		Not visible	• Available in pharmaceutical grade, compatible in cleanroom areas	Used amount either dissolved in aqueous solution or particles were too small to visually observe
Sodium carbonate		Not visible	• Available in pharmaceutical grade, compatible in cleanroom areas	
Glass, chipped from Pasteur capillary pipette	Glass shards (intrinsic)	• Large particle • Reflects light • Difficult to disperse • Fast sedimentation rate	• Available in pharmaceutical grade, compatible in cleanroom areas • Realistically simulates intrinsic particles from glass vial used during routine production	Chipping glass may generate fine glass particles in cleanroom area
Rubber, cut from bromobutyl stopper	Rubber particle(intrinsic)	• Large pellet • Difficult to disperse • Fast sedimentation rate	• Available in pharmaceutical grade, compatible in cleanroom areas • Realistically simulates intrinsic particles from bromobutyl stopper used during routine production	Challenging to cut a fine particle in LAF cabinet with tweezers and scalpel

Table 3. *Cont.*

Defect Materials	Simulates	Characteristics in Solution	Advantages	Disadvantages
Fiber, sterile cloth	Fiber (extrinsic)	• Small or large thread-like particle • Easy to disperse • Slow sedimentation rate	• Available in pharmaceutical grade, compatible in cleanroom areas • Realistically simulates extrinsic particles from sterile mat or cleaning/disinfection cloth used during routine production	• Fiber may eventually disintegrate over time, making the defect undetectable • Challenging to cut a fine fiber in LAF cabinet with tweezers and scissors
Fiber, paper towel		• Small thread-like particle • Easy to disperse • Slow sedimentation rate • Fully disintegrates	• Widely available • Easy to process	• Unstandardized quality, incompatible with higher-grade cleanroom areas • Tearing generates airborne particles • Quickly and fully disintegrates, making the defect undetectable
Dented aluminum crimp	Mechanical damage primary packaging	Not applicable	• Realistically simulates mechanical damage encountered during routine production • Defects can be introduced after production process outside LAF cabinet • Different damages can be introduced to simulate minor (cosmetic) or major (packaging integrity) damages to challenge personnel	None observed
Chipped plastic cap protecting vial septum	Mechanical damage primary packaging	Not applicable		

3.5. Manufacturing Qualificaiton Test Sets Under GMP Conditions

Based on the literature search, personnel interviews and feedback, and pre-GMP formulation studies (Figure 1), the developed manufacturing protocol was used to produce the final GMP QTSs complying with the specifications of an optimal QTS (Table 1). The pre-GMP formulation studies ensured that all selected defect types could be effectively tech transferred and reproduced in a GMP cleanroom setting. This approach allowed us to manufacture two GMP QTSs that simulated defects encountered during routine GMP productions while complying with GMP standards.

The final GMP QTSs both contained 100 glass containers manufactured in a LAF. Glass vials filled with WFI, capped with bromobutyl rubber stoppers and aluminum crimp sleeves, were used as containers. To address the needs of different product formulations, two QTSs were manufactured: one for clear solutions and another simulating colored solutions, specifically those similar to bevacizumab-800CW (Figure 3) [11]. The defect types introduced into these vials are detailed in Table 4 and the manufacturing protocol of the QTS containing the colored solution is given in the Supplementary Materials.

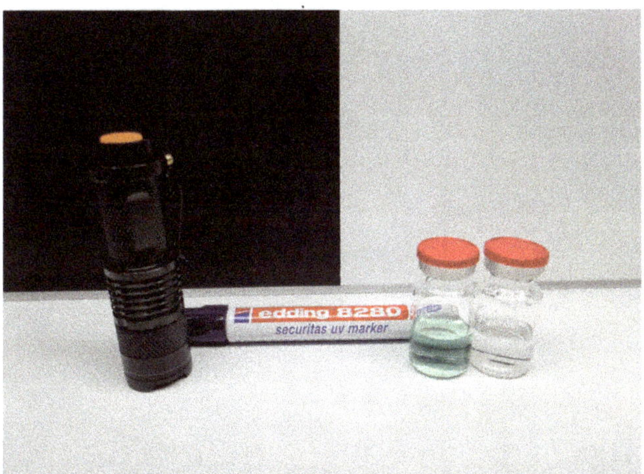

Figure 3. UV lamp and UV marker with two vials from the final GMP QTSs filled with either WFI + fluorescent dye IRDye 800CW (left vial, colored solution) or WFI (right vial, clear solution).

Table 4. The composition of the final GMP QTSs composed of 100 containers.

Defect	Simulates	Defect Classification	Frequency
Dent crimp seal	Cosmetic damage, mechanical stress	Minor	2%
Damaged plastic cap, rubber stopper exposed	Critically damaged product, loss of rubber septum sterility	Critical	2%
Rubber particle	Extrinsic particulate matter from bromobutyl rubber	Major	1%
Glass shard	Extrinsic particulate matter from glass vial	Major	2%
Small particulate matter	Extrinsic or intrinsic (protein aggregates, drug precipitates) particulate matter	Major	4% [a]
Fibers	Extrinsic particulate matter from sterile mat or cleaning/disinfection cloth	Major	4%
No defects	Drug products with no defects that should not unjustly be rejected	Not applicable	85%

[a] One container with MCC, one container with talc, one container with 0.005 mg/mL barium sulfate, and one container with 0.010 mg/mL barium sulfate. See also the Supplementary Materials.

The GMP QTSs included diverse defect materials—glass, rubber, fibers from Sontara® cloth, talc, MCC, and barium sulfate—selected based on their ability to simulate defects encountered during routine GMP productions (Figures 4 and 5). The inclusion of multiple defect types was selected to train and qualify personnel for a wide range of defects. The defects were categorized as critical, major, or minor.

Each container in the set was uniquely marked with a UV marker to bear either the number 1 (no defect) or 2–16 (defects), and this marking was designed to be easily discernible under a UV lamp (Figure 2). A comprehensive decoding table used by the trainer (a hospital pharmacist) of the personnel accompanied the set, providing a detailed description of the different defects along with their corresponding numbers for reference during the qualification procedure.

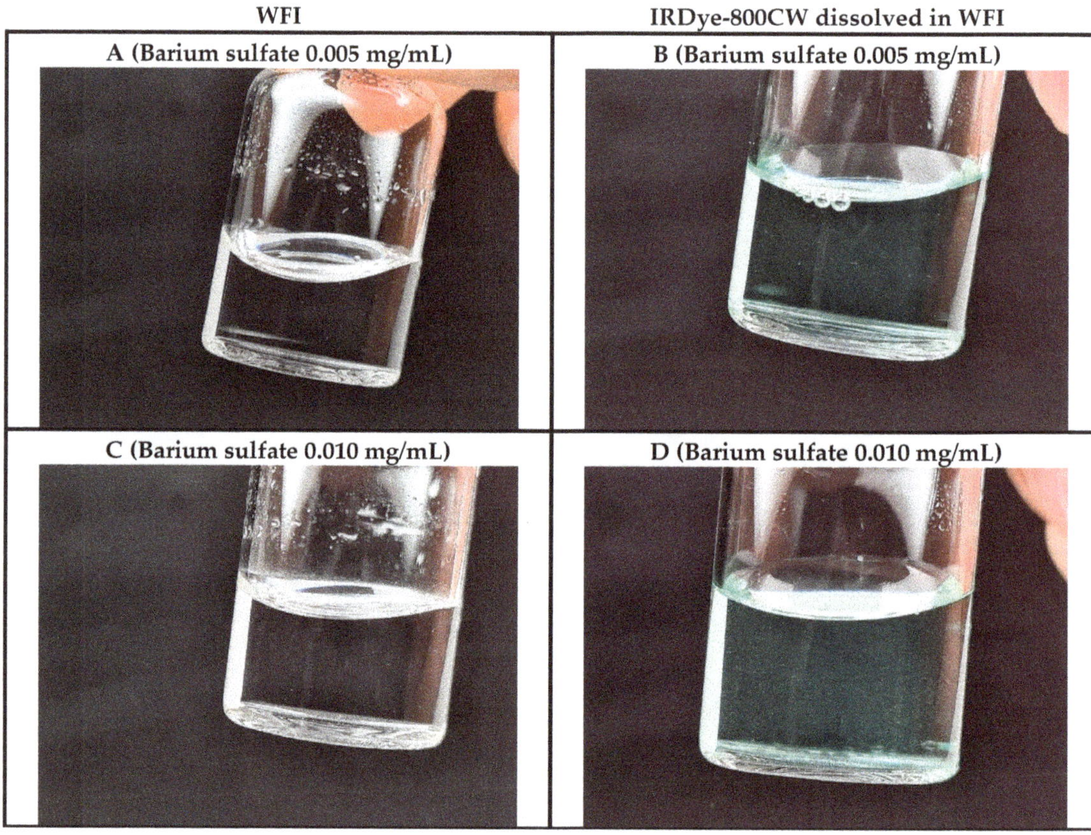

Figure 4. *Cont.*

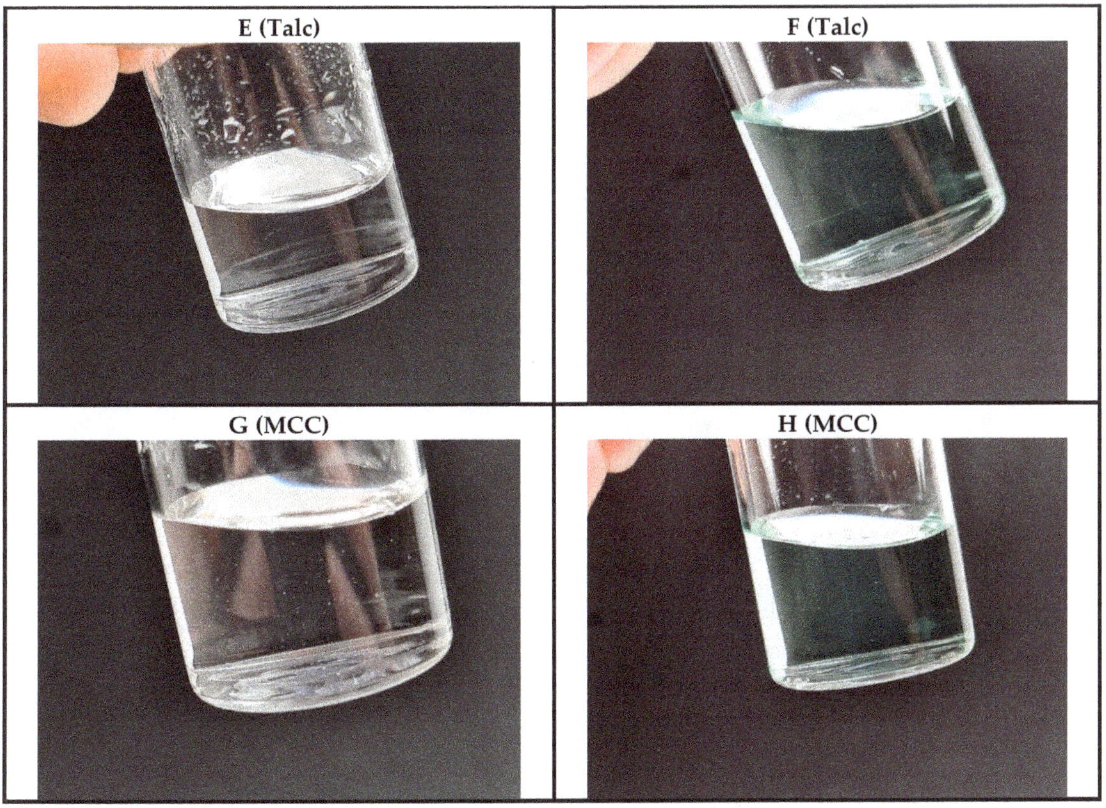

Figure 4. Representative images of the manufactured GMP QTSs containing either WFI (left, clear solution) or IRDye-800CW dissolved in WFI (right, colored solution) simulating small intrinsic and/or extrinsic particulate matter as defects. (**A**,**B**) Barium sulfate 0.005 mg/mL; (**C**,**D**) barium sulfate 0.010 mg/mL; (**E**,**F**) talc; (**G**,**H**) microcrystalline cellulose (MCC).

To ensure the validity of the introduced defects and the absence of defects in non-defective containers, a thorough four-eye consensus method was employed. This method was executed to guarantee that the defects were distinctly visible and that non-defective containers indeed were free of defects. The stability of the test set was validated over a two-year period using this consensus method.

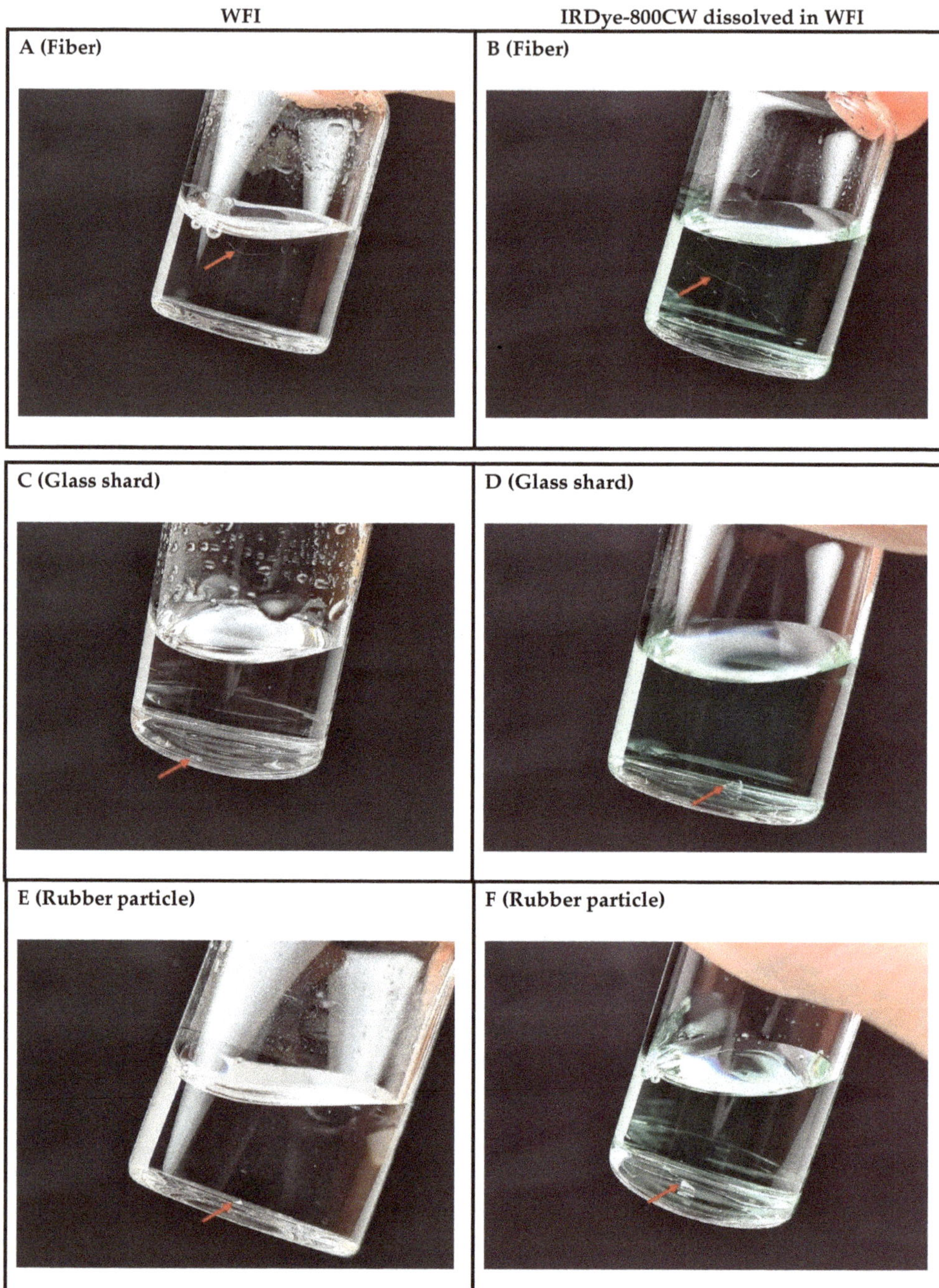

Figure 5. Representative images of the manufactured GMP QTSs containing either WFI (left, clear solution) or IRDye-800CW dissolved in WFI (right, colored solution) simulating either large intrinsic particulate matter or extrinsic particulate matter as defects. (**A**,**B**) Fibers; (**C**,**D**) glass shard; (**E**,**F**) rubber particle. The red arrows point at the particulate matter present in the vial.

3.6. Comparison Qualification Test Set Defects with Protein (Monoclonal Antibody) Aggregates

To assess whether the defects introduced into the GMP QTSs realistically simulated intrinsic particulate matter (e.g., protein aggregates), bevacizumab-800CW vials manufactured under GMP conditions were placed in an incubator for 48 h at 50 °C and at room temperature for an additional 7 days as a stress test to induce protein aggregates in the solution. After 48 h of storage at 50 °C, the bevacizumab-800CW vials contained detectable aggregates (Figure 6A), which showed similar particle characteristics (e.g., motion, particle size, and sedimentation rate) as the GMP QTS container containing a barium sulfate suspension of 0.005 mg/mL (Figure 6B). After an additional storage period of 7 days at room temperature, the bevacizumab-800CW vial contained more and visibly larger aggregates (Figure 6C), which showed similar particle characteristics as the GMP QTS container containing a barium sulfate suspension of 0.010 mg/mL (Figure 6D). Taken together, these results demonstrate that the barium sulfate suspension is suitable to simulate varying degrees of protein aggregates by using different barium sulfate concentrations.

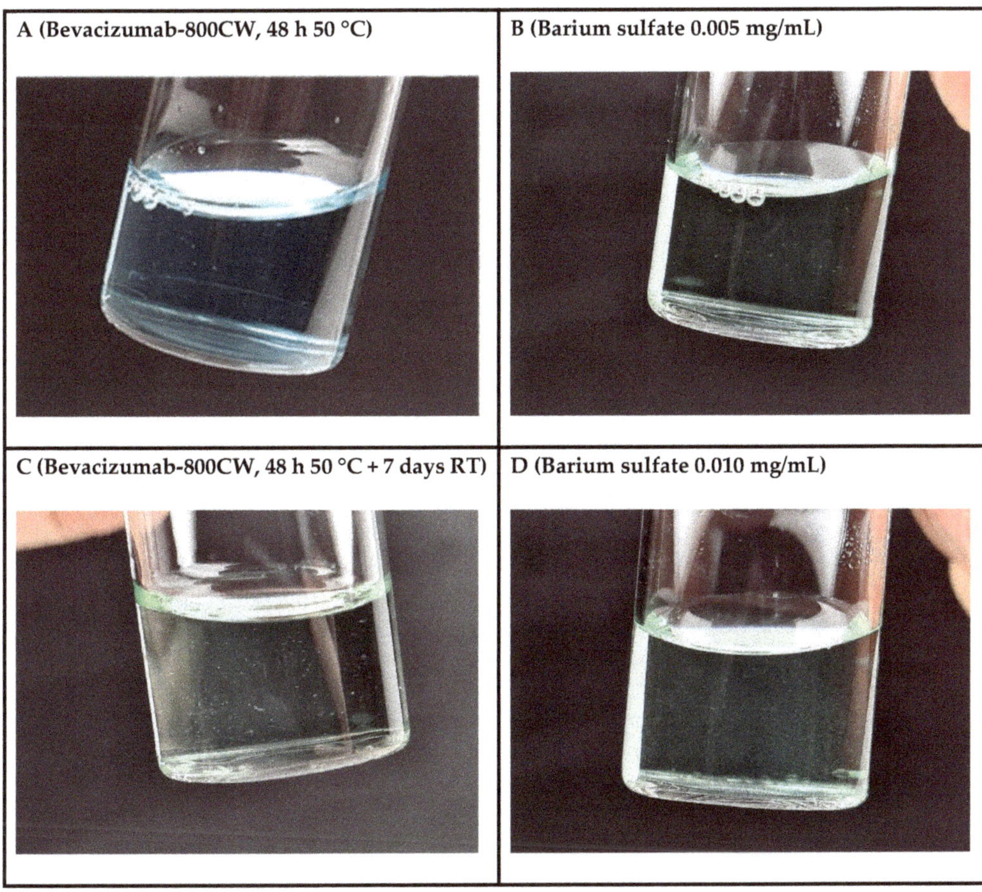

Figure 6. Barium sulfate containers from the GMP QTS simulated protein aggregates the best. (**A**) Bevacizumab-800CW stored at 50 °C for 48 h; (**B**) IRDye-800CW dissolved in WFI containing barium sulfate (0.005 mg/mL). (**C**) Bevacizumab-800CW stored at 50 °C for 48 h + 7 days at room temperature; (**D**) IRDye-800CW dissolved in WFI containing barium sulfate (0.010 mg/mL).

3.7. Evaluation of Qualification Test Sets for GMP Training and Qualification Purposes

The developed QTSs manufactured under GMP conditions were used for GMP training and formal visual inspection qualification procedures. Personnel stated that the GMP QTSs were a significant improvement for training and qualification purposes compared to using manufacturing rejects. Factors attributed to this improvement were a fully blinded qualification procedure, the use of fully representative containers and solutions in a representative batch size, the wide range of defects, the possibility to use less/more challenging defects, and the possibility to include new defects based on routine GMP productions and manufacturing reject trend analysis. Personnel also stated that the wide range of introduced defects simulated the wide range of intrinsic and particulate matter encountered during GMP productions.

Based on the experience and evaluation of the hospital pharmacist involved in the GMP training and formal visual inspection qualification procedures, the GMP QTSs were seen as a significant improvement compared to QTSs using manufacturing rejects. Besides the abovementioned factors stated by personnel, a significant factor attributing to this improvement was using a fully qualified GMP QTS in which the defects and non-defects were confirmed by the consensus method (Section 3.5), which ensured the validity of the introduced defects and the absence of defects in non-defective containers. Therefore, all qualification results could be interpreted unambiguously, which is considered to be an improvement compared to qualification procedures using manufacturing rejects (discussed in Section 4).

4. Discussion

The present study describes the development and feasibility of an adaptable and optimal QTS for personnel involved in visual inspection procedures of parenteral drug products manufactured under GMP conditions in hospital pharmacy compounding facilities. Although personnel qualification is required by GMP guidelines, no adaptable manufacturing protocols or formal guidelines for the development of an optimal and in-house manufactured QTSs are available in the current literature, which possibly points at unstandardized visual inspection qualification procedures between different production sites. The survey results from the five Dutch hospital pharmacies indeed showed that the used QTSs, procedures, and acceptance criteria differed between the production sites. To standardize the visual inspection qualification procedure and use a QTS that is not only representative for the defects and containers encountered during routine GMP productions but also compliant with guidelines on visual inspection of parental drug products, we developed an adaptable manufacturing protocol for an in-house manufactured GMP QTS based on these guidelines and personnel interviews. As a proof-of-concept, two QTSs were manufactured under GMP conditions, showing the feasibility and adaptability of the protocol. To the best of our knowledge, this is the first study presenting these data, and our developed manufacturing protocol may aid compounding facilities in the standardization, training, and qualification of personnel involved in visual inspection procedures.

The literature search identified key elements and attributes for an optimal QTS and visual inspection procedures, which we considered as relevant for an adaptable QTS protocol [1,7,9]. The interviews with GMP personnel further supported these findings, indicating the practical relevance of these key elements. Therefore, these key elements and attributes were used for the development of our protocol [1,8,10,12].

The literature search also identified one study describing a QTS manufacturing process [16]. However, we considered this method unsuitable for the development of our protocol since it did not comply with the key elements and attributes for an optimal QTS.

The survey among hospital compounding facilities revealed considerable variability in the qualification procedures and used test sets. Although standardized processes and qualification procedures are desired within GMP compounding facilities to ensure a consistent level of training quality, no practical protocols or guidelines are currently available for visual inspection test sets or procedures. Our developed GMP QTS manufacturing protocol addresses this gap by providing an in-house and adaptable manufacturing protocol for GMP compounding facilities that can be readily implemented.

The adaptability of the manufacturing protocol is particularly beneficial for hospital pharmacy compounding facilities, which generally operate with fewer resources, manufacture smaller batch sizes, but have larger product ranges than a given pharmaceutical company. Therefore, the protocol can be easily adapted to manufacture QTSs relevant for different products (e.g., different fill volumes, colored/turbid solutions, different primary packaging, et cetera) at low costs without the need to amass sufficient manufacturing rejects, which is especially challenging for products with smaller batch sizes. Moreover, the wishes, experience of personnel involved in visual inspection procedures, and manufacturing reject trend analyses can be used to further optimize the test set, and by extension, the training, qualification, and inspection procedures.

Using manufacturing rejects to develop QTSs can lead to a biased and incomplete number of defects present in the test set since the composition is fully dependent on rejects encountered during routine productions [9]. In addition, the interpretation of the visual inspection qualification results may be challenging in case manufacturing rejects are used for the QTSs. During the UMCG qualification procedures using manufacturing rejects, some personnel stated that containers coded as defects could not be identified as such, and containers coded as non-defects were identified as defects. A possible reason for this discrepancy could be that the defect was either too challenging for the personnel or that the defect, initially present, disappeared over time; for instance, in case the particulate matter dissolved or fully disintegrated after an extended period of storage. Another reason could be that a defect was introduced over time in containers that initially did not contain any defects; for instance, container damage due to frequent handling or the precipitation of the active pharmaceutical ingredient or excipients over time. The question then arises: are the current, discrepant observed qualification results true or not? This makes unambiguous interpretation of the qualification results challenging.

For the developed QTSs, insoluble and not readily disintegrating materials were used to introduce stable defects that are presumed to be present for an extended period of time. Furthermore, the consensus visual inspection method was employed and ensured that all introduced defects were accurately identified as such and confirms that the containers that did not contain any defects were indeed identified as such. This procedure can be seen as the qualification of the test set itself with the four-eye method, which warrants its validity and can be periodically repeated (e.g., annually). In case the QTS does not (or no longer) meets the desired criteria, a new QTS can be manufactured by the compounding facility. Based on our own experience, the developed GMP QTSs are stable at room temperature for at least two years.

Since no manufacturing rejects are required for the developed GMP QTSs, these rejects from the visual inspection procedure can possibly be used for preclinical research or process optimization procedures of the manufactured drug products. For instance, manufacturing rejects containing extrinsic particulate matter (e.g., fiber or glass shard) cannot be administered to patients but can be used to develop, validate, or optimize analytical methods of the drug product, which is of particular interest for expensive drug products such as fluorescent-labelled monoclonal antibodies [19] or neoantigen vaccines [20].

Besides personnel qualification, the adaptable manufacturing protocol for a QTS could be employed for the process development and optimization of (semi-)automated visual inspection technologies. With the possibility to manufacture different batch sizes containing any desired defect in any desired frequency, these QTSs could be used to calibrate, qualify, and validate these technologies. Depending on the process parameters and required accuracy of the systems, the manufacturing protocol can be adapted accordingly to yield a QTS that is suitable for system qualification and validation. However, to the best of our knowledge, the qualification and validation of (semi-)automated visual inspection technologies with in-house manufactured QTSs have not been described in the literature. Therefore, the application and feasibility of our developed QTS for (semi-)automated systems needs to be investigated.

Although we used a mixed methods study design, there are several limitations of the present study. First, the survey sample size was limited to five large Dutch hospital pharmacy compounding facilities. Therefore, the survey result did not present data of centralized compounding facilities or other, smaller hospital pharmacy compounding facilities in the Netherlands or abroad. Second, only experienced personnel of the UMCG were interviewed, and these data were used for the development and optimization of the QTS formulations. Third, for the formulation studies and the proof-of-concept, we only focused on clear and colored aqueous solutions in clear primary containers. However, it is expected that the motion characteristics as well as visibility of particulate matter differ in viscous or turbid solutions packaged in opaque or colored (e.g., amber) primary containers [9,15]. Finally, for proof-of-concept, we manufactured two GMP QTSs with a limited amount of containers containing small particulate matter (talc, MMC, 0.010 mg/mL, and 0.005 mg/mL). To further challenge personnel, serial dilutions of these formulations can be made with a resulting lower particle count, which yield QTS containers that are more challenging to detect during qualification procedures. These limitations should be considered and taken into account for the development of in-house manufactured QTSs by compounding facilities using the provided protocol (Supplementary Materials).

In conclusion, this study presents the development of a practical, feasible, and adaptable manufacturing protocol for a QTS for the qualification of personnel involved in the visual inspection of parental drug products manufactured under GMP conditions. Due to its adaptability, the qualification test set can be expanded and further customized and optimized based on specific wishes, personnel experiences, and manufacturing reject trend analyses. Together, our developed QTS manufacturing protocol has been proven to be a valuable addition to process standardization, training, and qualification of personnel.

Supplementary Materials: The following supporting information can be downloaded at https://www.mdpi.com/article/10.3390/pharmaceutics17010074/s1, Manufacturing protocol for the GMP QTS colored with fluorescent dye IRDye 800CW.

Author Contributions: Conceptualization, H.J.W., J.M.M. and B.G.; methodology, B.G. and K.R.K.; validation, J.v.Z., H.J.W., J.M.M. and B.G.; formal analysis, T.v.d.B.-B., H.P.S.H., K.R.K., H.H.W. and B.G.; investigation, T.v.d.B.-B., H.P.S.H., K.R.K. and B.G.; resources, J.v.Z., H.J.W., J.M.M. and B.G.; data curation, T.v.d.B.-B., H.P.S.H., K.R.K. and B.G.; writing—original draft preparation, T.v.d.B.-B., H.P.S.H., K.R.K. and B.G.; writing—review and editing, T.v.d.B.-B., H.P.S.H., H.H.W., J.v.Z., J.M.M., H.J.W. and B.G.; visualization, T.v.d.B.-B., H.P.S.H. and B.G.; supervision, J.M.M., H.J.W. and B.G.; project administration, T.v.d.B.-B., H.P.S.H., K.R.K. and B.G. All authors have read and agreed to the published version of the manuscript.

Funding: This research received no external funding.

Institutional Review Board Statement: This research did not require institutional review board statement.

Informed Consent Statement: This research did not require informed consent statements since no patients were included in this study.

Data Availability Statement: The data are contained within the article.

Acknowledgments: The authors thank I.R. den Toom for image editing.

Conflicts of Interest: The authors declare no conflicts of interest.

Appendix A. Ishikawa Diagram and Risk Assessment of Possible Causes and Sources of Defective Containers and/or Particulate Contamination

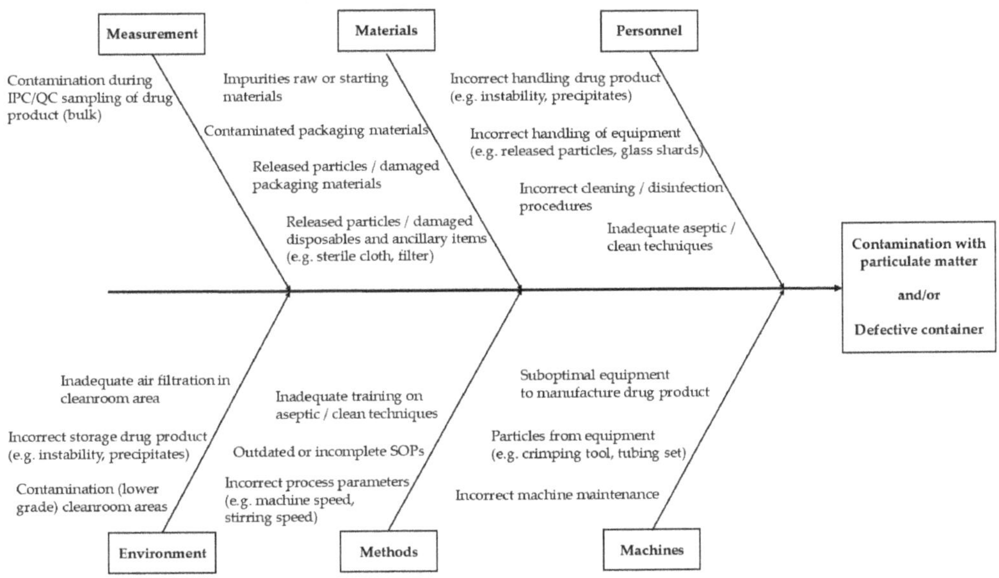

Appendix B. Questionnaire Survey National Hospital Pharmacy Compounding Facilities

Dear colleague,

Currently, we are in the process of developing and manufacturing a standardized qualification test set for the GMP visual inspection qualification procedures of personnel. We intend to manufacture the qualification test set in our compounding facility under GMP conditions, including containers with defects and particulate matter. We intend to manufacture the defective units by adding known particles (fibers, hairs, glass, particles, etc.).

Therefore, we are curious about the strategies employed by other hospital pharmacies. Could you please answer the following questions:

1. How do you qualify personnel involved in the visual inspection of parenteral drug products?
2. How do you develop the qualification test set consisting of containers with and without particles/defects?
3. How many defective containers does your qualification test set contains?
4. What are the particles/defects in the qualification test set?
5. What is your experience regarding the visual inspection qualification procedures of personnel?
6. What are your acceptance criteria for qualifying/disqualifying personnel, e.g., maximum number of missed defects, maximum number of compliant units that are rejected, etc.?

7. Is it possible to review your qualification procedure (confidential, of course)? If desired, we can also send ours.

We hope that you can assist us and look forward to your responses.
Kind regards,

Appendix C. Questionnaire for GMP Personnel Regarding the Visual Inspection

During the interview, detailed follow-up questions were asked to obtain more information about common particles and defects encountered during routine production.

1. Could you explain what visual inspection of parental drug products is?
2. Please describe the visual inspection procedure in detail.
3. Is there a four-eye check during the visual inspection?
4. What are common particles encountered during the visual inspection procedure?
5. Is the origin of these particles always clear or known?
6. What are particles that are difficult to detect during the visual inspection procedure?
7. What are common defects that are found during the visual inspection procedure, such as packaging integrity issues or (cosmetic) damages to the packaging?

References

1. EU GMP Annex 1. Available online: https://health.ec.europa.eu/system/files/2022-08/20220825_gmp-an1_en_0.pdf (accessed on 4 November 2024).
2. Le Brun, P.; Crauste-Manciet, S.; Krämer, I.; Smith, J.; Woerdenbag, H. *Practical Pharmaceutics*, 2nd ed.; Springer Nature Switzerland AG: Cham, Switzerland, 2023; pp. 797–798.
3. Borgonje, P.E.; Dunnewind, T.; Bosma, L.; Tokromo-Evegaars, M.; Meulenhoff, P.C.W.; Breukels, O. Testing of Parenteral Drug Products for Visible Particles: Comparison of the Ph. Eur. Method with an Alternative Method Using Polarised Light. *Eur. J. Hosp. Pharm.* **2024**, *31*, 447–449. [CrossRef] [PubMed]
4. US Pharmaceutical Convention. United States Pharmacopeia. In *Monograph ⟨1787⟩ Measurement of Subvisible Particulate Matter in Therapeutic Protein Injections*; USP-NF: Rockville, MD, USA, 2023.
5. Cash, P.W.; Narwal, R.; Levitskaya, S.V.; Krause, S.; Murphy, D.; Mazaheri, M. Semi-Quantitative Analysis of Inherent Visible Particles for Biopharmaceutical Products. *PDA J. Pharm. Sci. Technol.* **2016**, *70*, 134–142. [CrossRef] [PubMed]
6. European Directorate for the Quality of Medicines & HealthCare. Particulate Contamination: Visible Particles. In *European Pharmacopoeia (Ph.Eur.)*, 11.5 ed.; EDQM Council of Europe: Strasbourg, France, 2024. Available online: https://pheur.edqm.eu/home (accessed on 6 December 2024).
7. US Pharmaceutical Convention. United States Pharmacopeia. In *Monograph <1790> Visual Inspections of Injections*; NF-USP: Rockville, MD, USA, 2023.
8. FDA Inspection of Injectable Products for Visible Particulates Guidance for Industry DRAFT GUIDANCE. Available online: https://www-fda-gov.proxy-ub.rug.nl/media/154868/download (accessed on 4 November 2024).
9. Melchore, J.A.; Berdovich, D. Considerations for Design and Use of Container Challenge Sets for Qualification and Validation of Visible Particulate Inspection. *PDA J. Pharm. Sci. Technol.* **2012**, *66*, 273–284. [CrossRef] [PubMed]
10. British Pharmacopoeia SC I N. Particulate Contamination. In *BP 2024 (Ph. Eur. 11.5 Update)*; Medicines & Healthcare producs Regulator Agency; The Stationery Office Ltd. (TSO): Norwich, UK, 2024.
11. ter Weele, E.J.; Terwisscha van Scheltinga, A.G.T.; Linssen, M.D.; Nagengast, W.B.; Lindner, I.; Jorritsma-Smit, A.; de Vries, E.G.E.; Kosterink, J.G.W.; Lub-de Hooge, M.N. Development, Preclinical Safety, Formulation, and Stability of Clinical Grade Bevacizumab-800CW, a New near Infrared Fluorescent Imaging Agent for First in Human Use. *Eur. J. Pharm. Biopharm.* **2016**, *104*, 226–234. [CrossRef] [PubMed]
12. Parental Drug Association (PDA); Shabushnig, J.G. Visual Inspection of Injectable Products: More than Sorting Good from Bad.... Available online: https://www.scribd.com/document/711615516/PDA-Visual-Inspection-of-Injectable-Products (accessed on 4 November 2024).
13. Shire, S.J.; Shahrokh, Z.; Liu, J. Challenges in the Development of High Protein Concentration Formulations. *J. Pharm. Sci.* **2004**, *93*, 1390–1402. [CrossRef] [PubMed]
14. Andya, J.D.; Hsu, C.C.; Shire, S.J. Mechanisms of Aggregate Formation and Carbohydrate Excipient Stabilization of Lyophilized Humanized Monoclonal Antibody Formulations. *AAPS PharmSci* **2003**, *5*, 21–31. [CrossRef] [PubMed]

15. Melchore, J.A. Sound Practices for Consistent Human Visual Inspection. *AAPS Pharmscitech* **2011**, *12*, 215–221. [CrossRef] [PubMed]
16. Borchert, S.J.; Maxwell, R.J.; Davison, R.L.; Aldrich, D.S. Standard Particulate Sets for Visual Inspection Systems: Their Preparation, Evaluation, and Applications. *Parenter. Sci. Technol.* **1986**, *40*, 265–276.
17. Labonté, V.; Marion, A.; Virgilio, N.; Tavares, J.R. Gas-Phase Surface Engineering of Polystyrene Beads Used to Challenge Automated Particle Inspection Systems. *Ind. Eng. Chem. Res.* **2016**, *55*, 7362–7372. [CrossRef]
18. IPS-Group A/S Sontara® Micropure AP. Available online: https://ips-group.dk/product/sontara-micropure-ap/ (accessed on 7 March 2024).
19. Linssen, M.D.; Hooghiemstra, W.T.R.; Jorritsma-Smit, A.; Allersma, D.P.; Dijkstra, G.; Nagengast, W.B. Development and Characterisation of Antibody-Based Optical Imaging Probes for Inflammatory Bowel Disease. *Pharmaceuticals* **2021**, *14*, 922. [CrossRef] [PubMed]
20. Oosting, L.T.; Franke, K.; Martin, M.V.; Kloosterman, W.P.; Jamieson, J.A.; Glenn, L.A.; de Jager, M.W.; van Zanten, J.; Allersma, D.P.; Gareb, B. Development of a Personalized Tumor Neoantigen Based Vaccine Formulation (FRAME-001) for Use in a Phase II Trial for the Treatment of Advanced Non-Small Cell Lung Cancer. *Pharmaceutics* **2022**, *14*, 1515. [CrossRef] [PubMed]

pharmaceutics

MDPI

Article

Development and Characterization of Trihexyphenidyl Orodispersible Minitablets: A Challenge to Fill the Therapeutic Gap in Neuropediatrics

Camila Olivera [1,2,3], Oriana Boscolo [1,2], Cecilia Dobrecky [1,2,4], Claudia A. Ortega [5], Laura S. Favier [5], Valeria A. Cianchino [5], Sabrina Flor [1,2,3] and Silvia Lucangioli [1,2,3,]*

1 Departamento de Tecnología Farmacéutica, Facultad de Farmacia y Bioquímica, Universidad de Buenos Aires, Junin 956, Buenos Aires C1113AAD, Argentina; colivera@docente.ffyb.uba.ar (C.O.); sflor@ffyb.uba.ar (S.F.)
2 Instituto de Tecnología Farmacéutica y Biofarmacia (InTecFyB), Facultad de Farmacia y Bioquímica, Universidad de Buenos Aires, Junin 956, Buenos Aires C1113AAD, Argentina
3 Consejo Nacional de Investigaciones Científicas y Técnicas (CONICET), Godoy Cruz 2290, Buenos Aires C1414AAD, Argentina
4 Departamento de Farmacología, Facultad de Farmacia y Bioquímica, Universidad de Buenos Aires, Junin 956, Buenos Aires C1113AAD, Argentina
5 Área de Farmacotecnia, Ética y Legislación Farmacéutica, Departamento de Farmacia, Facultad de Química, Bioquímica y Farmacia, Universidad Nacional de San Luis, San Luis D5700HHW, Argentina
* Correspondence: slucangi@ffyb.uba.ar

Abstract: Background: Trihexyphenidyl (THP) has been widely used for over three decades as pediatric pharmacotherapy in patients affected by segmental and generalized dystonia. In order to achieve effective and safe pharmacotherapy for this population, new formulations are needed. **Objective:** The aim of this work is the development of trihexyphenidyl orodispersible minitablets (ODMTs) for pediatric use. **Methods:** Six different excipients were tested as diluents. The properties of powder mixtures were evaluated before direct compression and pharmacotechnical tests were performed on the final formulation. The determination of the API content, uniformity of dosage, and physicochemical stability studies were analyzed by an HPLC-UV method. **Results**: The developed ODMTs met pharmacopeia specifications for content, hardness, friability, disintegration, and dissolution tests. The physicochemical stability study performed over 18 months shows that API content remains within 90.0–110.0% at least for this period. **Conclusions:** These ODMTs will allow efficient, safe, and high-quality pharmacotherapy.

Keywords: trihexyphenidyl; orodispersible minitablets; pediatric pharmacotherapy; orphan formulation

1. Introduction

Trihexyphenidyl (THP) (1-cyclohexyl-1-phenyl-3-piperidin-1-ylpropan-1-ol) (Figure 1) [1] acts as an anticholinergic agent by intervening at the level of muscarinic receptors. While its most popular therapeutic use is for treating Parkinson's disease in adult patients, it has been widely used over three decades as pediatric pharmacotherapy in patients affected by segmental and generalized dystonia [2,3]. This neurological condition is characterized by sustained or intermittent muscle contractions, causing anormal movements or postures [4] that can be painful. The contractions they suffer from impact on patient autonomy and movement capacity, also affecting speech and participation in daily activities [5].

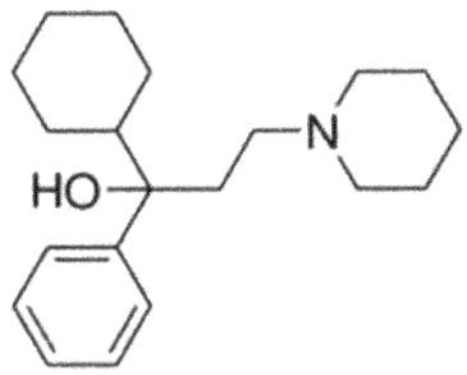

Figure 1. Trihexyphenidyl chemical structure.

THP is used as pharmacotherapy in children with extrapyramidal cerebral palsy (PCEP), where a variety of involuntary movements predominate, and it is characterized by postural instability secondary to defective regulation of muscle tone and coordination [6]. In this type of pathology affecting children, oral administration formulations are commonly used [7,8] and are considered preferable whenever possible. The pharmacokinetics and pharmacodynamics of the active substance differ between children and adults due to differences in their metabolic development. Therefore, when developing a formulation for pediatrics, dosing flexibility as well as easy administration and patient acceptability must be considered [9].

Hence, it is necessary to develop administration systems appropriate to the patient's age range while maintaining their safety, efficacy, and accessibility. In most cases, available conventional oral formulations are not intended to meet the requirements of this subgroup of the population [10]. Thanks to scientific and technological advances, new pharmaceutical forms have emerged with advantages in terms of administration convenience, dosing, and efficacy. Minitablets are relatively new solid pharmaceutical forms that present the advantages of conventional tablets and, additionally, are associated with ease and flexibility of dosing. Clinical studies demonstrate that the use of THP has improved symptoms associated with dystonia [2], which often manifest early in life.

The World Health Organization (WHO) and international regulatory agencies work to raise awareness and promote activities related to pediatric research in both academic and industrial settings [11].

In pursuit of achieving effective and safe pharmacotherapy in the pediatric population, the development of new formulations that meet their needs is required. The therapeutic requirements of pediatric patients, unlike adults, continuously change as their organism does [12]. Ensuring patient adherence to treatment is critical. Due to the swallowing difficulty that pediatric patients have, liquid formulations are usually prescribed, but the physicochemical and microbiological instability they present must be considered, as well as their high transportation and storage costs.

Orodispersible minitablets (ODMTs) emerge as a response to pediatric pharmacotherapy since, due to their small size and rapid disintegration, they are ingested without any difficulty [13–15]. They are defined as tablets with a diameter smaller than 3 mm [16] which, once placed in the oral cavity, disintegrate within a few seconds upon contact with saliva [17].

Processed and co-processed excipients are widely used in the development of orodispersible tablet formulations. After undergoing a co-processing technique, such as spray drying, the new excipients present advantages over their individual previous properties. Among them may be found particle shape and size uniformity, increased porosity, and decreased sensitivity to lubricants, improving flowability and compressibility [18]. These types of excipients can encompass diluents as well as superdisintegrants, glidants, and binders. A distinction should be made between different types of co-processed excipients based on their chemical characteristics. On one hand, there are those based on lactose, mannitol, sorbitol, and starch, and on the other hand, there are those based on cellulose such as microcrystalline cellulose and other derivatives. In this work, six different processed and co-processed excipients were tested for potential use in producing ODMTs by direct compression. There are databases that compile toxicological as well as clinical information about the use of different excipients in the pediatric population. The processed and co-processed excipients tested are widely used in the production of various pharmaceutical forms.

Pediatric patients with dystonia associated with cerebral palsy should start pharmacotherapy with a dose of 0.02–0.06 mg/kg of THP administered two to three times a day (up to a dose of 1–2 mg) with weekly increments of 0.05–0.1 mg/kg [19–21].

In order to fill the gap in pediatric therapeutics, THP ODMTs have been designed, developed, and characterized in response to the absence of pediatric formulation of the API in some pharmaceutical markets [22,23]. There is no literature yet describing the development of solid THP formulas specifically targeted at this population subgroup.

Currently, there is no available solid form of THP ODMTs destined for the pediatric population. The aim of this work was the development and characterization of an orphan formulation, as it is based on a known and studied drug but not commercially available in an appropriate preparation or dose [24].

2. Materials and Methods

2.1. Chemical and Reagents

Trihexyphenidyl hydrochloride (100.79 DB, MW 337.93) and magnesium stearate were purchased from Parafarm, Saporiti Drogstore, Buenos Aires, Argentina. StarLac® was acquired from Meggle Pharma, Wasserburg am Inn, Germany; and Disolcel® from Mingtai Chemical Co., Ltd., Taoyuan, Taiwan. Pharmaburst® was purchased from Unifarma s.a, Buenos Aires, Argentina; Mannogem 2080® from SPI Pharma, Wilmington, DE, USA; Cellactose 80®, Avicel C15® from FMC BioPolymer, Philadelphia, PA, USA; and Avicel RC 591® from Productos Destilados SAICyF, Buenos Aires, Argentina.

2.2. Equipment

Physicochemical Stability Study was performed working with an HPLC-UV (Thermo Fisher Scientific Vanquish HPLC) coupled to a diode array spectrophotometer detector (Waltham, MA, USA) using an XBridge™ C18 (5 μm, 4.6 × 150 mm) Hypersil GOLD C18 column. Chromatographic conditions were 30 °C column temperature, 20 μL injection volume at 215 nm, with a flow rate of 1.0 mL/min. The mobile phase consisted of methanol: 1% p/v ammonium acetate pH 6.5 (75:25) according to a method previously developed and validated in house.

2.3. ODMTs

2.3.1. Design and Preformulation Study

A direct compression technique was used for the development of THP ODMTs. The powder mixture was compressed using a SC-1 mini-press single-punch eccentric machine (Talleres Sanchez, Ciudad Autónoma de Buenos Aires, Argentina) tablet press with a 3 mm diameter round-shaped punch. The direct compression pathway was selected for the manufacture of the ODMTs since it involves the lowest number of steps in the production process that could be easily implemented in hospital facilities. ODMTs were characterized by determining their organoleptic properties, as well as pharmacotechnical parameters such as weight uniformity, disintegration time, friability, and hardness. The identification, quantification, and dose uniformity of the THP ODMTs were carried out through an HPLC-UV.

The requirements of dosage forms for the pediatric population include the use of as few excipients as possible in the final formulation. There are excipients in which a co-processing method is carried out in order to improve the properties of the individual excipients. The resulting co-processed excipients will have improved flowability and compressibility properties, as well as reduced moisture and lubricant sensitivity, improving tableting performance. The selection of the most suitable co-processed excipient is a critical point in the development and manufacture of ODMTs.

For the development of the ODMTs, six different excipients have been tested as diluents of the final formulation. After a search of the literature and market research for the most common excipients used in tablet production, with established safety, six co-processed excipients have been selected to evaluate rheological and pharmacotechnical parameters. The co-processed diluents are mentioned below: lactose/starch, fructose/starch, mannitol/sorbitol, lactose/cellulose, microcrystalline cellulose/guar gum, and microcrystalline cellulose/sodium carboxymethylcellulose [25].

For preformulation studies, characterization of the physical mixture has been carried out. Powder rheological properties such as angle of repose, bulk and tapped density, Carr's index, and Hausner ratio were determined in each powder blend. To evaluate drug-excipients physicochemical compatibility, FTIR analysis and scanning electron microscopy (SEM) studies were performed.

Once the best co-processed and active pharmaceutical ingredient (API) mixtures in terms of flowability, compressibility, and compatibility were defined, the final qualitative/quantitative formulation was optimized in terms of percentage of superdisintegrant, lubricant, and glidant.

The diluent/API ratio in the powder blend was evaluated. To verify the non-interaction, an estimated proportion of the rest of the excipients present in the final formulation was used (superdisintegrant, lubricant, and glidant). The blending was made by sieving the powders through a 35-mesh sieve and using a tumbling mixer (Erweka V mixer model AR 403), achieving powder homogeneity after 10 min of mixing confirmed by sampling analysis and energy-dispersive X-ray spectroscopy. Rheological pre-compression parameters were tested and compared. A codified numerical scale (USP 43) [26] was used to determine if the angle of repose, Carr's index, and Hausner ratio were bad, acceptable, good, very good, or excellent for each case.

2.3.2. Flowability, Density, and Compressibility Parameters

Angle of Repose (°)

Powder flowability was determined according to USP-43 [26] by calculating the angle of repose, where the blend is allowed to fall freely through a funnel at a specific height and size. The height of the funnel was adjusted in such a way that the bottom of the funnel just touched the tip of the powder. The angle of repose is determined by the horizontal plane and the inclination of the resulting cone, and its numerical value is indicative of powder flowability. The diameter and height of the powder cone was measured. This is a critical parameter in the process of tablet direct compression, especially when manufacturing tablets with a 3 mm diameter punch.

Angle of repose was determined by the following equation:

$$\tan \theta = h/r$$

where θ is angle of repose, h is the height, and r is the radius of the cone.

Bulk and Tapped Density

A powder blend was accurately weighed and placed in a 100 mL measuring cylinder using an Erweka-D63150. Bulk density (Bd) is determined by the following formula:

$$Bd = \text{powder weight}/\text{powder volume}$$

The determination of the tapped density (Td) is calculated in the same way as powder bulk density by determining the volume at 1250 and 500 taps, setting a speed of 300 taps/min according to USP method I [26] with a powder density tester. The following formula is used for calculation:

$$Td = \text{powder weight}/\text{tapped powder volume}$$

Hausner Ratio (Hr)

The Hausner ratio (Hr) is defined by the following formula and provides information on powder flowability.

$$Hr = \text{tapped density } (V_0)/\text{bulk density } (V_f)$$

Carr's Index (%)

Carr's index (CI) is related to the Hausner ratio as both provide powder compressibility characteristics.

$$CI\ (\%) = 100 \times [(V_0 - V_f)/V_0]$$

Each rheological parameter evaluated was determined in triplicate, and the average of each one was considered for choosing the best diluent that meets the necessary requirements and properties to perform direct compression.

2.3.3. Pharmaceutical Formula Optimization

For the development of the THP ODMTs, the following excipients were selected as part of the final formulation (Table 1): co-processed lactose and corn starch (Star-Lac®), magnesium stearate, sodium croscarmellose (DISOLCEL®), and colloidal silicon dioxide (AEROSIL®) using the direct compression (DC) method. Different proportions were tested in different combinations once the chosen diluent was defined. For the first stage, the final formula was based on the minitablets' pharmacotechnical properties in terms of hardness, friability, and disintegration.

Table 1. Qualitative–quantitative final formulation.

Function	%	Raw Material
API	12.50	Trihexyphenidyl
Diluent	80.50	Lactose + corn starch co-process
Superdisintegrant	5.00	Sodium croscaramellose
Glidant	1.00	Silicium dioxide
Lubricant	1.00	Magnesium stearate

Sodium croscarmellose, magnesium stearate, and silicium dioxide were incorporated as pharmaceutical excipients that provided superdisintegrant, lubricant, and glidant/adsorbent characteristics to the formulation, respectively. The proportion of sodium croscarmellose and silicium dioxide was evaluated, while magnesium stearate was established according to bibliographic data.

To optimize the mixing time, a sample collection was made at 4 different times by quarts. These samples were processed and analyzed by an HPLC-UV with a previously developed and validated method, and the RSD between the samples for each time was calculated. An RSD value of less than 2% suggests that the blend was homogeneous. Lubricant mixing time is a crucial parameter when magnesium stearate is used. Due to its hydrophobic properties, if the mixing time is not optimized, it could produce a coating layer over the active ingredient for excessive mixing that affects disintegration and dissolution time. Therefore, the lubricant mixing point was established at 1 min. Both parameters are fundamental when it comes to ODMTs.

2.3.4. Compatibility Study Confirmation

Attenuated Total Reflection–Fourier Transform Infrared Spectroscopy Analysis (ATR FTIR)

To evaluate API/pharmaceutical excipients' compatibility, an ATR FTIR analysis was carried out using a Nicolet iS50 spectrometer (Thermo Scientific, Waltham, MA, USA) with a one-reflection diamond crystal with 64 scans at a resolution of 4 cm^{-1}. This method allows a simple, fast, and efficient evaluation of possible physical interactions with no need for any previous sample preparation where a mechanical clamp is used to improve the contact between the powder and the equipment. The potential formulation powder mixture was tested by varying the diluent.

Scanning Electron Microscopy and Energy-Dispersive X-Ray Spectroscopy

Additional information related to possible incompatibilities is obtained by performing SEM on the API and API/excipient powder mixture using an FEI INSPECT s50 thermionic microscope operated between 0.1 kV and 30 kV. Images were obtained with an ETD (Everhart–Thornley detector) secondary-electron detector and a vCD backscattered electron detector. EDS analyses were obtained using an Octane Pro detector manufactured by EDAX (Pleasanton, CA, USA). The voltage used was 20 kV for EDS analysis. SE and BSE low-voltage imaging, i.e., near 5 kV, was used to avoid the use of Au or C sputtering. An aliquot of raw sample powder was sprinkled on the carbon tape for sample treatment.

By characterizing the morphological surface of the samples and by combining the mentioned techniques, useful information of polymorphic and crystalline habit changes that may occur can be obtained. Since THP has nitrogen in its chemical structure, nitrogen elemental distribution and mapping was carried out combining SEM with energy-dispersive spectroscopy. The homogeneity of the mixture can also be confirmed with additional studies performed using energy-dispersive X-ray spectroscopy.

2.4. Production of ODMTs

THP ODMTs were elaborated using a co-processed diluent (Star-Lac), sodium croscarmellose, silicium dioxide, and magnesium stearate by a direct compression technique. All mentioned excipients were accurately weighed and properly mixed, passing first through a No. 40 and 60 sieve for the lubricant. The direct blend characterization and mixing time were previously determined and optimized. Compression was carried out using a single 3 mm punch tablet press. The compression parameters were adjusted to obtain an ODMT batch of approximately 20 mg/minitablet weight.

2.5. ODMT Characterization

2.5.1. Pharmacotechnical Parameters

Weight Uniformity

Twenty ODMTs were randomly selected and individually weighed. The results were expressed as weight average and RSD.

Hardness

Twenty ODMTs were randomly selected, and hardness was evaluated using a YD-1 tablet hardness tester (Tianjin Guoming Medicinal Equipment Co., Ltd., Tianjin, China). The results were expressed as force average (N) and RSD.

Friability

Twenty ODMTs were randomly selected and weighed before and after placing them in the CS-4 Friabilometer USP (CS-4 Tablet Friability Tester, Tianjin Guoming Medicinal Equipment Co., Ltd., Tianjin, China) after 100 rotations at 25 rpm.

The percentage weight loss is calculated with the following formula:

$$\%F = (W_{initial} - W_{final})/W_{initial}) \times 100$$

where F is for friability measurement.

Disintegration Time

Six ODMTs were randomly selected and placed in 900 mL of distilled water maintained at 37 ± 0.5 °C. This test was carried out using a BJ-1 Disintegration Tester (Tianjin guoming medicinal equipment CO., Ltd., Tianjin, China), and the time average and RSD were calculated.

Wetting Time

Six ODMTs samples were each placed into a Petri dish over a colored paper filter. The time it takes for the colored solution to reach the upper part of the tablet is recorded as the wetting time. This provides important information relating to tablet disintegration.

2.5.2. In Vitro Dissolution Study and Dissolution Profile

The dissolution test and dissolution profile of the developed THP ODMTs were carried out using USP-43 [26] ERWEKA apparatus I (DT 126 light Series equipment, Frankfurt, Germany) at 100 rpm. The assay was adapted for the evaluation of ODMTs using four minitablets per basket, and 500 mL of acetate buffer pH 4.5 dissolution medium was placed in each vessel and the temperature maintained at 37 ± 0.5 °C. To perform the dissolution assay, an aliquot was withdrawn after 45 min and subsequently quantified. The amount of THP should be no less than 75% according to the USP 43 API monograph [27]. Additionally, the dissolution profile was determined, and aliquots were withdrawn at different times (1, 20, 30, 50, 60, 75, 90, 105, and 120 s and 4, 6, 8, 15, and 45 min) and subsequently quantified [28,29]. In all cases, quantification was carried out by HPLC-UV.

2.5.3. Physicochemical Stability Study

The physicochemical stability study was evaluated by determining the API content and dose uniformity (at time 0). Samples were kept at 25 °C ± 2 °C and at a relative humidity of 60% ± 5% (RH%). The ODMT content was analyzed using an HPLC-UV at 0, 3, 6, 9, 12, and 18 months. All determinations were made in duplicate.

3. Results and Discussion

3.1. ODMT Compounding

3.1.1. Design and Preformulation Study

There are currently no commercialized THP ODMTs. Suitable THP formulations for children are only found in some countries as liquid formulations (syrup). Recent studies show that young children prefer conventional minitablets to liquid formulations [30]. Acceptance evaluation performed in healthy adults demonstrates ODTs as the preferred dosage form for a given API [31,32]. A randomized controlled crossover trial in healthy volunteers compared conventional tablets, ODTs, and OD minitablets, and the latter were selected for being the easiest to take [33]. All the above demonstrate the benefits of developing this type of formulation as a novel drug delivery system for targeted populations.

The DC technique was used as the method of choice for the manufacture of the minitablets as only a few simple processes are involved, which makes it possible to transfer this technology to hospitals. Although direct compression has advantages compared to other compression techniques, when a small diameter punch is used, other considerations must be taken into account to achieve a successful product. Excipients with very good flowability that allow uniform API distribution are required. For this purpose, direct compression co-processed excipients were tested. These have improved quality characteristics compared to the excipients from which they are derived. Using spray drying to co-process both excipients, synergism is achieved, and a new diluent with fast disintegrating properties and good flowability is obtained. In this sense, favorable attributes of each excipient are maintained and improved after the process.

Excipients used in the manufacture of ODMTs must meet certain additional requirements that include good solubility, rapid disintegration without any residue, pleasant taste, and good mouthfeel.

As well as in common orodispersible tablets (ODTs), a diluent, disintegrant, and lubricant must be included in the formulation. Sodium croscarmellose was chosen as a superdisintegrant, silicium dioxide as glidant, and magnesium stearate as lubricant. To choose the best diluent for the development of ODMTs, six co-processed excipients have been tested.

3.1.2. Flowability, Density, and Compressibility Parameters

As previously explained, when using a 3 mm punch to produce minitablets, it should be ensured that the powder mixture presents excellent pre-compression parameters. Since the diluent has the highest proportion in the formulation, its flowability and compressibility properties must be considered as the determining factor in the production process.

For each physical mixture (diluent + API), three individual measurements were made to determine the Hausner ratio, Carr's index, and angle of repose. A color was assigned to the average of each parameter and classified as non-acceptable, acceptable, good, very good, or excellent. The results of each parameter according to the USP 43 numerical range [26] scale are color-coded and presented in Figure 2.

	Hausner Ratio ± SD	Carr's index (%) ± SD	Angle of repose (°) ± SD
Star-Lac®	1.15 ± 0.03	20.7 ± 1.16	30.0 ± 1.21
Pharmaburst®	1.32 ± 0.00	24.0 ± 0.00	32.1 ± 3.45
Mannogem 1080®	1.24 ± 0.01	22.0 ± 2.00	32.5 ± 1.21
Cellactose 80®	1.36 ± 0.01	27.3 ± 1.16	32.7 ± 0.81
Avicel C15®	1.38 ± 0.01	27.7 ± 0.58	42.6 ± 5.97
Avicel RC 591®	1.43 ± 0.01	30.0 ± 0.00	44.7 ± 3.63

SCALE
Bad
Acceptable
Good
Very good
Excellent

Figure 2. Color scale according to powder rheological parameter results obtained for each physical mixture (diluent + API).

As shown in Figure 2, the blend powder containing Star-Lac as the diluent was the one with the best pre-compression parameters obtained.

3.1.3. Pharmaceutical Formula Optimization

The final formulation of the THP ODMTs contains as few market-tested excipients as possible in order to ensure its safety. The selected superdisintegrant is commonly used in tableting and allows the minitablet to disperse immediately upon contact with saliva. Sodium croscarmellose is a cross-linked compound of sodium carboxymethylcellulose, which, through its mechanism, allows the tablet to swell and disintegrate rapidly, promoting the contact of liquid/saliva with the formulation. For orodispersible formulations, it is typically used in a range of 2–5%. Different percentages of sodium croscarmellose have been evaluated. Tablet disintegration and wetting time, as well as tablet hardness and friability, have been taken into account to decide the most effective amount of superdisintegrant to be added in the final powder mixture. Three tablet batches have been elaborated with 2.0, 3.5, and 5.0% of superdisintegrant, respectively (Table 2). In terms of wetting and disintegration time, the batch containing 5.0% of sodium croscarmellose presents a lower time value with respect to the batch containing 2.0% and 3.5%. Each test was carried out in sextuplicate on all the batches prepared (n = 6).

Table 2. Excipient composition for formulation optimization.

Excipient	Batch 1	Batch 2	Batch 3	Batch 4	Batch 5	Batch 6
Superdisintegrant (%)	2.0	3.5	5.0	-	-	-
Glidant/adsorbent (%)	-	-		0.5	1.0	1.5

The average of these parameters among batches did not show a significant difference and were within the established ranges. Thus, a concentration of 5% of sodium croscarmellose was used in the manufacture of ODMTs. Rapid disintegration and tablet size are the most important parameters in order to deliver a solid form to pediatric patients, ensuring treatment adherence and easy administration.

The proportion of magnesium stearate was established according to a literature search, where 1.0% was the common quantity used, which allows the clean release of the tablet without cracking and reduces the friction between the metal surface and the solid dosage form. As a good mixing practice, the lubricant was incorporated as a final step of the mixing of the powder. Due to its hydrophobic characteristics, a long lubricant mixing time would generate a hydrophobic layer over the API that could negatively affect its dissolution time, delivery, and absorption and consequently influence the treatment effectiveness.

In the case of silicon dioxide, a range between 0.5, 1.0, and 1.5% was tested by evaluating its blend powder pre-compression parameters in the other three batches (Table 2). The amount of 1.0% was set as the minimum that gave the best blend flowability to the mixture.

It is known that the effect of powder mixing time can directly impact on the homogeneity of the blend, as well as the disintegration and dissolution time. A poor homogeneity of the mixture refers to a poor distribution of the API that can ultimately affect the patient's treatment. Therefore, the uniformity of the mixture must be ensured, and for this reason, a mixing time test was carried out applying the quartering technique. In order to optimize the mixing time, the powder mixture was divided into four equal fractions at different times, and the RSD of the API concentration among these was evaluated. Figure 3 depicts that at low mixing times, the calculated RSD is high. As mixing continues, the RSD value reaches a minimum. From this point on, the increase in the calculated RSD values is indicative of powder heterogeneity. The selected mixing time corresponds to the lowest point of the graph obtained from RSD vs. mixing time.

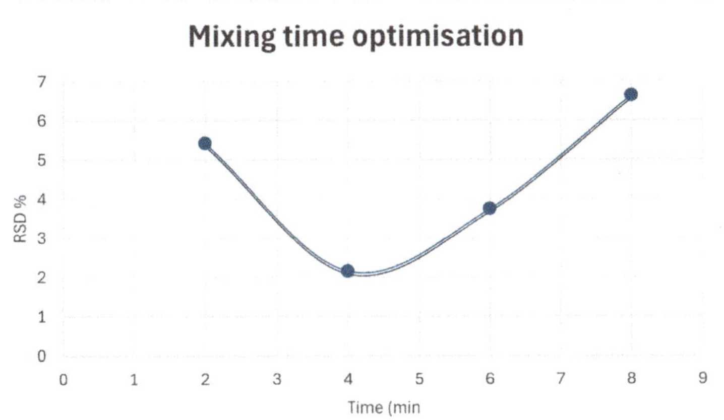

Figure 3. Mixing time optimization.

The images obtained from the elemental composition (Figure 4) show a uniform distribution of the API, which can be confirmed by the distribution of nitrogen and chloride (the only source of which is THP) throughout the area analyzed.

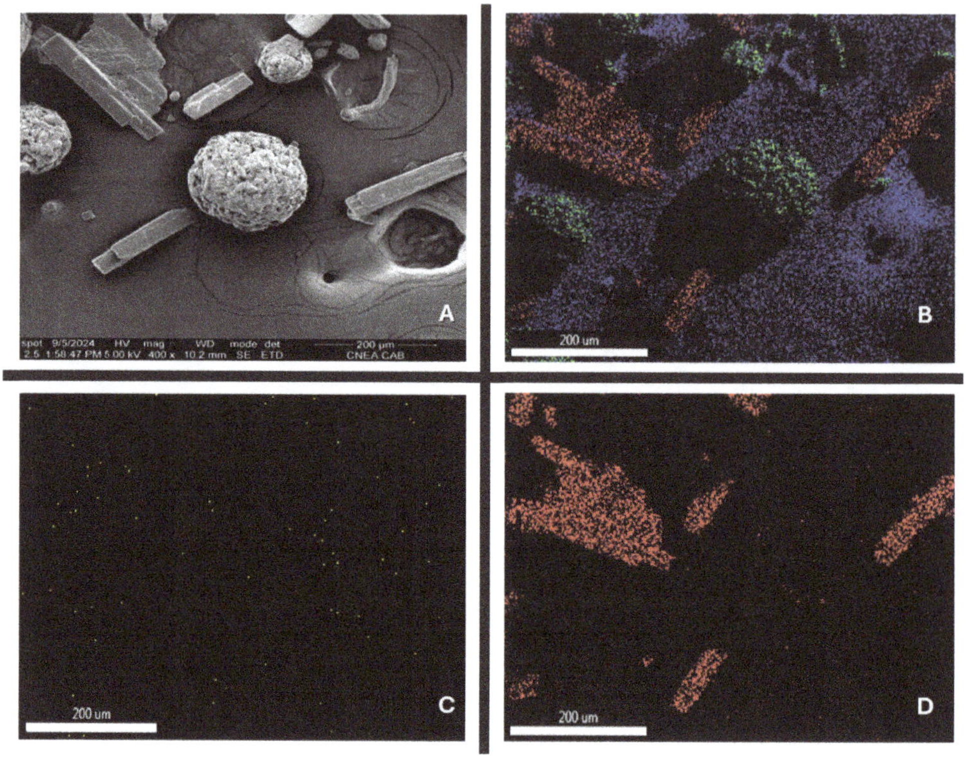

Figure 4. (**A**) Contrast image API/excipient blend 400×; (**B**) API/excipient blend elemental mapping; (**C**) nitrogen mapping; (**D**) chloride mapping.

3.1.4. Compatibility Studies

As a preliminary step, different screening methods have been employed on the API, excipients, and powder mixtures. Once ATR-FTIR on all samples was carried out, rheological data were evaluated, and the best API/excipient blend was selected.

To complement the preliminary data and confirm the non-interaction between the excipients of the selected mixture, additional studies employing SEM analysis have been carried out.

Attenuated Total Reflection–Fourier Transform Infrared Spectroscopy Analysis

The excipients were tested alone, and in each mixture, the IR spectra obtained were analyzed for possible interactions.

THP characteristic functional peaks at 3294 cm^{-1} (for OH stretching), 2926 cm^{-1} (for aromatic C-H stretch), 969 cm^{-1} (for C-N), and 698 cm^{-1} (for C-H bending) are observed. The characteristic peaks present in the individually obtained spectra are found at the same wavelengths in the excipient's mixture as a sum of spectra (Figure 5), indicating that there is no interaction between excipients and the active ingredient.

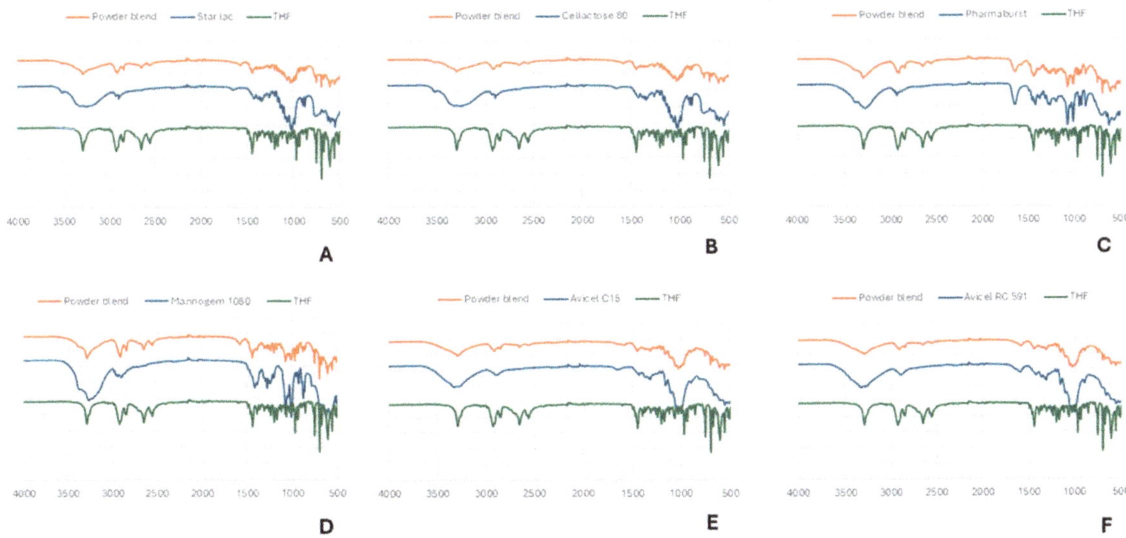

Figure 5. ATR-FTIR analysis of THP and its respective co-process excipient and powder blend. (**A**) Star Lac; (**B**) Cellactose 80; (**C**) Pharmaburst; (**D**) Mannogem 1080; (**E**) Avicel C15; (**F**) Avicel RC 591.

Scanning Electron Microscopy and Energy-Dispersive X-Ray Spectroscopy

Figure 6 depicts the surface morphology of THP ODMTs. Figure 6A shows that the selected diluent has a spherical shape, which makes it an excellent DC excipient. A detailed distribution of the API and excipient can be observed in Figure 6C,D, where there is no significant difference between their particle sizes, which corresponds to the short mixing time needed to achieve mixture homogeneity. Conversely, a difference in their morphology can be observed, which could explain the segregation of the excipients at longer mixing times.

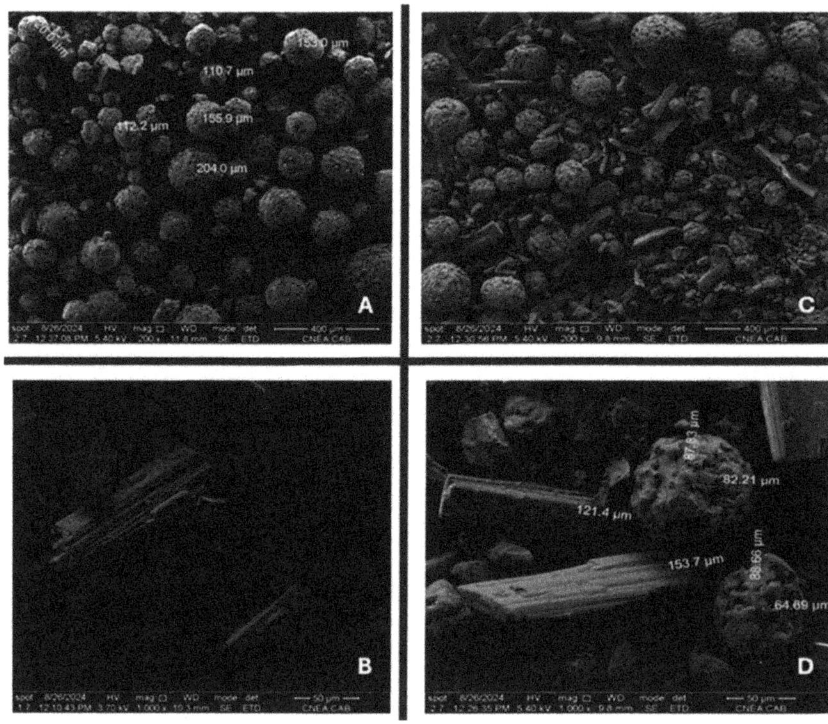

Figure 6. Scanning electron micrographs of (**A**) Star-Lac, (**B**) THP, (**C**) API/excipient blend 200×, and (**D**) API/excipient blend 1000×.

3.2. ODMTs Characterization

3.2.1. Pharmacotechnical Parameters

Due to the absence of international guidelines for ODMTs, requirements for conventional tablets were selected instead. During the production of THP ODMTs, pharmacotechnical tests such as weight uniformity, hardness, friability, and disintegration were performed according to USP-43 [26]. The disintegration time was less than 30 s. This is partly due to the presence of sodium croscarmellose, as previously mentioned, which favors the entry of liquid, causing it to swell thus facilitating disintegration. This result is consistent with previously published work on ODTs containing sodium croscarmellose [34].

Conventional THF tablet formulations show higher disintegration times, ranging from 54 s to 1.23 min [35].

There is no consensus regarding disintegration time limits for ODTs. While the FDA guideline for ODTs recommends a disintegration time of less than 30 s, the European Pharmacopeia states less than 180 s [36]. USP ODT monographs show disintegration times between 30 and 60 s, but there are no established limits for ODTs [26]. The developed formulation shows disintegration times that comply with the more stringent criteria.

The short wetting time obtained is closely related to disintegration time. A summary of pharmacotechnical parameters is shown in Table 3.

Table 3. Post-compression pharmacotechnical parameters.

Weight Uniformity (mg ± SD)	Hardness (Newton ± SD)	Friability (%)	Disintegration (s ± SD)	Wetting Time (s ± SD)
20.6 ± 0.6	30.9 ± 4.3	<1	29.5 ± 1.1	<1 min

3.2.2. In Vitro Dissolution Study and Dissolution Profile

The dissolution profile of the THP ODMTs provides information on how the formulation will perform in vivo. As shown in Figure 7 (percentage dissolution vs. time plot), it was observed that 2 min after the start of the test, 100% of the THP was dissolved (Q = 70% according to USP 43 [37]).

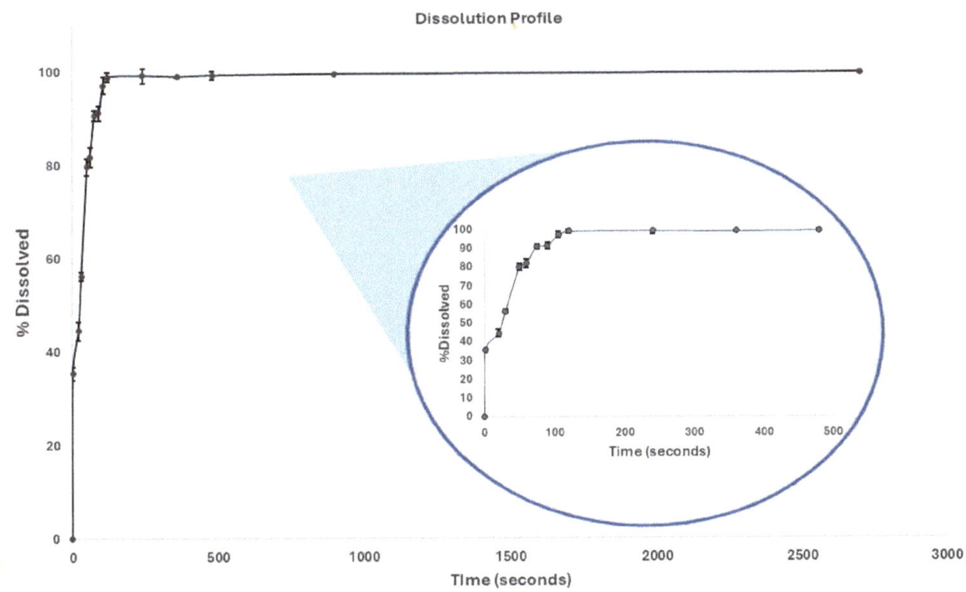

Figure 7. THP ODMT dissolution profile.

3.2.3. Physicochemical Stability Study

A physicochemical stability study was performed over the course of 18 months. Content (as shown in Table 4) and THP dose uniformity remain within USP specification (90.0–110.0% of the labeled value) [37], and content uniformity values are within the established range (85.0–115.0% of the labeled value) and have an RSD of less than 2% [38]. Our findings suggest that the optimized formulation is physically and chemically stable over the studied period.

Table 4. Determination of THP ODMTs.

Months	API Content (% ± RSD)	API Content (mg ± SD)
0	96.98 ± 0.1	2.42 ± 0.01
3	98.50 ± 0.2	2.46 ± 0.13
6	104.40 ± 0.1	2.61 ± 0.14
9	105.90 ± 0.1	2.65 ± 0.11
12	100.70 ± 0.1	2.52 ± 0.03
18	102.20 ± 0.1	2.56 ± 0.05

4. Conclusions

The powder mixture obtained using Star-Lac as the co-process diluent was the one that showed the best pre-compression results. The final formulation complies with API content and post-compression parameters (average weight, hardness, friability, and disintegration time) according to pharmacopeial guidelines.

In conclusion, a novel formulation of direct compressed THP ODMTs intended for pediatric administration was successfully designed, developed, optimized, and characterized, and within 18 months, it was physiochemically stable. This will provide the sole treatment alternative for segmental and generalized dystonia in pediatric patients due to the lack of a pharmaceutical formulation available in the market.

Author Contributions: Conceptualization, C.O. and S.L.; methodology, C.O. and S.L.; software, S.F. and L.S.F.; validation, S.F., L.S.F. and C.O.; formal analysis, S.F., C.A.O. and S.L.; investigation, C.O., S.F. and V.A.C.; resources S.L.; data curation, C.O., S.F., O.B. and C.D.; writing—original draft preparation, C.O.; writing—review and editing, C.O. and C.D.; visualization, C.D., S.F. and S.L.; supervision, S.L.; project administration, S.L.; funding acquisition, S.L. All authors have read and agreed to the published version of the manuscript.

Funding: This research was financed by UBACyT 20020220300155BA project, University of Buenos Aires.

Institutional Review Board Statement: Not applicable.

Informed Consent Statement: Not applicable.

Data Availability Statement: The data presented in this study are available on request from the corresponding author.

Acknowledgments: The authors thank the financial support from the University of Buenos Aires and CONICET. The authors thank Juan Manuel Lázaro Martinez for his contribution to ATR FTIR analysis.

Conflicts of Interest: The authors declare no conflicts of interest.

References

1. National Library og Medicine, PubChem. Trihexyphenidyl Hydrochloride. Available online: https://pubchem.ncbi.nlm.nih.gov/compound/66007 (accessed on 4 January 2023).
2. Burke, R.E.; Fahn, S.; Marsden, C.D. Torsion Dystonia: A Double-Blind, Prospective Trial of Highldosage Trihexyphenidyl. *Neurology* **1986**, *36*, 160–164. [CrossRef] [PubMed]
3. Marsden, C.D.; Marion, M.H.; Quinn, N. The treatment of severe dystonia in children and adults. *J. Neurol. Neurosurg. Psychiatry* **1984**, *47*, 1166–1173. [CrossRef]
4. Phukan, J.; Albanese, A.; Gasser, T.; Warner, T. Primary dystonia and dystonia-plus syndromes: Clinical characteristics, diagnosis, and pathogenesis. *Lancet Neurol.* **2011**, *10*, 1074–1085. [CrossRef] [PubMed]
5. Baker, L.B.; Harvey, A.R.; Egberts, K.J.; Reddihough, D.S.; Scheinberg, A.; Williams, K. Trihexyphenidyl for dystonia in cerebral palsy. *Cochrane Database Syst. Rev.* **2016**, *2016*, CD012430. [CrossRef]
6. Foley, J. The athetoid syndrome: A review of a personal series. *J. Neurol. Neurosurg. Psychiatry* **1983**, *46*, 289–298. [CrossRef] [PubMed]
7. Pranzatelli, M.R. Oral pharmacotherapy for the movement disorders of cerebral palsy. *J. Child Neurol.* **1996**, *11*, 13–22. [CrossRef]
8. Pidcock, F.S.; Hoon, A.H.; Johnston, M.V. Trihexyphenidyl in posthemorrhagic dystonia: Motor and language effects. *Pediatr. Neurol.* **1999**, *20*, 219–222. [CrossRef] [PubMed]
9. Claudio González, Q.F. Pharmacology in the Pediatric Patient. *Rev. Medica Clin. Las Condes* **2016**, *27*, 652–659. [CrossRef]
10. Lopez, F.L.; Ernest, T.B.; Tuleu, C.; Gul, M.O. Formulation approaches to pediatric oral drug delivery: Benefits and limitations of current platforms. *Expert Opin. Drug Deliv.* **2015**, *12*, 1727–1740. [CrossRef] [PubMed]
11. Gupta, A.; Khan, M.A. Challenges of pediatric formulations: A FDA science perspective. *Int. J. Pharm.* **2013**, *457*, 346–348. [CrossRef] [PubMed]

12. Thabet, Y.; Klingmann, V.; Breitkreutz, J. Drug Formulations: Standards and Novel Strategies for Drug Administration in Pediatrics. *J. Clin. Pharmacol.* **2018**, *58*, S26–S35. [CrossRef] [PubMed]
13. Stoltenberg, I.; Breitkreutz, J. Orally disintegrating mini-tablets (ODMTs)—A novel solid oral dosage form for paediatric use. *Eur. J. Pharm. Biopharm.* **2011**, *78*, 462–469. [CrossRef] [PubMed]
14. Comoglu, T.; Dilek Ozyilmaz, E. Orally disintegrating tablets and orally disintegrating mini tablets–novel dosage forms for pediatric use. *Pharm. Dev. Technol.* **2019**, *24*, 902–914. [CrossRef] [PubMed]
15. Tumuluri, V. *Pharmaceutical Mini-Tablets: A Revived Trend*; Elsevier Inc.: Amsterdam, The Netherlands, 2020; Volume 3. [CrossRef]
16. Lennartz, P.; Mielck, J.B. Minitabletting: Improving the compactability of paracetamol powder mixtures. *Int. J. Pharm.* **1998**, *173*, 75–85. [CrossRef]
17. Hirani, J.J.; Rathod, D.A.; Vadalia, K.R. Orally disintegrating tablets: A review. *Trop. J. Pharm. Res.* **2009**, *8*, 161–172. [CrossRef]
18. Dominik, M.; Vraníková, B.; Svačinová, P.; Elbl, J.; Pavloková, S.; Prudilová, B.B.; Šklubalová, Z.; Franc, A. Comparison of Flow and Compression Properties of Four Lactose-Based Co-Processed Excipients: Cellactose® 80, CombiLac®, MicroceLac® 100, and StarLac®. *Pharmaceutics* **2021**, *13*, 1486. [CrossRef] [PubMed]
19. Hoon, A.H., Jr.; Freese, P.O.; Reinhardt, E.M.; Wilson, M.A.; Lawrie, W.T., Jr.; Harryman, S.E.; Pidcock, F.S.; Johnston, M.V. Age-dependent effects of trihexyphenidyl in extrapyramidal cerebral palsy. *Pediatr. Neurol.* **2001**, *25*, 55–58. [CrossRef]
20. Sanger, T.D.; Bastian, A.; Brunstrom, J.; Damiano, D.; Delgado, M.; Dure, L.; Gaebler-Spira, D.; Hoon, A.; Mink, J.W.; Sherman-Levine, S.; et al. Prospective open-label clinical trial of trihexyphenidyl in children with secondary dystonia due to cerebral palsy. *J. Child Neurol.* **2007**, *22*, 530–537. [CrossRef] [PubMed]
21. Rice, J.; Waugh Mary-Clare, M.C. Pilot study on trihexyphenidyl in the treatment of dystonia in children with cerebral palsy. *J. Child Neurol.* **2009**, *24*, 176–182. [CrossRef]
22. Drugs.com®. Trihexyphenidyl Hydrochloride Oral Solution Shortage. Available online: https://www.drugs.com/drug-shortages/trihexyphenidyl-hydrochloride-oral-solution-1080 (accessed on 5 March 2024).
23. Ashp Pharmacist Advancing Healthcare®. Trihexyphenidyl Hydrochloride Oral Solution. Available online: https://www.ashp.org/drug-shortages/current-shortages/drug-shortage-detail.aspx?id=1080&loginreturnUrl=SSOCheckOnly (accessed on 5 March 2024).
24. Morri, M.; Casabonne, C.; Leonardi, D.; Vignaduzzo, S. Orphan Formulations for Pediatric Use: Development and Stability Control of Two Sildenafil Citrate Solutions for the Treatment of Pulmonary Hypertension. *AAPS PharmSciTech* **2020**, *21*, 221. [CrossRef]
25. Singh, S.; Nwabor, O.F.; Ontong, J.C.; Kaewnopparat, N.; Voravuthikunchai, S.P. Characterization of a novel, co-processed bio-based polymer, and its effect on mucoadhesive strength. *Int. J. Biol. Macromol.* **2020**, *145*, 865–875. [CrossRef]
26. United States Pharmacopeia. Powder Flow ⟨1174⟩. USP-NF. 2024. Available online: https://doi.usp.org/USPNF/USPNF_M99885_02_01.html (accessed on 6 February 2024).
27. United States Pharmacopeia. Clorhidrato de Trihexifenidilo. USP-NF. 2024. Available online: https://doi.usp.org/USPNF/USPNF_M85480_04_02.html (accessed on 6 February 2024).
28. Henestrosa, C.; Olivera, C.; Flor, S.; Lucangioli, S.; Vacatello, A.; Ortega, C.A.; Favier, L.S.; Cifuente, D.A. A Novel Development of Levothyroxine Sodium Orodispersible Mini Tablets for the Treatment of Pediatrics Hypothyroidism. *Recent Adv. Drug Deliv. Formul.* **2023**, *17*, 152–159. [CrossRef] [PubMed]
29. Ortega, C.A.; Favier, L.S.; Cianchino, V.A.; Cifuente, D.A. New Orodispersible Mini Tablets of Enalapril Maleate by Direct Compression for Pediatric Patients. *Curr. Drug Deliv.* **2020**, *17*, 505–510. [CrossRef]
30. Klingmann, V.; Spomer, N.; Lerch, C.; Stoltenberg, I.; Frömke, C.; Bosse, H.M.; Breitkreutz, J.; Meissner, T. Favorable acceptance of mini-tablets compared with syrup: A randomized controlled trial in infants and preschool children. *J. Pediatr.* **2013**, *163*, 1728–1732. [CrossRef]
31. Slavkova, M.; Breitkreutz, J. Orodispersible drug formulations for children and elderly. *Eur. J. Pharm. Sci.* **2015**, *75*, 2–9. [CrossRef]
32. Dowson, A.; Bundy, M.; Salt, R.; Kilminster, S. Patient preference for triptan formulations: A prospective study with zolmitriptan. *Headache* **2007**, *47*, 1144–1151. [CrossRef] [PubMed]
33. Hayakawa, Y.; Uchida, S.; Namiki, N. Evaluation of the ease of taking mini-tablets compared with other tablet formulations in healthy volunteers. *Eur. J. Pharm. Sci.* **2016**, *84*, 157–161. [CrossRef] [PubMed]
34. Pabari, R.M.; Ramtoola, Z. Effect of a disintegration mechanism on wetting, water absorption, and disintegration time of orodispersible tablets. *J. Young Pharm.* **2012**, *4*, 157–163. [CrossRef]
35. Bhatt, P.; Kumar, A. Comparative study of preformulation and in vitro evaluation of sustained release marketed formulation of trihexyphenidyl hcl tablets. *World J. Pharm. Pharm. Sci.* **2018**, *7*, 1463–1478. [CrossRef]

a popular alternative to powders in the USA, they are less frequently or rarely compounded in European countries [11–21].

Whereas pediatric topical oral gels (for example, to treat inflammation or infection in the oral cavity) are widely available, oral gels are less common as alternatives to tablets or syrups [22–24]. Commercial oral pediatric hydrogel dosage forms registered as medicinal products have already been introduced as attractive alternatives for dietary supplements with vitamins. Like any soft food, semisolid oral hydrogels may assess ease of swallowing without mixing powders with food, which always creates the risk of incompatibility. Thus, oral administration of hydrogels is a new trend in pediatric therapy and brings positive recommendations with respect to safety, good palatability, and flexibility of dosage by measured volume. Hydrogels could be an attractive dosage form because of their smooth structure, which improves the child's feelings during administration, better taste masking, and less risk of liquid spilling from the spoon. They may be easily packed into single-dose sachets or in tubes. A dose from the latter may be measured using spoons or oral syringes.

If the active substance is suspended in the gel, the homogeneity during the whole time of storage should be assured by the proper viscosity of the carrier because, in contrast to liquid suspensions, the sediment cannot be restored by shaking. There is some risk that the high viscosity of the formulation may reduce the bioavailability of the drug or delay its absorption, but the same risk exists when mixing a child's medicine with food. Although there is a lack of research on this topic, it is definitely possible to consider it, especially when drug absorption is rapid. On the other hand, absorption from a tablet is determined by its disintegration, while in a gel, the medicinal substance is in the form of already small particles.

Valsartan (VAL) and candesartan cilexetil (CC) are used in the treatment of hypertension and belong to the therapeutic category of angiotensin II receptor blockers. Commercially available are tablets with CC (4, 8, 16, and 32 mg—Atacand and generic products). CC is slowly absorbed from the gastrointestinal tract, with a t_{max} of 3–4 h [25,26]. The activity, safety, and pharmacokinetics data of CC were studied in children from 1 to 17 years of age, with a dose for children between 1 and 6 years of 0.2 mg/kg/day (the usual dose ranges from 0.05 to 0.4 mg/kg/day) and from 6 years of age and older (weight < 50 kg) of 4–8 mg once daily (the usual dose ranges from 2 to 16 mg/day) [25–31]. According to the Atacand FDA leaflet, preparation of oral suspension by dispersing tablets in commercially available suspending media (Ora-Sweet SF, Ora-Plus, or Ora-Blend) is recommended [25]. The physicochemical properties of CC and VAL are presented in Table 1.

Table 1. Physicochemical characteristics of candesartan cilexetil (CC) and valsartan (VAL) [32–35].

Parameter	CC	VAL
Water solubility (25 °C)	pH 1.2—0.037 mg/mL pH 7.4—0.126 mg/mL	Water—0.18 mg/mL pH 8—16.8 mg/mL
pK_a	5.9	4.7
logP	6.1	1.5
BCS classification	II	II or III

Tablets with VAL (40, 80, 160, and 320 mg—Diovan and generic products) are indicated for adults and children 6–16 years old [36–39]. For younger children from 1 year old, the Diovan solution is recommended with a starting dose of 1 mg/kg up to a maximum dose of 4 mg/kg once daily (with dose adjustment based on blood pressure response and tolerability). For children older than 6 years of age and < 35 kg weight, 20 mg once daily (7 mL solution) is recommended, and for > 35 kg weight, 40 mg (14 mL solution) is advised [40]. Absorption from the solution is faster than from tablets (t_{max} is 1–2 h for a solution and 2–4 h for tablets). The systemic exposure to valsartan (AUC) is 60% higher with the suspension or solution compared to tablets, and when switching between forms, the dose of VAL may need to be adjusted [40,41]. Unfortunately, the availability of this product in the form of a solution is very limited in many European countries, and the off-label use of VAL in tablets is very common.

Suspension-type syrups compounded from Diovan tablets (VAL concentration 4 mg/mL) and Ora-type media can be stored in a glass bottle for either up to 90 days at temperatures below 30 °C or up to 75 days at refrigerated conditions [41]. Syrups prepared with Atacand tablets, with CC concentrations of 1 mg/mL or 2 mg/mL, should be used within 30 days (up to 100 days when unopened) when stored at room temperature [25,42–44]. For simpler suspending media, based on sucrose, stability of the suspensions for 3 or 4 weeks at room temperature was declared [21].

The aim of the current study was to develop hydrogels as alternative formulations to VAL and CC liquid suspensions. The new compounded formulations are proposed for easier drug administration, as described above. The chemical stability of the drugs in the gel vehicles was evaluated by using a HPLC method. Physical stability and the rheological properties of the final formulations were investigated at different temperatures during the time. The results obtained should allow gel vehicles to be considered a new dispersing medium for active substances, including when the drugs are obtained by manipulating tablets or capsules. The proposed extemporaneous formulations could also represent a valuable alternative to Ora® products when they are not available on the market.

The study did not include the impact on the bioavailability of the drug in terms of both crushing tablets and incorporation in a viscous medium. The tested active substances belong to BCS class II and are sparingly soluble in water, and the risk of changing bioavailability should be taken into consideration. However, a similar risk occurs when combining medicines with food, which is a common practice in administering drugs to children.

2. Materials and Methods

2.1. Materials

Hydroxyethylcellulose (HEC) (Natrosol 250 HR was purchased from A.C.E.F., Piacenza, Italy), sodium salt of carmellose (high-viscosity carboxymethylcellulose, CMC) (Sigma Aldrich, St. Louis, MO, USA), and carbomer (CAR) dedicated to oral use (Carbopol 974 P NF, Noveon, Cleveland, OH, USA) were used as gelling agents. Other chemical substances and solvents used in hydrogels were of pharmacopoeial quality: methylparaben (Fluka, Steinheim, Germany), glycerol (Amara, Krakow, Poland), potassium sorbate, and sorbitol (POCH, Avantor Performance Materials Poland, Gliwice, Poland).

Oral pediatric hydrogels were prepared with tablets obtained from a local pharmacy. For VAL hydrogels, Diovan® (Novartis, Nürnberg, Germany) coated tablets were used at a strength of 160 mg. The tablets contain the following excipients: microcrystalline cellulose, polyvinylpyrrolidone, colloidal silica, magnesium stearate, hypromellose, titanium dioxide, polyethylene glycol 8000, and iron oxides. For CC preparation, Atacand® (Astra Zeneca, Södertälje, Sweden) uncoated tablets with a strength of 16 mg were used, composed of the following excipients: calcium carboxymethylcellulose, hydroxypropylcellulose, lactose monohydrate, magnesium stearate, corn starch, polyethylene glycol 8000, and iron oxides.

Reagents used for high-performed liquid chromatography (HPLC) analysis, that is, acetonitrile (POCH, Gliwice, Poland), methanol (J.T.Baker, Deventer, Netherlands), and ortho-phosphoric acid (Fluka, Steinheim, Switzerland), were of HPLC grade. The

VAL and CC substances used for the calibration curve were donated by Polpharma (Starogard, Poland).

2.2. Preparation of Hydrogels

The composition of the placebo hydrogels is shown in Table 2. Methylparaben and potassium sorbate were used as preservatives. To increase palatability, sucrose, sorbitol, and glycerol were used as sweetening agents. Additionally, glycerol was added as a humectant. Hydrogel media were compounded by dissolving the following excipients in purified water: methylparaben, potassium sorbate, sorbitol, and sucrose. Afterward, glycerol was added, and using a mechanical stirrer, the polymer was dispersed and dissolved to form a hydrogel.

Table 2. Composition of placebo gels (% *w/w*).

Excipient	HEC	CMC (Sodium Salt)	CAR
Polymer	2.0	2.0	0.75
Sucrose		10.0	
Glycerol		5.0	
Sorbitol		4.0	
Potassium sorbate		0.10	
Methylparaben		0.10	
Water		to 100.0	

In the case of CAR, after the polymer was dispersed, neutralization with a 20% solution of sodium hydroxide (6.1 M) was performed to produce a hydrogel [45,46].

VAL and CC were incorporated into hydrogel carriers at concentrations of 4 mg/g and 1 mg/g, respectively. The following is required for 100 g of the gel: 2.5 tablets of Diovan containing 160 mg of VAL and 6.25 tablets of Atacand with a dose of CC 16 mg. Hydrogel formulations were prepared by mixing the pulverized tablets (787 mg of Diovan and 777 mg of Atacand) with the hydrogel medium. The suspension was prepared in a mortar by trituration of the powder with portions of the hydrogel media. The oral hydrogels were stored in plastic containers.

2.3. Short-Term Stability Studies

The short-term stability studies were carried out for the preparations stored at 25 °C and 4 °C for a period of up to 35 days. Every 7 days, the gels were analyzed by visual and microscopic observations, pH, viscosity, and other mechanical parameters were measured, and VAL and CC content was assayed. Microscopic observation was carried out using an optical microscope (Moticon, Wetzlar, Germany) with a camera (Motic BA 400).

2.4. Analysis of Viscosity, Rheology, and Texture of Oral Hydrogels

A cone/plate viscometer was employed (Brookfield RVDV-III Ultra Rheometer with Rheocalc software, manufactured by Brookfield Engineering Lab., Middleborough, MA, USA), and the dynamic viscosity of the hydrogels was measured as a relationship between shearing stress and shear rate. Rheological behavior was evaluated on the basis of a flow curve (a plot of viscosity to shear rate) and a hysteresis loop (a plot of shear stress to shear rate) [47,48]. The measurements were carried out at a temperature of 25.0 °C ± 0.1 °C controlled with a thermostatic water bath.

Additionally, some other mechanical parameters of the hydrogels were measured using a TA.XT Plus Texture Analyzer (Stable Micro Systems, Godalming, UK) equipped with A/BE Back Extrusion Ring (Ø 40 mm) and Texture Exponent software [49]. The following operating parameters were set: Pre-test speed of a probe 1.5 mm/s, test and post-test speed 2.0 mm/s, penetration distance of the probe in the sample was 5 mm, and trigger force of the probe was 10 g. The relationship between time and measured force was obtained, and the example curve is presented in Figure 1. The following mechanical parameters were measured: firmness [g], minimum adhesive force [g], adhesiveness [g·s], and cohesiveness [g·s] [48–54]. The analysis was performed at an ambient temperature. Each sample was measured in triplicate with empirically established 1-h time intervals between individual measurements (time necessary for hydrogel structure reconstitution).

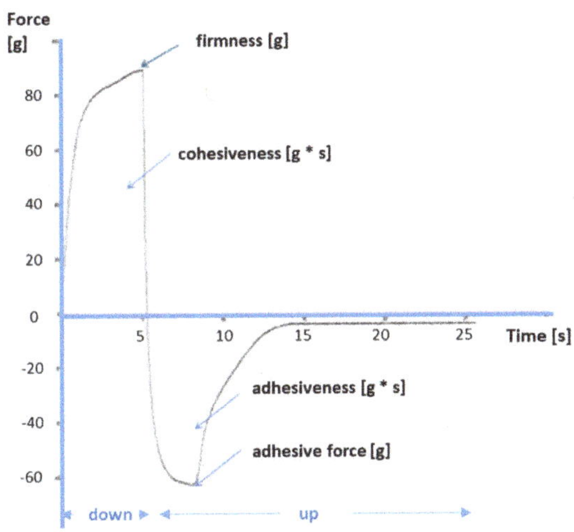

Figure 1. The curve and mechanical parameters of hydrogels were tested in a texture analyzer with a downstream and upstream movement of the probe.

2.5. HPLC Analysis of the Drug Content

To determine the VAL and CC content in the prepared oral hydrogels, HPLC was carried out using an Agilent HPLC system (Agilent Technologies, Waldbronn, Germany). Previously described and validated methods were employed [21,55–60]. The specificity and accuracy of the method for the analysis of oral hydrogels were confirmed. An isocratic separation on an Eclipse XDB—C18 column (4.6 × 150 mm, 5 μm) at 25 °C was performed with mobile phases: a mixture of a phosphate buffer pH 2.7 (0.065 M) with acetonitrile (55:45; *v*/*v*) for VAL and a mixture of a phosphate buffer pH 3.0 (0.05 M), methanol, and acetonitrile (30:20:50; *v*/*v*) for CC. The flow rate of the mobile phase was 1 mL/min, the UV detector was set at 215 nm, and the injected sample volumes were 20 μL. The retention times for VAL and CC were around 5 min and 13 min, respectively.

The three independent samples from each hydrogel were analyzed in triplicate. The 1.0 g sample of hydrogel was diluted to 10.0 mL with methanol. The solution was thoroughly shaken by hand for 5 min and then centrifuged for 15 min at 4000 rpm. The supernatant (1.0 mL) was diluted to 10.0 mL with a mobile phase to obtain solutions at concentrations of 10 μg/mL and 40 μg/mL for CC and VAL, respectively.

The concentration of the drugs in gels was calculated from calibration curves obtained from the analysis of standard solutions in mobile phases within the concentration range of

5–15 μg/mL and 10–80 μg/mL for CC and VAL, respectively. The linearity of the curve was confirmed by a correlation coefficient greater than 0.999. Interday precision for CAN and VAL was 4.52% and 1.15%, respectively (CV—coefficient of variation).

3. Results and Discussion

For the preparation of hydrogels, popular hydrophilic viscosity-increasing polymers were used, namely carbomer (CAR) and cellulose derivatives: hydroxyethylcellulose (HEC) and carmellose sodium (CMC). These polymers are excipients with wide uses and functions in the technology of pharmaceutical dosage forms (solid, semisolid, and liquid). They are commonly used in pediatric liquid dosage forms (syrups and suspensions) as thickening agents to prevent sedimentation of the dispersed phase. CMC is the most common, and CAR or HEC are used less frequently in liquid preparations for children, while they are very often applied as gelling agents in topical gels for children administered in oral cavities (pain relief, local anesthetics, and antifungal drugs). Based on adult safety and toxicity data, HEC, CMC, and CAR are considered safe for oral use in children, although only stronger data confirming the efficacy and safety in children have been published for CMC (STEP database) [61,62].

Among the three tested polymers, HEC is a non-ionic compound, while CAR and CMC are present in an ionic form, with pK_a 6.0 and 4.3, respectively [63–66]. The polymers used in the study are classified as high (CMC and HEC) or medium-high viscosity types gel-forming polymers.

The prepared hydrogels contained humectants (glycerol), sweeteners (sucrose and sorbitol), and preservatives. To ensure microbial stability, the addition of preservatives was necessary. The most frequently used are esters of p-hydroxybenzoic acid (parabens): methylparaben and propylparaben or potassium sorbate [67]. A combination of both was used based on previous findings that this combination was suitable for compounded syrups [21]. Sorbitol and glycerol concentrations are 4% and 5%, respectively, which is lower than in many syrups, and these compounds in such amounts should not be problematic regarding drug bioavailability [21,68–70].

The gels were prepared with VAL and CC at concentrations of 4 mg/mL and 1 mg/mL, as proposed for compounded syrups [18]. The concentration of crushed tablets in both gels was approximately 0.8%.

The density of the preparations is close to 1.0 g/mL (1.01–1.08 g/mL), which means that in practice, the dose measured in mass corresponds with the dose measured by volume. This allows for volume dose measurement using an oral syringe, which can also be a packaging container for the compounded gel. For children between 1 and 6 years, the doses are in the range of 3–6.5 mL for VAL and 0.5–4.0 mL for CC gels.

3.1. Visual and Microscopic Observations

The organoleptic assessment allowed us to propose optimum concentrations of the polymers in the gel. Depending on the polymer type, the following concentrations resulted in satisfying and visually similar consistency: 2.0% *w*/*w* for HEC and CMC and 0.75% *w*/*w* for CAR. The taste of the gels was pleasant.

The drug-containing gels prepared from tablets were suspension-type formulations that were non-transparent due to both insoluble active substances and excipients (silica, microcrystalline cellulose, magnesium stearate, and titanium dioxide). The gels prepared from the Atacand® tablets were pink due to the tablet dye color (iron oxides). Figure 2 presents hydrogels prepared from VAL and CC tablets. Visual observation of the preparations showed no changes in color, odor, or taste upon 35 days of storage at a temperature of 25 °C or 4 °C.

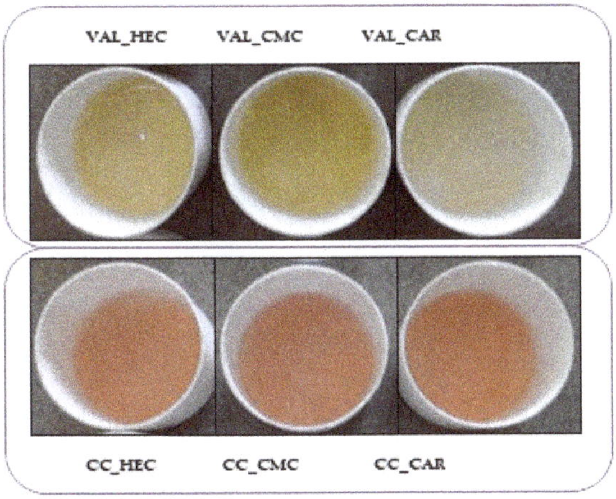

Figure 2. Hydrogels are prepared from valsartan (VAL) and candesartan cilexetil (CC) tablets using hydrogel carriers with hydroxyethylcellulose (HEC), carmellose sodium (CMC), and carbomer (CAR).

VAL and CC belong to the II BCS class and have poor solubility in water: 0.18 mg/mL and 0.10 mg/mL, respectively [32,33]. Therefore, it may be assumed that they are present in the gels in the suspended phase, together with other insoluble tablet excipients.

Homogenous suspension-type formulations with all three hydrogel media were easily prepared using a classical method with manual trituration of pulverized tablets with the vehicle in a mortar. The coating in the Diovan tablets was easily pulverized, and there was no need to sieve it or remove it in any other way.

The size of the suspended tablet particles was 10–25 µm and was similar to the VAL and CC preparations. The microscopic analysis during the stability study period (35 days) showed no evidence of recrystallization, and no particles greater than 30 µm were observed.

3.2. pH Measurements

The pH of the drug-free hydrogels was 6.5, 7.1, and 6.3 for HEC, CMC, and CAR, respectively. After the addition of CC, a significant change in pH ($p < 0.05$) occurred only in the CAR gel, where the pH increased to 6.8. The addition of VAL tablet mass caused a decrease in pH value below 6.0, with a significant drop ($p < 0.05$) in VAL_HEC gel (pH 4.7) and VAL_CMC gel (pH 5.1). The pH of VAL dispersion in water is 4.0, so it may be assumed that the observed decrease in pH in VAL hydrogels is caused by VAL partially dissolving in hydrogel media. During storage, no change in pH was noted for VAL hydrogels, and only a small drop in pH (by 0.2–0.3 units) was observed in the CC formulations after 28 days, independent of storage temperature. Changes in pH values during storage were considered significant for a difference of $\pm$ 0.5 units from the initial value.

3.3. Viscosity, Rheology and Consistency

The physical properties of the formulations were evaluated as important features, not only for handling and easy administration of the gels but also for detecting any quality changes upon storage.

Viscosity and rheology, together with other mechanical properties, such as firmness, cohesiveness, and adhesiveness, should be taken into consideration if desirable application properties and patient acceptability of semiliquid or semisolid preparations are evaluated. These are also important factors that influence the accuracy of the dosage when spoons or syringes are used as dosing devices.

Figure 1 presents an exemplary graph obtained as a result of the gel analysis performed using a texture analyzer.

Figure 3 presents the mechanical parameters (absolute values) of the hydrogels, determined as described above. Despite the similar consistency of all gels evaluated visually, placebo gels prepared with HEC were characterized by the lowest firmness, cohesiveness, and adhesiveness, while CMC and CAR were similar in their physical texture parameters but with larger cohesiveness of CMC.

Results of the mechanical analysis showed that the addition of the VAL or CC tablets to HEC, CMC, and CAR hydrogel media generally resulted only in a rather slight increase in the majority of the mechanical parameters. Small but significant changes were noted in the CAR hydrogels: in the presence of VAL, firmness and adhesive force were reduced, and in the presence of CC, an increase in adhesiveness and cohesiveness was observed, but firmness was unchanged. Atacand® tablets with CC contain calcium carboxymethylcellulose, and this excipient could be responsible for these changes because calcium ions might interact with ionic polymers, while HEC gels were insensitive [70].

Figure 3 also presents the characteristics of the preparations stored for up to 35 days at 25 °C. There was no significant effect on changes in mechanical parameters depending on the storage temperature (similar values for the samples at 4 °C were obtained). As a rule, an increase in the measured mechanical parameters is observed during storage; however, significantly larger changes were found in the gels with CC, especially in the CMC_CC. Similar results were observed by Chalah et al. [71], who noted a sharp increase in consistency for 2% CMC during storage. The observed time-related changes may have resulted from the influence of excipients included in the tablet mass (i.e., their slow dissolution and swelling). Very high values of firmness (807 g on the 35th day of storage) were also noted in the VAL_CMC gel, while the other parameters measured in this gel were stable. Observed changes did not influence; however, the application properties and organoleptic effects, such as thinning or thickening of gels after the addition of powdered tablets, were not noted.

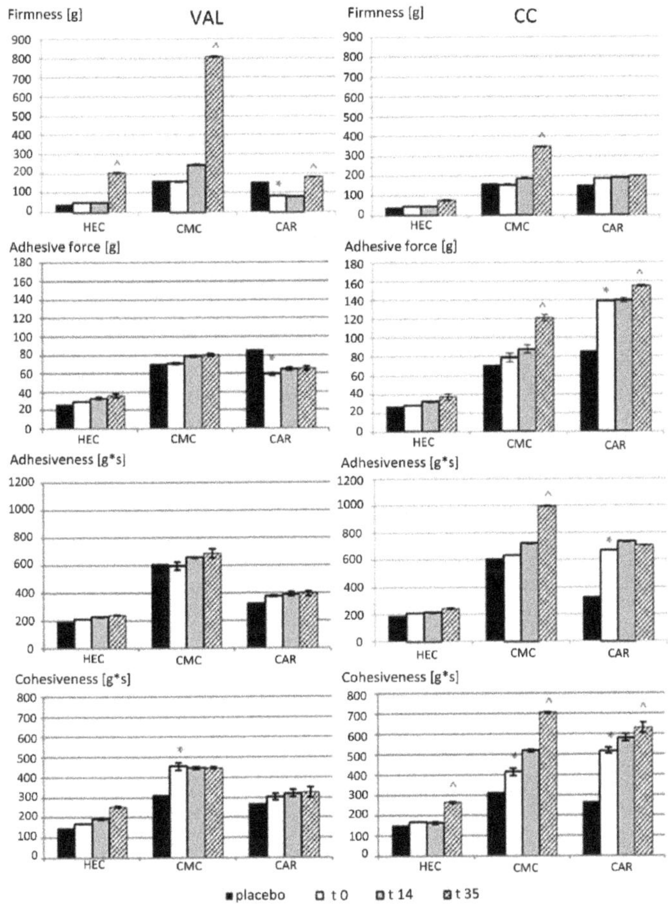

Figure 3. The mechanical properties of hydrogels prepared with VAL and CC tablets using hydrogel media (HEC, CMC, and CAR) and stored at 25 °C for 35 days. The mechanical parameters at t0 for the placebo hydrogels are also presented. * Statistical significance was demonstrated after the addition of the tablet mass ($p < 0.05$). ^ Statistical significance was demonstrated in relation to time t0, ($p < 0.05$).

The gels were also tested using a rheometer to determine their dynamic viscosity and rheology. It is difficult to present rheological measurements in a single number, as the graphs show a non-linear relationship between the response and the continuously changing mechanical forces applied. In Table 3, the values of viscosity recorded at the particular shear rate, that is, 8 s^{-1}, are presented, and Figure 4 shows the hysteresis loops recorded as a relationship between shear stress and shear rate. It was shown that benzalkonium chloride or sodium benzoate, in high concentrations of 0.1% *w/v*, affects the rheological parameters in carbomer's gel, reducing their viscosity and causing turbidity [70,72]. Considering that the addition of substances that prevent the growth of microorganisms is necessary, both the type and concentration of preservative added must be taken into account. No decrease in viscosity of the gels with carbomer and CC or VAL tablets was observed (Table 3).

Table 3. Changes in viscosity (measured at a shear rate 8 s^{-1}) of HEC, CMC, and CAR gels prepared with VAL and CC, stored for 35 days at 25 °C.

Gel	API	t = 0 [mPas]	t = 35 Days [mPas]	Viscosity Change [%]
HEC	---	8100	-----	
	VAL	8186	11,056	135
	CC	8244	7781	94
CMC	---	15,900	-----	
	VAL	12,907	16,173	125
	CC	16,785	20,278	121
CAR	---	9900	------	
	VAL	9178	9939	108
	CC	10,291	10,377	101

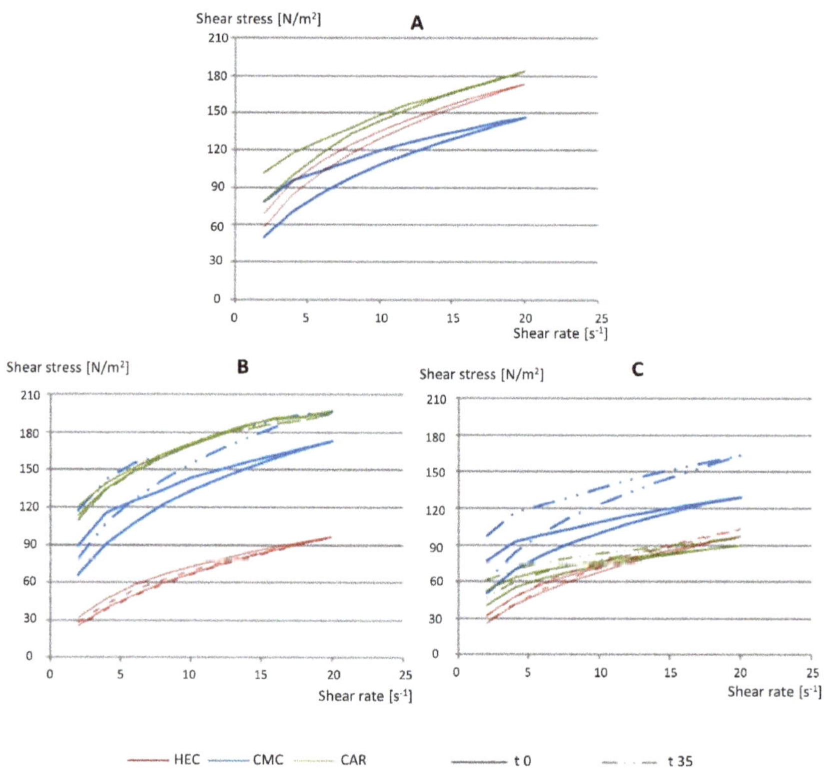

Figure 4. The representative hysteresis loops for HEC, CMC, and CAR gels were recorded for placebo gels at t0 (**A**) and gels with candesartan cilexetil (**B**) and valsartan (**C**) tablets after preparation (t0) and 35 days of storage at 25 °C.

The viscosity of the CMC gel measured with a rheometer was the highest, while HEC and CAR demonstrated similar viscosity (Table 3). The strongest thixotropic properties, measured by the size of the hysteresis loop, were also observed for the CMC gel (Figure 4). Such a difference was not observed when the measurements were performed with a texture analyzer (Figure 3). This means that mechanical measurements depend heavily on the measuring technique and the parameters determined. Finally, the results may be treated as complementary, and careful interpretation is required [48,49].

The solid phase of the VAL or CC tablets added to the gels resulted in only minor changes in their viscosity (Table 3). This could be expected, as the content of the solid particles in the gel was only 0.8%. After 35 days of storage, the changes observed in viscosity were not greater than 35%, which is not a large difference for this parameter.

No significant change in rheology was observed when CC was added to CAR gel, or VAL was mixed with CMC gel. In addition, only a small increase in shear stress was noted in the CMC gel with CC. On the other hand, in the case of both drugs, a significant reduction in shear stress was observed for the HEC gels, and this effect was also found when VAL was added to the CAR gel. Thixotropy (the area of the hysteresis loop) did not change. During storage for 35 days, a small increase in the gel structure, measured by shear stress, was noted only in the drug-loaded CMC gels, and this effect was not related either to the type of active substance added or to the temperature of storage (4 °C or 25 °C).

It may be concluded that changes in the physical characteristics of the gels in the presence of the added active substances in the form of the pulverized tablets (<1% content of solids) do not change the rheological behavior of the gels, or the change is too small to have an impact on the gel's applicability.

3.4. Chemical Stability of VAL and CC in Oral Hydrogels

The exemplary chromatograms of VAL_CMC and CC_CMC gels are presented in Figure 5. The determined changes in drug content in the gels during 35 days of storage are presented in Figure 6 (CV percentage was less than 3%). The short-term stability studies confirmed satisfying the chemical stability of VAL in all gels during storage, either at 25 °C or 4 °C. Surprisingly, a significant decrease in CC content was observed in all investigated hydrogels stored for longer than 14 days. The change was not related either to the temperature of storage or to the type of carrier. In addition, analysis of the chromatograms did not reveal any degradation products (Figure 5). Because the loss of CC measured in the gels after 21 and 35 days was around 10%, a storage time of no longer than 14 days may be recommended for CC preparations. The reason for the lower results may be the interaction of CC with the polymer, preventing complete recovery during sample preparation for analysis. During storage, stronger adsorption of the polymer on the CC particles could have occurred, and extraction with methanol, leading to precipitation of the polymer at the interface, could have resulted in the encapsulation of some of the solid CC particles and their poor dissolution. Thus, the same extraction method of CC from the samples at later time points was inefficient. Because the results of the determination of CC in the residue after centrifugation of the methanol solution were ambiguous, a change of the extraction solvent or sonication of the samples might be a suitable solution for this analytical problem. Ultimately, taking into account the observed changes in consistency, especially in the case of the CMC medium, we cannot recommend a storage time of CC gels longer than 14 days.

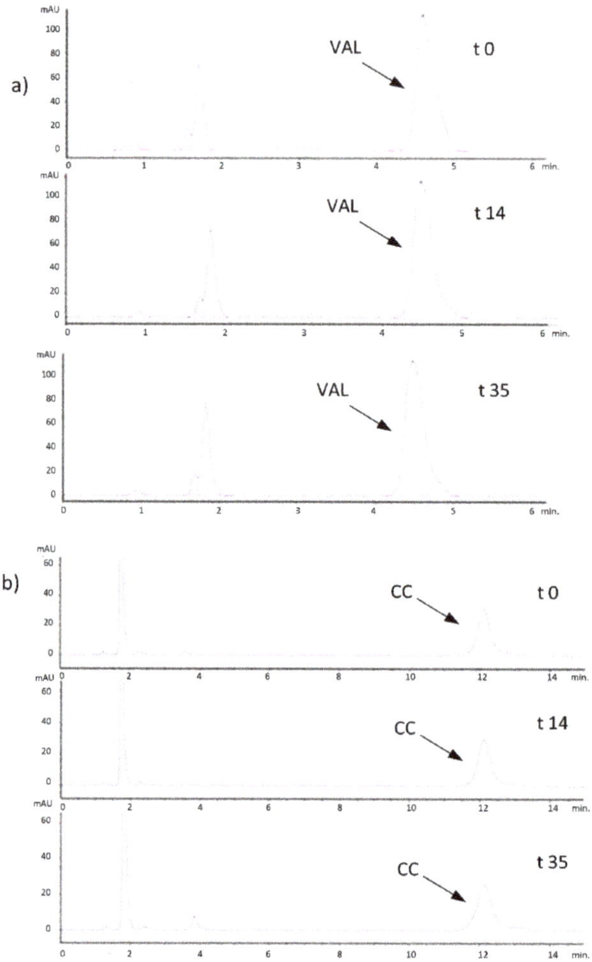

Figure 5. Chromatograms of VAL (**a**) and CC (**b**) in CMC gels: after preparation (t0) and after 14 and 35 days of storage at 25 °C.

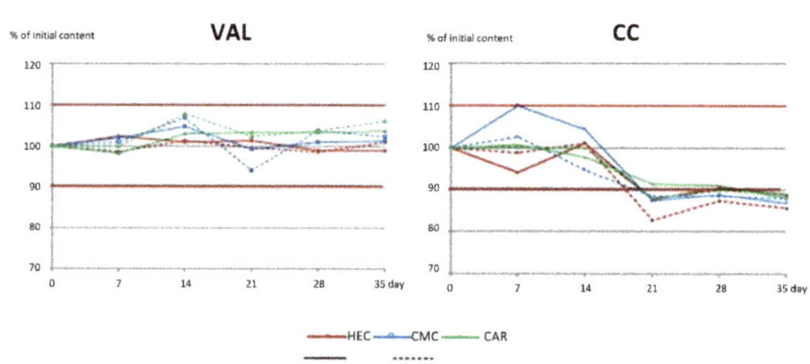

Figure 6. Stability (% of the initial content) of VAL and CC in oral hydrogels prepared with HEC, CMC, and CAR, stored at 25 °C and 4 °C for 35 days.

4. Conclusions

Semi-solid oral formulations appear to be a promising extemporaneous pediatric dosage form, and they were characterized as carriers for two hypotensive drugs used off-label in pediatrics: VAL and CC, which are available in tablets indicated for adults. Preferred mechanical and rheological properties eliminate the risk of spillage and ensure homogeneity of suspended particles during storage.

The three polymers tested, HEC, CMC, and CAR, can be used as bases for oral hydrogels, with sugars improving palatability and preservatives ensuring microbial quality. Despite the similar consistency assessed organoleptically, the gels differed in viscosity and rheological properties, but this did not matter during application, and the addition of powdered tablets did not significantly change these properties. According to USP pharmacopeia [73], the beyond-use-date of preserved water containing compounded preparations is 35 days, and during such period, the physicochemical stability of the obtained VAL gels was confirmed, but due to the lack of recovery of the entire CC dose during quantitative analysis of gels stored longer, the recommended storage time for CC preparations is 14 days.

Because of the possible interaction of the active substance with the polymer or other excipients, the use of the proposed oral gels as universal bases for pharmaceutical substances suspended in the form of powdered tablets should be assessed individually, depending on the specific commercial tablets. Since all the studied properties of gels with VAL and CC were similar for all the hydrogel media used, only on the basis of observation of organoleptic properties was the CAR gel considered the most advantageous.

CAR gel has one important feature that can be taken into account—at an acidic pH, such as that in the stomach, the gel transforms into a sol, which should be beneficial for the release and absorption of the active substance. Reduced drug release may be a concern for HEC and CMC gels, especially for drug substances belonging to class II or IV BCS. However, there is a lack of research on this topic, although the common mixing of pediatric drugs with highly viscous food also poses a risk of reduced bioavailability.

Author Contributions: Conceptualization, M.T., M.S. and K.W.; Methodology, M.T., M.S. and K.W.; Software, M.T. and M.S.; Validation, M.T. and M.S.; Formal Analysis, M.T., M.S. and K.W.; Investigation, M.T., M.S. and K.W.; Resources, M.T. and M.S.; Data Curation, M.T.; Writing—Original Draft preparation, M.T., M.S. and K.W.; Writing—review and editing, M.T., M.S. and K.W.; Visualization, M.T. and M.S.; Supervision, M.S. All authors have read and agreed to the published version of the manuscript.

Funding: This research received no external funding.

Informed Consent Statement: Informed consent was obtained from all subjects involved in the study.

Data Availability Statement: The original contributions presented in the study are included in the article; further inquiries can be directed to the corresponding author/s.

Acknowledgments: We are thankful to Polpharma (Starogard, Poland) for kindly donating materials.

Conflicts of Interest: The authors declare no conflicts of interest.

References

1. Thabet, Y.; Klingmann, V.; Breitkreutz, J. Drug formulations: Standards and novel strategies for drug administration in pediatrics. *J. Clin. Pharmacol.* **2018**, *58*, S26–S35. [CrossRef] [PubMed]
2. Malkawi, W.A.; AlRafayah, E.; AlHazabreh, M.; AbuLaila, S.; Al-Ghananeem, A.M. Formulation challenges and strategies to develop pediatric dosage forms. *Children* **2022**, *9*, 488. [CrossRef] [PubMed]

3. WHO. Development of Paediatric Medicines: Points to Consider in Formulation. *WHO Tech. Rep. Series.* **2012**, *970*, 197–225. Available online: https://www.who.int/publications/m/item/trs970-annex-5-development-of-paediatric-medicines-points-to-consider-in-formulation (accessed on 12 September 2024).
4. Alessandrini, E.; Brako, F.; Scarpa, M.; Lupo, M.; Bonifazi, D.; Pignataro, V.; Cavallo, M.; Cullufe, O.; Enache, C.; Nafria, B.; et al. Children's preferences for oral dosage forms and their involvement in formulation research via EPTRI (European Paediatric Translational Research Infrastructure). *Pharmaceutics* **2021**, *13*, 730. [CrossRef]
5. Lopalco, A.; Denora, N. Paediatric formulation: Design and development. *Int. J. Mol. Sci.* **2020**, *21*, 7118. [CrossRef]
6. Zanden, T.M.; Mooij, M.G.; Vet, N.J.; Neubert, A.; Rascher, W.; Lagler, F.B.; Male, C.; Grytli, H.; Halvorsen, T.; de Hoog, M.; et al. Benefit-risk assessment of off-label drug use in children: The Bravo framework. *Clin. Pharmacol. Ther.* **2021**, *110*, 952–965. [CrossRef]
7. Petkova, V.; Georgieva, D.; Dimitrov, M.; Nikolova, I. Off-label prescribing in pediatric population—Literature review for 2012–2022. *Pharmaceutics* **2023**, *15*, 2652. [CrossRef]
8. Richey, R.H.; Shah, U.U.; Peak, M.; Craig, J.V.; Ford, J.L.; Barker, C.E.; Nunn, A.J.; Turner, M.A. Manipulation of drugs to achieve the required dose is intrinsic to paediatric practice but is not supported by guidelines or evidence. *BMC Pediatr.* **2013**, *13*, 81. [CrossRef]
9. Andersson, Å.; Lindemalm, S.; Eksborg, S. Dividing the tablets for childrenGood or bad? *PHME* **2016**, *7*, 23–27. [CrossRef]
10. Orubu, E.S.; Tuleu, C. Medicines for children: Flexible solid oral formulations. *Bull. World Health Organ.* **2017**, *95*, 238–240. [CrossRef]
11. Richey, R.H.; Hughes, C.; Craig, J.V.; Shah, U.U.; Ford, J.L.; Barker, C.E.; Peak, M.; Nunn, A.J.; Turner, M.A. A systematic review of the use of dosage form manipulation to obtain required doses to inform use of manipulation in paediatric practice. *Int. J. Pharm.* **2017**, *518*, 155–166. [CrossRef] [PubMed]
12. Woods, D.J. Extemporaneous Formulations of Oral Liquids a Guide. Available online: https://pharma7roro.wordpress.com/wp-content/uploads/2010/06/extemprep1.pdf (accessed on 31 July 2024).
13. Patel, S.; Scott, N.; Patel, K.; Mohylyuk, V.; McAuley, W.J.; Liu, F. Easy to swallow "Instant" jelly formulations for sustained release gliclazide delivery. *J. Pharm. Sci.* **2020**, *109*, 2474–2484. [CrossRef] [PubMed]
14. Mohylyuk, V.; Patel, K.; Scott, N.; Richardson, C.; Murnane, D.; Liu, F. Wurster fluidised bed coating of microparticles: Towards scalable production of oral sustained-release liquid medicines for patients with swallowing difficulties. *AAPS PharmSciTech* **2019**, *21*, 3. [CrossRef] [PubMed]
15. Dashevskiy, A.; Mohylyuk, V.; Ahmed, A.R.; Kolter, K.; Guth, F.; Bodmeier, R. Micropellets coated with Kollicoat® Smartseal 30D for taste masking in liquid oral dosage forms. *Drug Dev. Ind. Pharm.* **2017**, *43*, 1548–1556. [CrossRef] [PubMed]
16. Silva, M.R.M.; Dysars, L.P.; Santos, E.P.; Ricci Júnio, E. Preparation of extemporaneous oral liquid in the hospital pharmacy. *Braz. J. Pharm. Sci.* **2020**, *56*, 18358. [CrossRef]
17. Stegemann, S. Patient centric drug product design in modern drug delivery as an opportunity to increase safety and effectiveness. *Expert Opin. Drug Deliv.* **2018**, *15*, 619–627. [CrossRef]
18. Timpe, C.; Stegemann, S.; Barrett, A.; Mujumdar, S. Challenges and opportunities to include patient-centric product design in industrial medicines development to improve therapeutic goals. *Br. J. Clin. Pharmacol.* **2020**, *86*, 2020–2027. [CrossRef]
19. O'Brien, F.; Clapham, D.; Krysiak, K.; Batchelor, H.; Field, P.; Caivano, G.; Pertile, M.; Nunn, A.; Tuleu, C. Making medicines baby size: The challenges in bridging the formulation gap in neonatal medicine. *Int. J. Mol. Sci.* **2019**, *20*, 2688. [CrossRef]
20. Menditto, E.; Orlando, V.; De Rosa, G.; Minghetti, P.; Musazzi, U.M.; Cahir, C.; Kurczewska-Michalak, M.; Kardas, P.; Costa, E.; Lobo, J.M.S.; et al. Patient centric pharmaceutical drug product design—The impact on medication adherence. *Pharmaceutics* **2020**, *12*, 44. [CrossRef]
21. Musko, M.; Sznitowska, M. Use of compounded dispersing media for extemporaneous pediatric syrups with candesartan cilexetil and valsartan. *Acta Pharm.* **2014**, *64*, 463–474. [CrossRef]
22. Passariello, A.; Nocerino, R.; Terrin, G.; Cecere, G.; De Marco, G.; Micillo, M.; Pezzella, V.; Cosenza, L.; Malamisura, M.; Maddalena, Y.; et al. Acceptability and efficacy of a gel hypotonic oral rehydration solution in children with acute gastroenteritis. *Eur. J. Gastroenterol. Hepatol.* **2015**, *27*, 523–526. [CrossRef] [PubMed]
23. Mawazi, S.M.; Al-Mahmood, S.M.A.; Chatterjee, B.; Hadi, H.A.B.; Doolaanea, A.A. Carbamazepine gel formulation as a sustained release epilepsy medication for pediatric Use. *Pharmaceutics* **2019**, *11*, 488. [CrossRef] [PubMed]
24. Edwards, T.; Liu, G.; Hegarty, J.E.; Crowther, C.A.; Alsweiler, J.; Harding, J.E. Oral dextrose gel to prevent hypoglycaemia in at-risk neonates. *Cochrane Database Syst. Rev.* **2021**, *5*, 5, Erratum in *Cochrane Database Syst Rev.* **2023**, *1–38*. [CrossRef]
25. FDA. Atacand, Drug Information. Available online: https://www.accessdata.fda.gov/drugsatfda_docs/label/2020/020838s041lbl.pdf (accessed on 30 July 2024).

26. Schaefer, F.; Zurowska, A.; Gimpel, C.; Van Hoeck, K.; Drozdz, D.; Montini, G.; Bagdasorova, I.V.; Sorof, J.; Sugg, J.; Teng, R.; et al. Candesartan in children with hypertension investigators. Efficacy, safety and pharmacokinetics of candesartan cilexetil in hypertensive children from 1 to less than 6 years of age. *J. Hypertens.* **2010**, *28*, 1083–1090. [CrossRef]
27. Stat Pearls. Candesartan Information. Available online: https://www.ncbi.nlm.nih.gov/books/NBK519501/ (accessed on 30 July 2024).
28. HIP. Study to Characterize the Long-Term Clinical Experience of Atacand in Hypertensive Children Ages 1 to <11 Years (Hypertension in Pediatrics). Available online: https://www.astrazenecaclinicaltrials.com/study/D2451C00006/ (accessed on 30 July 2024).
29. EMA. Atacand, Drug Information. Available online: https://www.ema.europa.eu/en/medicines/human/referrals/atacand (accessed on 30 July 2024).
30. MedLibrary, Candesartan Cilexetil Drug Information. Available online: https://medlibrary.org/lib/rx/meds/candesartan-cilexetil/page/3/#ID_4CCA141E-2679-47D6-B3E3-C57F1413B855 (accessed on 30 July 2024).
31. Redon, J.; Seeman, T.; Pall, D.; Suurorg, L.; Kamperis, K.; Erdine, S.; Wühl, E.; Mancia, G. Narrative update of clinical trials with antihypertensive drugs in children and adolescents. *Front. Cardiovasc. Med.* **2022**, *9*, 1042190. [CrossRef]
32. Siddiqui, N.; Husain, A.; Chaudhry, L.; Alam, M.S.; Mitra, M.; Bhasin, P.S. Pharmacological and pharmaceutical profile of valsartan: A review. *J. Appl. Pharm. Sci.* **2011**, *1*, 12–19. Available online: https://japsonline.com/admin/php/uploads/54_pdf.pdf (accessed on 31 July 2024).
33. Darwhekar, G.N.; Jain, D.K.; Chouhan, J. Biopharmaceutical classification of candesartan and candesartan cilexetil. *Asian J. Pharm. Life Sci.* **2012**, *2*, 295–302. Available online: https://api.semanticscholar.org/CorpusID:55243030%7D (accessed on 31 July 2024).
34. Candesartan Cilexetil Characteristics. PubChem Information. Available online: https://pubchem.ncbi.nlm.nih.gov/compound/Candesartan-cilexetil (accessed on 29 August 2024).
35. Valsartan Characteristics. PubChem Information. Available online: https://pubchem.ncbi.nlm.nih.gov/compound/valsartan (accessed on 29 August 2024).
36. Diovan FDA Information, Actualisied 2021. Available online: https://www.fda.gov/drugs/development-approval-process-drugs/drug-approvals-and-databases (accessed on 30 July 2024).
37. Lou-Meda, R.; Stiller, B.; Antonio, Z.L.; Zielinska, E.; Yap, H.K.; Kang, H.G.; Tan, M.; Glazer, R.D.; Valentin, M.A.; Wang, L. Long-term safety and tolerability of valsartan in children aged 6 to 17 years with hypertension. *Pediatr. Nephrol.* **2019**, *34*, 495–506. [CrossRef]
38. Schaefer, F.; Coppo, R.; Bagga, A.; Senguttuvan, P.; Schlosshauer, R.; Zhang, Y.; Kadwa, M. Efficacy and safety of valsartan in hypertensive children 6 months to 5 years of age. *J. Hypertens.* **2013**, *31*, 993–1000. [CrossRef]
39. Schaefer, F.; Litwin, M.; Zachwieja, J.; Zurowska, A.; Turi, S.; Grosso, A.; Pezous, N.; Kadwa, M. Efficacy and safety of valsartan compared to enalapril in hypertensive children: A 12-week, randomized, double-blind, parallel-group study. *J. Hypertens.* **2011**, *29*, 2484–2490. [CrossRef]
40. Diovan 3 mg/mL Oral Solution—Summary of Product Characteristics. Available online: https://www.medicines.org.uk/emc/product/5991/smpc#gref (accessed on 30 July 2024).
41. Diovan® (Valsartan) Tablets, for Oral Use. Patient Information Approved by the U.S. Food and Drug Administration. 2021. Available online: https://www.novartis.com/us-en/sites/novartis_us/files/diovan.pdf (accessed on 31 July 2024).
42. Candesartan Extemporaneous Syrups, Drug Monograph. Available online: https://publications.aap.org/pediatriccare/drug-monograph/18/4996/Candesartan?autologincheck=redirected (accessed on 30 July 2024).
43. Candesartan Extemporaneous Syrups, Formula Preparation. Available online: https://compoundingtoday.com/Formulation/SearchByKeyword.cfm (accessed on 31 July 2024).
44. Candesartan Extemporaneous Syrup, Formula Preparation. Available online: https://medilib.ir/uptodate/show/17058 (accessed on 31 July 2024).
45. Younes, M.; Aquilina, G.; Engel, K.H.; Fowler, P.; Frutos Fernandez, M.J.; Fürst, P.; Gürtler, R.; Gundert-Remy, U.; Husøy, T.; Manco, M.; et al. Safety evaluation of crosslinked polyacrylic acid polymers (carbomer) as a new food additive. *EFSA J.* **2021**, *19*, 06693. Available online: https://efsa.onlinelibrary.wiley.com/doi/pdf/10.2903/j.efsa.2021.6693 (accessed on 31 July 2024).
46. Carbopol® 934P NF Polymer Characteristic, Lubrizol Pharmaceuticals. Available online: https://www.lubrizol.com/Health/Pharmaceuticals/Excipients/Carbopol-Polymer-Products/Carbopol-934P-NF-Polymer (accessed on 30 July 2024).
47. Malkin, A.Y.; Derkach, S.R.; Kulichikhin, V.G. Rheology of gels and yielding liquids. *Gels* **2023**, *9*, 715. [CrossRef] [PubMed]
48. Wróblewska, M.; Słyż, J.; Winnicka, K. Rheological and textural properties of hydrogels, containing sulfur as a model drug, made using different polymers types. *Polimery* **2019**, *64*, 208–2015. [CrossRef]
49. Texture Analysis, Back Extrusion Ring (A/BE). Available online: https://textureanalysisprofessionals.blogspot.com/2015/02/texture-analysis-in-action-back.html (accessed on 31 July 2024).

50. Tomczykowa, M.; Wróblewska, M.; Winnicka, K.; Wieczorek, P.; Majewski, P.; Celińska-Janowicz, K.; Sawczuk, R.; Miltyk, W.; Tryniszewska, E.; Tomczyk, M. Novel gel formulations as topical carriers for the essential oil of Bidens tripartita for the treatment of candidiasis. *Molecules* **2018**, *23*, 2517. [CrossRef]
51. Hurler, J.; Engesland, A.; Poorahmary Kermany, B.; Škalko-Basnet, N. Improved texture analysis for hydrogel characterization: Gel cohesiveness, adhesiveness, and hardness. *J. Appl. Polym. Sci.* **2012**, *125*, 180–188. [CrossRef]
52. Wróblewska, M.; Szekalska, M.; Hafner, A.; Winnicka, K. Oleogels and bigels as topical drug carriers for ketoconazole—Development and in vitro characterization. *Acta Pol. Pharm.* **2018**, *75*, 777–786. Available online: https://ptfarm.pl/download/?file=File/Acta_Poloniae/2018/3/777.pdf (accessed on 31 July 2024).
53. Wróblewska, M.; Szymańska, E.; Winnicka, K. The Influence of tea tree oil on antifungal activity and pharmaceutical characteristics of Pluronic® F-127 gel formulations with ketoconazole. *Int. J. Mol. Sci.* **2021**, *22*, 11326. [CrossRef]
54. Brookfield Ametek. Food and Beverage Applications. Available online: https://www.brookfieldengineering.com/brookfield-university/learning-center/application-notes/texture-applications/food-and-beverage/cheese-triangles (accessed on 31 July 2024).
55. *European Pharmacopoeia*, 11th ed.; Council of Europe: Strasburg, France, 2023.
56. El-Gizawy, S.M.; Abdelmageed, O.H.; Omar, M.A.; Deryea, S.M.; Abdel-Megied, A.M. Development and validation of HPLC method for simultaneous determination of amlodipine, valsartan, hydrochlorothiazide in dosage form and spiked human plasma. *Am. J. Anal. Chem.* **2012**, *3*, 422–430. [CrossRef]
57. Madhavi, K.; Navamani, M.; Prasanthi, C. Simple analytical method for the simultaneous estimation of hydrochlorothiazide and candesartan by RP-HPLC. *Int. J. Appl. Pharm.* **2017**, *9*, 34–38. [CrossRef]
58. Revathi, R.; Saravanan, V.S.; Ethiraj, T.; Marreddy, J.L. RP-HPLC Analysis for quantitation of candesartan cilexetil in solid dosage forms. *Asian J. Pharm. Anal.* **2013**, *3*, 115–118. Available online: https://ajpaonline.com/AbstractView.aspx?PID=2013-3-4-2 (accessed on 31 July 2024).
59. Sharma, T.; Moitra, S.; Si, S.; Sankar, D. Development and validation of a HPLC method for the determination of valsartan and its degradation products in pharmaceutical formulation. *Int. J. Pharm. Pharm. Sci.* **2012**, *4*, 503–505. Available online: https://www.innovareacademics.in/journal/ijpps/Vol4Issue2/3530.pdf (accessed on 31 July 2024).
60. Vinzuda, D.U.; Sailor, G.U.; Sheth, N.R. RP-HPLC Method for Determination of Valsartan in Tablet Dosage Form. *Int. J. Chem. Tech. Res.* **2010**, *2*, 1461–1467. Available online: https://sphinxsai.com/july-sept_2010_vol2.3/chemtech/chemtechvol2.3july-sept210/CT=16%20(1461-1467).pdf (accessed on 31 July 2024).
61. STEP Database. Available online: https://step-db.ucl.ac.uk/eupfi/appDirectLink.do?appFlag=login (accessed on 31 July 2024).
62. Salunke, S.; Brandys, B.; Giacoia, G.; Tuleu, C. The STEP (Safety and Toxicity of Excipients for Paediatrics) database: Part 2—The pilot version. *Int. J. Pharm.* **2013**, *457*, 310–322. [CrossRef] [PubMed]
63. PubChem. Carmellose Sodium Characteristic. Available online: https://pubchem.ncbi.nlm.nih.gov/compound/Carmellose-sodium (accessed on 29 August 2024).
64. Carmellose Sodium Characteristic. Available online: https://www.chembk.com/en/chem/carmellose%20sodium#:~:text=carmellose%20sodium%20-%20Physico-chemical%20Properties%20Molecular%20Formula,C6H7O2%20(OH)2CH2COONa%20Molar%20Mass%20265.204%20Density%201,6%20g/cm3 (accessed on 29 August 2024).
65. UPICHEM. Carbomer 947P NF Characteristic. Available online: https://www.upichem.com/products/carbomer-974p-nf/#:~:text=Molecular%20Weight:,72.02%20g/mol (accessed on 29 August 2024).
66. Carbomer Properties. Pharmaceutical Polymers Typical Properties and Specifications. Available online: https://www.lubrizol.com/-/media/Lubrizol/Health/Literature/Pharmaceutical-Polymers-Typical-Properties-and-Specifications.pdf (accessed on 29 August 2024).
67. Rowe, R.C.; Sheskey, P.J.; Cook, W.G.; Fenton, M.E. *Handbook of Pharmaceutical Excipients*, 7th ed.; Pharmaceutical Press: London, UK, 2014.
68. Biopharmaceutics Classification System-Based Biowaivers. Available online: https://database.ich.org/sites/default/files/M9_Guideline_Step4_2019_1116.pdf (accessed on 29 August 2024).
69. Truffin, D.; Häusler, O.; Martin, M.; Cotier, S.; Laparre, J.; Ramnath, M. Polyols permeability on Caco-2 cells and their effects on transport of low-permeability drugs. *Future Pharmacol.* **2023**, *3*, 229–237. [CrossRef]
70. Trissel, L.A. *Stability of Compounded Formulations*, 5th ed.; American Pharmacists Association: Washington, DC, USA, 2012.
71. Chalah, K.; Benmounah, A.; Mahdad, M.; Kheribet, R. Rheological study of sodium carboxymethyl-cellulose: Effect of concentration and molecular weight. *Mater. Today Proc.* **2022**, *53*, 185–190. [CrossRef]
72. Aodah, A.H.; Bakr, A.A.; Booq, R.Y.; Rahman, M.J.; Alzahrani, D.A.; Alsulami, K.A.; Alshaya, H.A.; Alsuabeyl, M.S.; Alyamani, E.J.; Tawfik, E.A. Preparation and evaluation of benzalkonium chloride hand sanitizer as a potential alternative for alcohol-based hand gels. *Saudi Pharm. J.* **2021**, *29*, 807–814. [CrossRef]
73. *The United States Pharmacopeia and National Formulary*; Pharmacopeia Convention: Rockville, MD, USA, 2022.

pharmaceutics

MDPI

Article

Liquid- and Semisolid-Filled Hard Gelatin Capsules Containing Alpha-Lipoic Acid as a Suitable Dosage Form for Compounding Medicines and Dietary Supplements

Jelena Jovičić-Bata [1], Nemanja Todorović [1,*], Veljko Krstonošić [1], Ivan Ristić [2], Zorana Kovačević [3], Milana Vuković [1] and Mladena Lalić-Popović [1,4]

[1] Department of Pharmacy, Faculty of Medicine Novi Sad, University of Novi Sad, 21000 Novi Sad, Serbia; jelena.jovicic-bata@mf.uns.ac.rs (J.J.-B.); veljko.krstonosic@mf.uns.ac.rs (V.K.); milana.vukovic@mf.uns.ac.rs (M.V.); mladena.lalic-popovic@mf.uns.ac.rs (M.L.-P.)
[2] Faculty of Technology Novi Sad, University of Novi Sad, 21000 Novi Sad, Serbia; ivan.ristic@uns.ac.rs
[3] Department of Veterinary Medicine, Faculty of Agriculture, University of Novi Sad, 21000 Novi Sad, Serbia; zorana.kovacevic@polj.edu.rs
[4] Centre for Medical and Pharmaceutical Investigations and Quality Control (CEMPhIC), Faculty of Medicine Novi Sad, University of Novi Sad, 21000 Novi Sad, Serbia
* Correspondence: nemanja.todorovic@mf.uns.ac.rs

Abstract: Liquid-filled hard gelatin capsules may have pertinent advantages both for therapeutic effect and extemporaneous preparations of medicines. Alpha lipoic acid is a substance used in medicines and dietary supplements and there is a need for creating an appropriate formulation which would be suitable for each individual patient or consumer. Based on its biopharmaceutical and physical chemical characteristics, eight different capsule formulations were designed and characterized. Silicon dioxide was added to form a semisolid content and prevent leakage. The formulation filled with alpha lipoic acid solution in polyethylene glycol 400 showed the best performance. Although the addition of silicon dioxide to the formulation with polyethylene glycol 400 led to a change in both flow character and viscosity, the release rate did not show a statistically significant decrease (more than 85% of content was released after 5 min testing). Applied technique is a simple and an appropriate approach for compounding and could be used for other substances with similar properties.

Keywords: thioctic acid; dissolution test; rheology; FTIR; colloidal silicon dioxide; polyethylene glycol (PEG-400); extemporaneous formulations; dosage forms and excipients; compounding technologies

1. Introduction

Alpha-lipoic acid (ALA, thioctic acid) is a sulfur-containing organic acid, produced in the mitochondria of plant and animal species from octanoic acid and cysteine as a source of sulfur. Due to its amphiphilic properties, ALA is ubiquitous, present in cell membranes and cytosol [1]. There are indications that Western diets do not provide ample amounts of ALA [2]. The endogenous synthesis of ALA regulated by lipoic acid synthase in humans is possibly insufficient [3], dependent on lipoic acid synthase activity [4] and decreases with age [3,5]. Exogenous sources of ALA are therefore required. The naturally occurring, biologically active form of ALA is its R-enantiomer, but commercial preparations of ALA often contain a mixture of R and S-enantiomers (Figure 1). S-enantiomer is a byproduct of ALA industrial synthesis with no known negative health effects [6,7]. R-enantiomer might be slightly better absorbed and cleared from the body slower than the S-form [2]. Additionally, isolated R-form is more expensive.

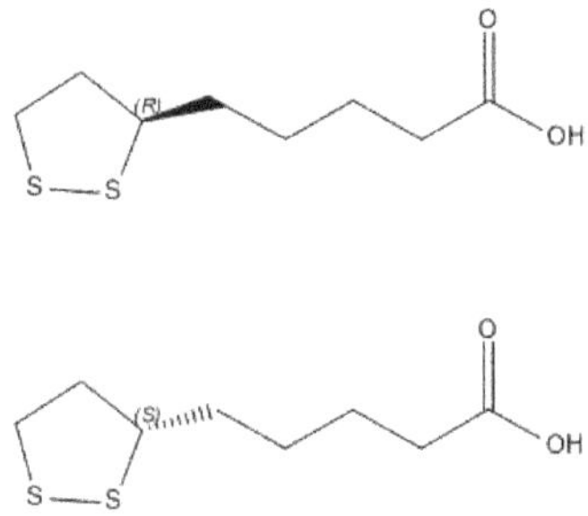

Figure 1. Chemical structure of alpha-lipoic acid (ALA); the levorotatory isomer S-(−)-ALA and the dextrorotatory isomer R-(+)-ALA.

In the human body, the fraction of ALA covalently bound to proteins is an important part of several mitochondrial enzyme complexes engaged in energy production [8,9]. Unbound ALA acts as a "universal antioxidant" [6], active inside and outside of cells, both in its oxidized and reduced (dihydrolipoic acid/DHLA) forms [10]. ALA scavenges reactive oxygen species (ROS), regenerates other antioxidants such as glutathione, vitamin C and vitamin E, chelates selected metal ions, affects the activity of several redox enzyme systems and possibly modulates some signaling pathways including the insulin pathway [11, 12]. ALA has also been shown to display anti-inflammatory actions by suppressing the production of pro-inflammatory proteins [13–18].

ALA is available to consumers in various oral dosage forms, e.g., capsules, both soft and hard, immediate release tablets, film-coated gastroresistant tablets [19,20], and is registered both as medicines and dietary supplements (DS). These products differ significantly. In most countries, DS are regulated as food and are freely available for purchase. Strict conforming to pharmacopeial standards in terms of quality testing enforced on medicines by pharmacopeias (e.g., dissolution testing, disintegration testing, and friability) are usually not matched by DS regulations. DS can be registered and marketed without quality testing and their efficacy being established.

Doses of ALA in DS range from 10 mg to 600 mg, the latter being a dose equal to the one used in medicines. Daily doses of ALA used in treatment of diabetes neuropathy are usually 300 to 1800 mg, but the optimal doses for other potential "indications" have not been established. Clinical studies of ALA assessed the use of 100 to 2400 mg of ALA per day in different disorders [21]. Furthermore, there are indications that the dosing of ALA should be adjusted in patients with severe renal function impairment [22]. It should be noted that ALA can trigger insulin autoimmune syndrome (IAS). Namely, a sulfhydryl compound like ALA can help dissociate S-S bonds within insulin molecules and expose specific insulins' amino acid sequence (Ile-Leu-Gln), which acts as an antigen, thereby provoking an allergic reaction [23]. The development of IAS is strongly connected to sulfhydryl with specific genotypes in the blood type marker Human Leucocyte Antigen (HLA). Furthermore, Gullo et al. estimated that increased use of ALA in food supplements led to an increased frequency of IAS in Italy [24].

ALA is a weak acid with a pKa value between 4.76 and 5.4 [25]. As a lipophilic compound, it has a logP value of 2.11 [26]. ALA preparations should be taken on an empty stomach, 30 min before or 2 h after a meal, as food has been shown to impair its absorption [27]. Due to ALA properties, formulation of its dosage forms presents a challenge for the pharmaceutical industry. Namely, it is poorly soluble in water, unstable in the presence of gastric acid, and extensively metabolized in the liver, which results in its bioavailability of only about 30% [3]. It is classified as a class II substance in the biopharmaceutics classification system (BCS) [20,28]. The bioavailability of ALA is better in the presence of substances that increase its solubility and in the form of liquid formulations [29,30]. Hence, the formulation characteristics of its dosage forms can significantly affect its bioavailability and, consequently, its effects.

Taking into account the general risk of IAS and data from animal studies, the calculated upper safe dose per person per day is 42 mg [31]. Although higher doses have not been linked to serious adverse effects, the European Food Safety Authority suggests that 150–200 mg of ALA per day causes safety concerns [32–34]. Though there is plethora of oral dosage forms with ALA on the market worldwide, there is a need for a specific strength or dosage that might not be commercially available. Also, the removal of some ingredients that patients are allergic to might be required.

However, ALA is chemically unstable under light and heat. The decomposition of ALA is accompanied by an unpleasant odor due to the sulfur it contains. At temperatures that are greater than its melting point (59–62 °C), immediate polymerization occurs [35]. Thus, the US Food and Drug Administration categorized ALA into category 1 in section 305B of the FD&C Act, which are bulk drug substances that have physical and chemical properties that could have an impact on the performance of the compounded product. ALA is also under consideration to be allowed for use in compounding by 503A facilities [36].

Thus, the aim of this work was the preparation of custom-made simple dosage forms with ALA and their complete characterization. Compounding was performed using hard gelatin capsules that are suitable in pharmaceutical practice. Two formulations contained solid powder filling, three formulations were liquid, and three were compounded as semisolid formulations.

2. Materials and Methods

2.1. Materials

The following chemicals were used in the experiment: USP-grade alpha-lipoic acid (ALA, Farmalabor, Canosa di Puglia, Italy), CapsuLac® 60 (Meggle, Wasserburg am Inn, Germany), Excipient II (Farmalabor, Canosa di Puglia, Italy; composition: pregelatinized corn starch, magnesium stearate, micronized silicon dioxide, micronized talc), absolute ethanol (Zorka Pharma-Hemija, Šabac, Serbia), polyethylene glycol 400 (PEG 400, Alfa Aesar, Kandel, Germany), caprylic/capric triglycerides (Comcen, Belgrade, Serbia), colloidal silicon dioxide (Centrohem, Stara Pazova, Serbia), hard gelatin capsules size 0 (Farmalabor, Canosa di Puglia, Italy; composition: indigo FD&C Blue 2 (E132), titanium dioxide, and yellow iron oxide (E172), gelatin). Methanol (Lachner, Neratovice, Czech Republic) was used for the content determination test. The dissolution rate was tested in a 0.5% sodium lauryl sulfate (SLS, Centrohem, Stara Pazova, Serbia) water solution. Purified water used in all experiments was obtained by distillation (AC-L8, Optic Ivymen System, J.P. Selecta, Barcelona, Spain) at the Department of Pharmacy, Faculty of Medicine Novi Sad.

2.2. Capsules Formulation

Capsules were compounded according to the standard operating procedure of the Pharmaceutical Technology Laboratory at the Department of Pharmacy, Faculty of Medicine Novi Sad. A manual capsule-filling machine (Farmalabor, Canosa di Puglia, Italy) with a size 0 capsule kit (V = 0.68 mL) was used. The loading capacities were determined for the powder components after standard filling with pure substances (n = 20) and they were 261.70 ± 29.43 mg, 479.07 ± 6.75 mg, and 443.29 ± 13.70 mg for ALA, CapsuLac® 60, and Excipient II, respectively.

Three solid-filled capsule formulations were compounded for comparation with new liquid- and semisolid-filled capsules. Formulation F_0 contained only 100 mg of ALA. Formulations F_1 and F_2 contained CapsuLac® 60 and Excipient II as fillers and 100 mg of ALA. Masses of fillers were calculated using Equation (1):

$$m = C - D, \quad (1)$$

where m is the mass of the filler needed to compound one capsule, C is the experimentally determined loading capacity of the filler, and D is the dose of ALA needed to compound one capsule (100 mg).

The masses of pure substances required for the compounding of 50 capsules were sifted through a test sieve 355 μm on a sieve shaker (AS 200 control, Retsch, Haan, Germany) and weighed on a technical balance (Radwag, Radom, Poland). Mixing was conducted on a powder mixer (Pharmalabor, Canosa di Puglia, Italy) for 20 min, at maximum mixing speed (5/5, 130 rpm) and using a mixing container whose volume was approximately half filled with the powder. The composition of the solid-filled capsules is shown in Table 1.

Table 1. Composition of the solid-filled capsules.

Formulation	Ingredient		
	ALA	CapsuLac® 60	Excipient II
F_0	100 mg	/	/
F_1	100 mg	q.s. *	/
F_2	100 mg	/	q.s.

* q.s.—quantum satis.

Additionally, three liquid-filled and three semisolid-filled (with the addition of colloidal silicon dioxide) formulations were compounded.

Formulations with liquid filling (F_3, F_4 and F_5) were compounded by measuring the ALA needed to compound 50 capsules (5 g) and dissolving in a required volume of absolute ethanol, PEG 400 or caprylic/caprylic triglycerides. The required volume corresponded to 70% of the capsule volume, i.e., 476 μL per capsule (23.8 mL for 50 capsule size 0). Mixing was performed on a magnetic stirrer (Boeco, Hamburg, Germany) at room temperature for 2 h. After mixing, clear yellow solutions were obtained with absolute ethanol and PEG 400, while mixing ALA with caprylic/caprylic triglycerides resulted in obtaining a suspension. Using an automatic pipette (Brand, Wertheim, Germany), 476 μL of the resulting solution or suspension was transferred to the open capsules on the manual capsule filling machine and the capsules were closed. Before sealing the capsules, silicon dioxide was added in semisolid-filled capsule formulations (F_6, F_7 and F_8) to the full volume with shaking on a vibrating plate (Retsch, Hahn, Germany). The composition of the capsules with liquid and semisolid matrix are shown in Table 2.

Table 2. Composition of the liquid- and semisolid-filled capsules.

Formulation	Ingredient				
	ALA	Absolute Ethanol	PEG 400	Caprylic/Capric Triglycerides	Silicon Dioxide
F_3	100 mg	ad 476 μL	/	/	/
F_4	100 mg	/	ad 476 μL	/	/
F_5	100 mg	/	/	ad 476 μL	/
F_6	100 mg	ad 476 μL	/	/	q.s.*
F_7	100 mg	/	ad 476 μL	/	q.s.
F_8	100 mg	/	/	ad 476 μL	q.s.

* q.s.—quantum satis.

2.3. *Flowability*

The flowability determination of ALA, CapsuLac® 60, Excipient II, and the mixture for the preparation of formulations F_1 and F_2 was performed on a compaction apparatus (Jolting volumeter, stav II, J. Engelsmann AG, Ludwigshafen, Germany). A measuring cylinder of 10 mL was used, and the mass of the sample was 2 g. Bulk volume and tapped volume after 10, 100, 500, 900, and 1250 impacts were recorded. All measurements were performed in triplicate, and results are presented as mean ± standard deviation. The flowability of the powder was estimated based on the values of the Compressibility Index and the Hausner Ratio, which were calculated according to the guidelines given in the 11th European Pharmacopoeia (Ph. Eur. 11) [37], as shown in Equations (2) and (3):

$$\text{Compressibility Index} = 100 \times \frac{V_0 - V_f}{V_0}, \quad (2)$$

$$\text{Hausner Ratio} = \frac{V_0}{V_f} \quad (3)$$

where V_0 is the unsettled apparent volume and V_f is the final tapped volume.

Additionally, for the same substances and mixtures, the angle of repose (α) was determined according to the recommendations given in Ph. Eur. 11. (Equation (4)). The test was performed in triplicate, and the results are presented as mean $\pm$ standard deviation [37].

$$\tan(\alpha) = \frac{\text{height}}{0.5 \times \text{base}} \quad (4)$$

2.4. Uniformity of Mass

Uniformity of mass was conducted according to Ph. Eur. 11. Twenty randomly selected capsules were weighed on an analytical balance (Radwag, Radom, Poland) before and after careful emptying of the capsule filling. From the difference in the two values, the average value of twenty measurements was calculated. It was observed whether the individual masses deviated more than the permitted percentage deviation (7.5%, average masses greater than 300 mg) [37].

2.5. Assay

The filling of 10 individual capsules was carefully dissolved in 10 mL of methanol. The samples were exposed to ultrasonic waves for 15 min without heating (Bandelin Sonorex, Berlin, Germany). The content in the prepared samples was determined spectrophotometrically (G1103A, Agilent Technologies, Santa Clara, CA, USA) [38]. The absorbance of the solution was measured at 330 nm. The dependence of absorbance on ALA concentration was linear in the concentration range 0.078125–2.5 mg/mL ($R^2 = 0.99988$). The content is expressed as a percentage of the declared (theoretical) value.

2.6. Fourier Transform Infrared Spectroscopy

The infrared spectra were obtained using a Fourier transform infrared spectrophotometer (FTIR) IRAffinity-1S (Shimadzu, Tokyo, Japan). Measurements were carried out using ATR (attenuated total reflection) in the range 4000–400 cm^{-1}, with a resolution of 4 cm^{-1}.

2.7. In Vitro Dissolution Study

The selection of the medium for testing the dissolution rate was based on the study of the solubility and stability of ALA. Solubility was tested in water, pH 1.2 and pH 6.8 mediums without and with addition of sodium lauryl sulfate (SLS) in the concentrations of 0.1, 0.25, and 0.5%. Solubility was tested in triplicate after 24 h in a thermostatic water bath with a shaker (WSB-18, Witeg Labortechnik, Wertheim, Germany) at a temperature of 37 °C. The stability of the solution was tested by re-measuring the content in the samples after an additional 24 h at a temperature of 37 °C. As a medium, a 0.5% aqueous solution of sodium lauryl sulfate (SLS) was chosen.

The dissolution rate test was performed using a basket apparatus on a dissolution rate test device (DT 800 LH, Erweka®, Heussenstam, Germany). The volume of the medium was 500 mL, at a temperature of 37 °C, and at a rotation speed of 100 rpm. Sampling was performed at 5, 15, 25, 35, 45, and 60 min from the start of the test. The samples were filtered prior to analysis through membrane filter size 0.45 µm (Sartorius Lab Instruments, Göttingen, Germany). The concentration of ALA at the observed time points was determined by the aforementioned spectrophotometric method.

2.8. Rheological Properties

HAAKE MARS rheometer (Thermo Scientific, Karlsruhe, Germany) was used for the investigation of rheological behavior. Measurements were performed 24 h after compounding at room temperature (25 ± 0.1 °C) using cylinder CC25 DIN/Ti for liquid samples and plate–plate PP35 Ti measuring geometry with a gap of 1.000 mm for semisolid samples. Continual increase in shear rate from 0.005 to 200 s^{-1} during 120 s was carried out with the purpose of conducting the hysteresis loop test. Afterwards, the shear stress was constant for 60 s at 200 s^{-1} and lastly, it decreased to 0 s^{-1} during the next 120 s.

Linear viscoelastic region (LVR) was determined by amplitude sweep test where storage (G′) and viscous modulus (G″) were recorded versus shear stress (0.01–10 Pa) at constant frequency of 1 Hz. Frequency sweep tests were performed based on the strain, selected as middle of LVR. G′ and G″ moduli were recorded versus frequency (0.1–10 Hz) at constant shear stress.

3. Results

3.1. Flowability

As expected, pure ALA has the worst flowability according to all three observed parameters. Interestingly, the combinations of ALA and selected diluents have a better flowability than pure diluents according to the Hausner Ratio and Compressibility Index. Excipient II has poor flowability compared to CapsuLac® 60. Consequently, the formulations containing Excipient II (F_2) are characterized by worse flowability compared to the formulation containing CapsuLac® 60 (F_1). The values of the Compressibility Index, Hausner Ratio, and angle of repose of pure substances and tested mixtures F_1 and F_2 are shown in Table 3.

Table 3. Character of flowability of tested powdery substances and mixtures.

Substance/ Mixture	Hausner Ratio		Compressibility Index (%)		Flow Character According to Hausner Ratio and Compressibility Index	Angle of Repose		Flow Property According to Angle of Repose
	Mean	SD	Mean	SD		Mean	SD	
ALA	1.51	0.01	33.63	0.30	Very poor	49.09	0.55	Poor
CapsuLac® 60	1.31	0.02	23.80	1.21	Passable	32.87	1.43	Good
Excipient II	1.43	0.04	30.26	2.11	Poor	36.71	0.79	Fair
F_1	1.14	0.03	12.08	2.22	Good	39.74	0.29	Fair
F_2	1.29	0.01	22.43	0.37	Passable	41.22	0.36	Passable

3.2. Uniformity of Mass and Assay

Uniformity of mass as well as content uniformity are in accordance with the requirements of Ph. Eur. 11. The F_2 formulation has a greater mass variation compared to F_1 formulation, which may be related to the worse flowability. The results of uniformity of mass and assay of the prepared formulations are shown in Table 4.

Table 4. Results of uniformity of mass and assay test.

Formulation	Uniformity of Mass (%)		Assay (%)	
	Min	Max	Mean	SD
F_1	98.42	102.03	96.61	1.38
F_2	95.37	102.21	97.79	2.05
F_3	98.33	105.98	98.93	0.97
F_4	95.72	106.11	98.09	2.45
F_5	95.19	107.27	98.17	1.09
F_6	97.43	104.68	96.05	0.84
F_7	95.63	104.95	101.18	3.01
F_8	96.44	104.99	99.82	2.17

3.3. *Fourier Transform Infrared Spectroscopy*

The FTIR spectra of ALA and other ingredients with appropriate formulations are shown in Figure 2. The band in ALA spectrum at 2926 cm^{-1} corresponds to the methylene stretching and does not change after the ALA formulation. Also, bands at 2850 and 2920 cm^{-1} for symmetric and asymmetric ν(C–H) vibrations, respectively, are presented in pure ALA and all formulations. A prominent band at 1687 cm^{-1} is associated with the C=O stretching vibrations from the carbonyl group of ALA as shown in Figure 2. The OH stretching from the –COOH group presents at 1465, 1427, and 1247 cm^{-1} from ν(C–O)/δ(OH) out-of-plane, with strong absorption at 929 from δ(OH) out-of-plane. The position of these characteristic bands of –OH group in ALA did not change in the spectra of the F_1 and F_2 formulations as shown in Figure 2a. However, the S–S and C–S bands were observed at 673 cm^{-1} from ν(C–S) and at 499 and 451 cm^{-1} from ν(S–S) [39,40]. Figure 2a illustrates that there was no typical band appearance or disappearance of ALA in the F_1 and F_2 formulation, demonstrating the existence of ALA. In F_1, peaks from lactose are presented at 3260 cm^{-1} from OH vibration, 1070 to 1030 cm^{-1} from C–O–C and C–OH groups of the lactose. Other lactose peaks overlap with intensive peaks of ALA. In the F_2 formulation, characteristic peaks from corn starch are presented at 3250 cm^{-1} from O-H stretching, C–O–C asymmetric stretching at 1149 cm^{-1} and 1078 and 1014 cm^{-1} originated from C–O stretching. These peaks are presented in F_2 without shifting.

In the F_3 and F_6 formulations, shifting of the characteristic ALA peaks is observed as follows: C=O carbonyl from 1687 to 1714 cm^{-1}, as well as peaks from ν(C–O)/δ(OH) out-of-plane from 1465, 1427 and, 1247 cm^{-1} in pure ALA to 1456, 1417, and 1271 cm^{-1} in formulation, which confirmed the formation of a supramolecular structure with ethanol. The formation of a complex structure is also confirmed by the disappearance of the strong absorption at 929 cm^{-1} from δ(OH) out-of-plane in pure ALA. Other characteristic peaks of ethanol are present in the F_3 and F_6 formulation at 879 and 1045 cm^{-1} from C–C–O stretching, 1085 cm^{-1} from C–O stretching, CH_3 rocking and at 3332 cm^{-1} from the OH group in ethanol.

In the F_4 and F_7 formulation, shifting of the C=O carbonyl from 1687 (in pure ALA) to 1728 cm^{-1} confirms the interaction of PEG and ALA. PEG characteristic peaks presented in the F_4 and F_7 formulation at 3456 cm^{-1} are ascribed to O–H stretching. The absorption at 1456 cm^{-1} was designated to the C–H bending vibrations of the –CH_2 group; the peak at 941 cm^{-1} was associated with the –CH out-of-plane bending vibrations of PEG. The C–O–C ether stretching absorption band at 1095 cm^{-1} overlapped with peaks from ALA ν(C–O)/δ(OH) out-of-plane (at 1465, 1427 and 929 cm^{-1}).

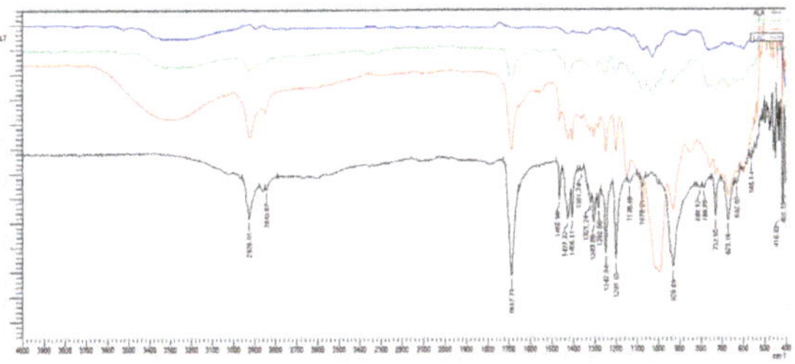

(**a**) ALA, F_1, F_2, CapsuLac® 60

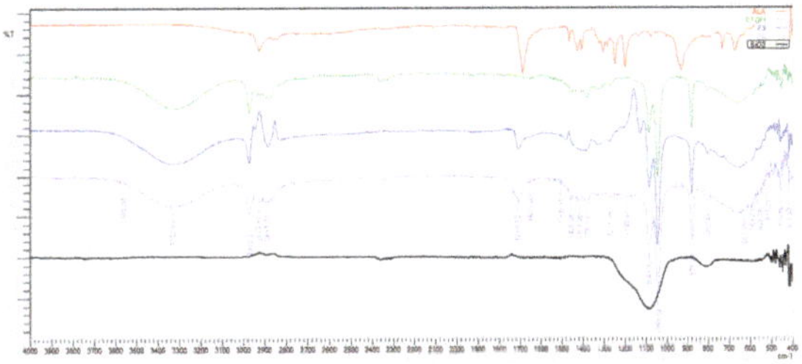

(**b**) ALA, F_3, F_6, absolute ethanol, SiO_2

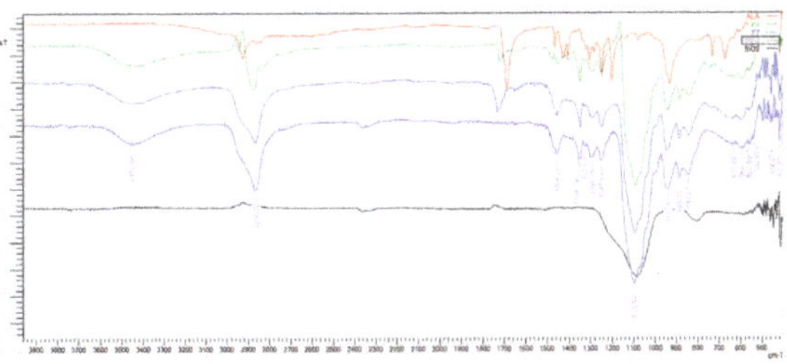

(**c**) ALA, F_4, F_7, PEG 400, SiO_2

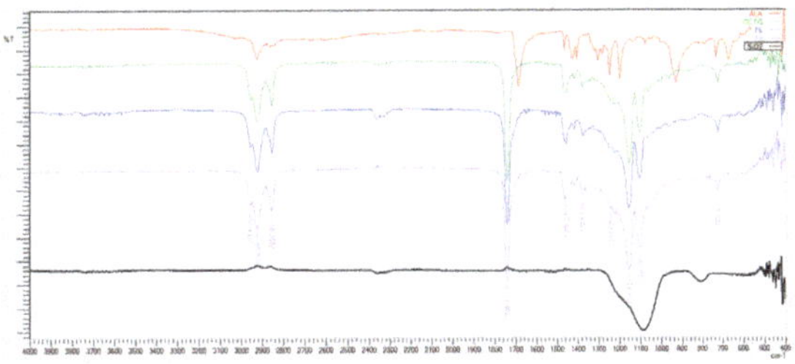

(**d**) ALA, F_5, F_8, caprylic/capric triglycerides, SiO_2

Figure 2. The FTIR spectra of (**a**) solid-filled capsules; (**b**) capsules with absolute ethanol; (**c**) capsules with PEG 400; and (**d**) capsules with caprylic/capric triglycerides.

The formation of a supramolecular structure of ALA with caprylic/capric triglycerides filler is confirmed by FTIR spectra, as shown in Figure 2d. In the F_5 and F_8 spectra, characteristic peaks from ALA disappear and the formulation spectra are the same as caprylic/capric triglycerides filler. A characteristic peak at 1741 cm^{-1} from carbonyl C=O, as well as peaks at 1103 and 153 cm^{-1}, originating from C–O–C ester group vibration, are present in the spectra of pure caprylic/capric triglycerides and both formulations F_5 and F_8.

The peaks from SiO_2 are not noticeable in any spectrum of the obtained formulations, as can be clearly seen in Figure 2. This is due to the absence of the peak at 1085 cm^{-1} originating from the Si–O–Si asymmetric stretching vibration and 804 cm^{-1} from the in-plane bending vibrations of geminal groups.

3.4. *In Vitro Dissolution Study*

The solubility of ALA in all tested media (distilled water, pH 1.2 media, and pH 6.8 phosphate buffer) with and without SLS was sufficient to provide sink conditions for the dissolution of 100 mg ALA in 500 mL of media (the solubility is higher than the concentration obtained by dissolving the triple dose in the medium). The concentration of ALA was unchanged after 24 h of storage at 37 °C ($p < 0.05$). The solubility results are shown in Figure 3.

Capsules with pure ALA have a similar dissolution rate compared to ones with CapsuLac® 60 as a diluent. However, using Excipient II as a diluent slows the release of ALA from the investigation solid-filled capsules, as shown in Figure 4a.

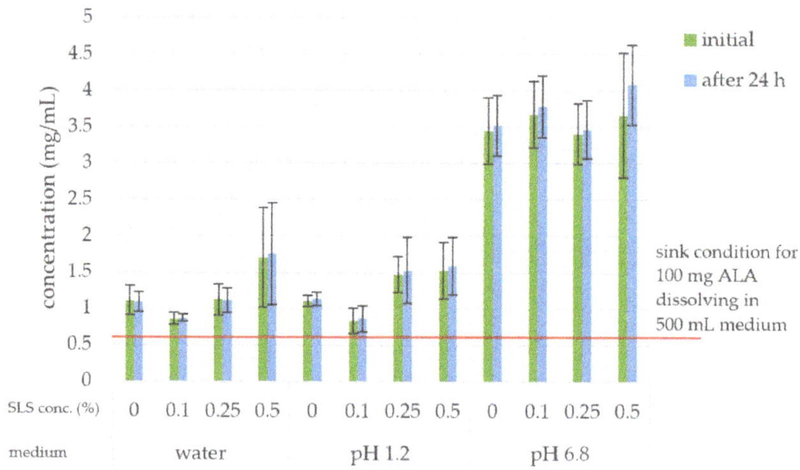

Figure 3. The solubility of ALA after 24 h in tested media (initial), and the results of repeated measurement of concentrations after an additional 24 h in order to test stability.

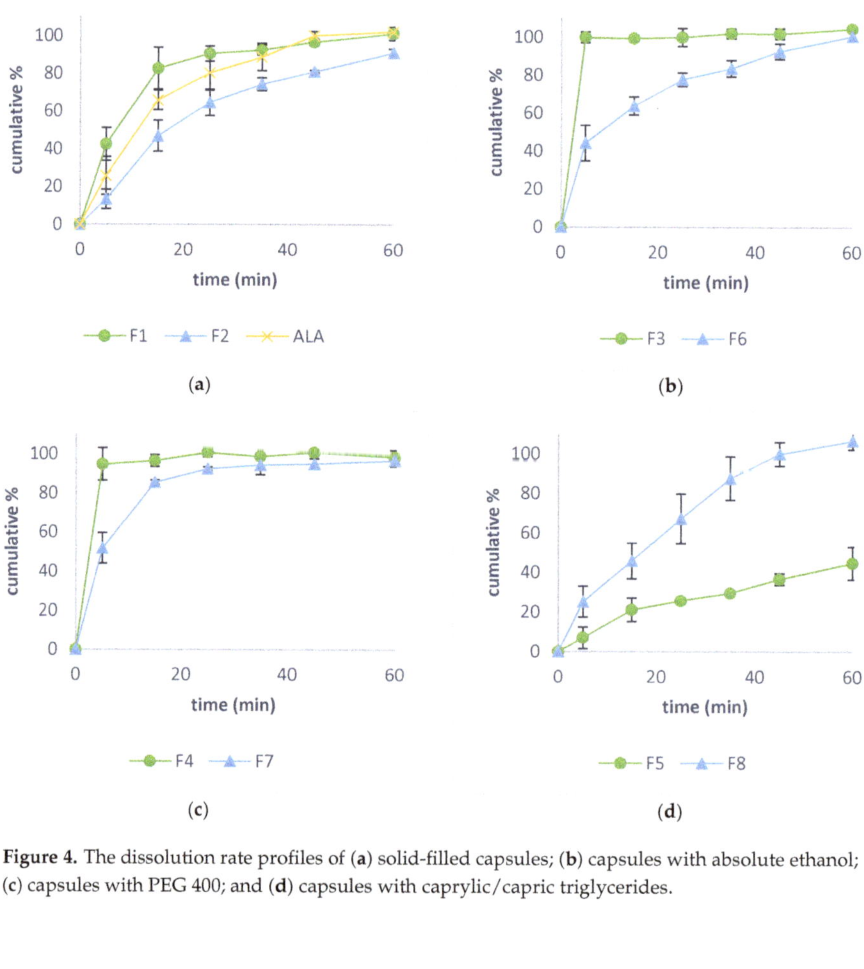

Figure 4. The dissolution rate profiles of (**a**) solid-filled capsules; (**b**) capsules with absolute ethanol; (**c**) capsules with PEG 400; and (**d**) capsules with caprylic/capric triglycerides.

The release of ALA from the formulation filled with solutions (F_3 and F_4) is practically instantaneous and after 5 min the complete release of the contents is achieved. As expected, the addition of silicon dioxide to the formulations results in slower release due to increased viscosity. The mentioned effect is more pronounced in the formulation with ethanol (F_6), where 63.86% of the content was released after 15 min, than in the formulation with PEG 400, where 85.37% of the content was released in the same time. The dissolution rate of ALA from the formulation filled with suspension (F_5) was the slowest (only 44.77% after 60 min). Interestingly, the addition of silicon dioxide to formulation F_5 (F_8) led to an improvement of ALA release rate (complete content after 60 min was dissolved), contrary to the previous two formulations with liquid contents. The dissolution rates curves are presented in Figure 4.

3.5. Rheological Properties

The linear dependence of shear stress on shear rate in pure PEG 400 and ALA solution in PEG 400 indicates their Newtonian behavior. The R-squared value of 1 was attained when experimentally determined curves were fitted via the equation of Newton's law. The measured viscosity of PEG 400 is 87.6 ± 0.6 mPa·s. The character of the flow behavior was not changed after the addition of ALA, but the viscosity was increased to 102.9 ± 1.7 mPa·s as presented in Figure 5a.

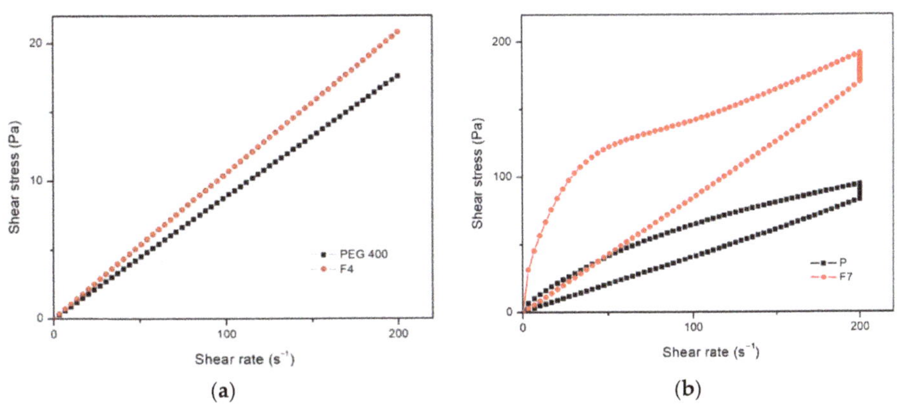

Figure 5. Rheograms of shear stress versus shear rate of (**a**) ALA solution in PEG 400 (F_4) and pure PEG 400; (**b**) ALA silicon dioxide gel formulation in PEG 400 (F_7) and corresponding placebo formulation without ALA (P).

The addition of silicon dioxide to PEG 400 led to a change in both flow character and viscosity. Non-Newtonian, time-dependent, thixotropic flow behavior was observed in the placebo gel formulation (P). The same as in pure PEG 400, the addition of ALA (F_7) to the placebo gel formulation increased the viscosity without changing the flow type, as shown in Figure 5b. Thixotropy is more pronounced in formulation F_7, considering the area of the hysteresis loop. The area of the hysteresis loop is significantly larger in formulation F_7 (10430 ± 151 Pa·s), compared to the placebo gel formulation P (3701 ± 11.79 Pa·s).

In the placebo gel formulation, which consisted only of PEG 400 and silicon dioxide (P), G' dominates over G'' at low frequencies. The cross-over at about 2.15 Hz occurs and after that, G'' continues to be dominant. In the semisolid formulation with ALA (F_7), G' is more pronounced compared to G'' for the entire observed range of frequencies (Figure 6).

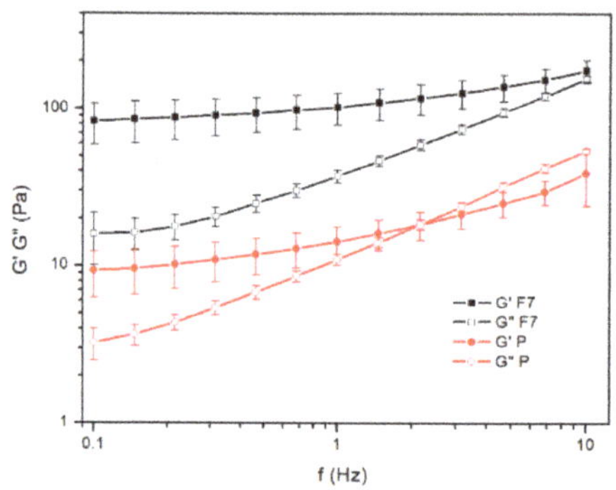

Figure 6. Effect of ALA on changes in G′ and G″ modulus versus frequency.

G″ to G′ ratios (tan δ) are from 0.19 ± 0.02 to 0.90 ± 0.11 for F_7 formulation and from 0.36 ± 0.07 to 1.49 ± 0.57 for placebo (P) formulation without ALA indicating their weak gel structures.

4. Discussion

ALA is a specific compound as it has authorized formulations of drugs as well as food supplements and it is used as a potential therapeutic agent for many chronic diseases with potential epidemiological, economic and social impact. Authorized formulations contain multiple excipients and usually dose above 200 mg. Taking into account the prolonged use of ALA formulations and its pleiotropic effect, there is a need for the compounding of simplified formulations. As indicated before, ALA is a poorly soluble molecule; thus, in the literature, there are various techniques used to increase ALA solubility, but they have some drawbacks and disadvantages. Many solubility enhancement techniques are costly processes that are often difficult to carry out and have poor manufacturability. In this research, simple formulations were prepared, suitable for compounding.

Powder formulations in this study were prepared by mixing ALA with CapsuLac® 60 or Excipient II as fillers. As expected, the type of filler influenced flowability and dissolution properties of ALA. An interesting finding was that the addition of ALA to solid fillers (i.e., CapsuLac® 60 and Excipient II) improved their flowability. Though, ALA has very poor flowability (Hausner Ratio (1.51) and Compressibility Index (33.63%), Table 3) and when added to diluents, it impacts their flowability. Another interesting result is that ALA increases the flowability of both diluents, though their chemical composition and particle size and shape is different. Flowability is a critical quality attribute in hard capsules formulations, and this effect of ALA is seen as positive, thus there is no need for the determination of the percolation threshold [41]. As expected, since ALA did not have a negative impact on flowability, both formulations ensure the adequacy of the uniformity of mass and the assay tests. However, smaller variations were observed in formulation F_1, which had better flowability. The individual masses of the capsules varied in the range of 98.42–102.03% in the F_1 formulation, while in the F_2 formulation they were in the range of 95.37–102.21% in relation to the average mass. Similar results were obtained in the assay test, where smaller standard deviations were observed in formulation F_1 (1.38%) than in formulation F_2 (2.05%). The suitability of using CapsuLac® 60 and Excipient II as fillers in capsule compounding has been previously confirmed. CapsuLac® 60 and Excipient II have proven to be excipients that provide adequate flowability and compliance with pharmacopeial requirements in terms of mass and content variation, as in the example of pantoprazole low-dose capsules compounding [42].

The dissolution rate of formulations where CapsuLac® 60 was used as filler was faster than those with Excipent II. This was also noticed in our previous study [42]. Also, it is notable that, compared to pure ALA, mixture with Excipient II decreased the dissolution rate, but mixture with CapsuLac® 60 increased the dissolution rate. The reason for this might be the composition of fillers. Namely, Excipient II contains pregelatinized corn starch and micronized silicon dioxide, which first forms a gel structure in dissolution medium and then dissolves. FTIR spectra did not detect any interaction with the investigated fillers. The shells were not expected to interact with the content. Also, the rapid and complete disintegration and dissolution of gelatin shells in tested conditions has been well documented in previously published studies [43,44].

Additionally, though ALA's lack of gastric stability has been implied in other studies [30,45], in our study ALA was stable in pH 1,2 medium at 37 °C with and without SLS (0.1%, 0.25%, and 0.5%) for 24 h. Also, ALA was stable at 37 °C for 24 h in water and pH 6.8 buffer, with and without SLS.

Liquid formulations were prepared because, according to the literature, bioavailability could be markedly increased when ALA is orally administered in the liquid form rather than a solid dosage form. Higher plasma concentrations and accelerated absorption of ALA is expected from liquid formulations [30,45]. Both types of vehiculum and whether ALA is dissolved or suspended have an impact on dissolution rate. Formulations with absolute ethanol (F_3) and PEG 400 (F_4) released the entire ALA content in the first 5 min. Formulations where ALA was suspended (i.e., with caprylic/caprylic triglycerides, F_5) showed significant retardation in dissolution rate, compared to formulations F_3 and F_4 where ALA is dissolved. F_5 released only 7% of ALA content after 5 min. The lipophilicity of the medium and slower mixing with the aqueous dissolution medium, as well as the lower affinity of ALA to migrate can be the reasons for the slow release obtained. Additionally, the surface area available for dissolution is smaller in suspension formulations, and the particle size is one of the key factors affecting the dissolution process [46].

An increase in viscosity was observed in all formulations where silicon dioxide was added (F_6, F_7 and F_8), but the effects on dissolution rate were not equal. Namely, an increase in viscosity was expected to be inversely proportional to the dissolution rate [47]. When silicon dioxide is added to formulations in which ALA is dissolved, the aforementioned deceleration of release occurs, as shown in Figure 2a,b. However, after adding silicon dioxide to the formulation with PEG 400, 85.37% of the ALA content was released after 5 min. Although a decrease in the dissolution rate of ALA is observed, it is not statistically significant considering the guidelines given by the European Medicines Agency (EMA). According to these guidelines, for fast-release formulations where more than 85% of the content is released within 15 min, no mathematical considerations are needed and their release profiles can be considered similar [48]. Consequently, it can be concluded that the observed increase in viscosity in the formulation with PEG 400 (F_4) after the addition of silicon dioxide (F_7) did not lead to a statistically significant decrease in the dissolution rate of ALA. Interestingly, the release profile improved when silicon dioxide was added to the formulation in which ALA was suspended. The reason for this may be the stabilization of the suspension, which prevents the agglomeration of ALA particles, as well as increased wetting. It could be concluded that PEG 400 was most suitable as the vehicle for liquid compounding.

Based on the results of previously published studies [49–52], the viscosity of ALA solution in PEG 400 is suitable for filling hard gelatin capsules. The moderate viscosity of the solution of ALA in PEG 400 is desirable due to the avoidance of loss caused by splashing during the filling process. Also, the addition of silicon dioxide after and not before filling capsules provided a viscosity increase after precise dose filling and problems that were observed with high viscosity filling materials was avoided. Silicon dioxide contains colloidal, nanometer-sized primary particles with superficial silanol groups, which makes it possible to build hydrogen bonds with PEG 400 and form cross-linked gel networks [53]. The addition of ALA in the system with silicon dioxide and PEG 400 showed G' dominating over G'' in the entire tested frequency range, without the characteristic cross-over observed with the placebo (P) formulation. A potential reason why the elastic part dominates over the viscous part in formulation F_7 could be the high concentration of ALA and its contribution to the increase in viscosity (Figure 5a). The presence of ALA in the formulation contributes to the increase in elastic (gel) properties. However, the ratio of G″ to G′ (tan δ) are higher than 0.1 and the F_7 formulation cannot be considered as a true rather than as a weak gel [54–56]. The obtained rheological behavior can be considered as a desirable one, because it did not statistically significantly affect the dissolution rate of ALA. Based on all the above, it is concluded that the applied capsule filling technique is suitable for compounding.

5. Conclusions

This research aimed to provide a thorough and complete characterization of compounded hard gelatin capsules containing ALA dose of 100 mg. Capsules with liquid and semisolid content were proven to be suitable for compounding as ones with conventional solid content filing. All formulations complied to pharmacopeial requirements. However, dissolution profiles were faster in formulations filled with liquid content compared to solid-filled formulations. Although the addition of silicon dioxide led to an increase in viscosity and a change in rheological behavior, the release rate did not decrease significantly. PEG 400 (formulation F_4) proved to be the most adequate liquid medium for compounding since ALA was completely dissolved in it and FTIR analysis did not indicate interactions. Subsequently adding silicon dioxide (formulation F_7) in order to form semisolid content is adequate for preventing content leaking without impacting the filling process.

Author Contributions: Conceptualization, J.J.-B., M.L.-P., and N.T.; methodology, M.L.-P. and J.J.-B.; software, V.K. and I.R.; validation, V.K., N.T., and M.L.-P.; formal analysis, M.V.; investigation, N.T.; resources, M.L.-P.; data curation, Z.K., M.V., and I.R.; writing—original draft preparation, N.T., I.R., Z.K., and J.J.-B.; writing—review and editing, M.L.-P., V.K., and J.J.-B.; visualization, I.R., M.V., and N.T.; supervision, M.L.-P.; project administration, N.T. and Z.K.; funding acquisition, M.L.-P. All authors have read and agreed to the published version of the manuscript.

Funding: This research received no external funding.

Institutional Review Board Statement: Not applicable.

Informed Consent Statement: Not applicable.

Data Availability Statement: The original contributions presented in the study are included in the article, further inquiries can be directed to the corresponding author.

Acknowledgments: This study was supported by the Ministry of Education, Science, and Technological Development, Republic of Serbia (project 451-03-66/2024-03/200114).

Conflicts of Interest: The authors declare no conflicts of interest.

References

1. Rochette, L.; Ghibu, S.; Muresan, A.; Vergely, C.; Alpha, C.V. Alpha-lipoic acid: Molecular mechanisms and therapeutic potential in diabetes. *Can. J. Physiol. Pharmacol.* **2015**, *93*, 1021–1027. [CrossRef] [PubMed]
2. Shay, K.P.; Moreau, R.F.; Smith, E.J.; Smith, A.R.; Hagen, T.M. Alpha-lipoic acid as a dietary supplement: Molecular mechanisms and therapeutic potential. *Biochim. Biophys. Acta (BBA) Gen. Subj.* **2009**, *1790*, 1149–1160. [CrossRef] [PubMed]
3. Goraca, A.; Huk-Kolega, H.; Piechota, A.; Kleniewska, P.; Ciejka, E.; Skibska, B. Lipoic acid-biological activity and therapeutic potential. *Pharmacol. Rep.* **2011**, *63*, 849–858. [CrossRef] [PubMed]
4. Padmalayam, I.; Hasham, S.; Saxena, U.; Pillarisetti, S. Lipoic acid: Synthase (LASY): A novel role in inflammation, mitochondrial function, and insulin resistance. *Diabetes* **2009**, *58*, 600–608. [CrossRef] [PubMed]
5. Du, G.; Qiao, Y.; Zhuo, Z.; Zhou, J.; Li, X.; Liu, Z.; Li, Y.; Chen, H. Lipoic acid rejuvenates aged intestinal stem cells by preventing age-associated endosome reduction. *EMBO Rep.* **2020**, *21*, e49583. [CrossRef] [PubMed]
6. Salehi, B.; Berkay Yılmaz, Y.; Antika, G.; Boyunegmez Tumer, T.; Fawzi Mahomoodally, M.; Lobine, D.; Akram, M.; Riaz, M.; Capanoglu, E.; Sharopov, F.; et al. Insights on the use of α-lipoic acid for therapeutic purposes. *Biomolecules* **2019**, *9*, 356. [CrossRef]
7. Wang, J.Q.; Ling, X.; Wang, H.J.; Chen, F.E. α-Lipoic acid chemistry: The past 70 years. *RSC Adv.* **2023**, *13*, 36346–36363. [CrossRef] [PubMed]
8. Bustamante, J.; Lodge, J.K.; Marcocci, L.; Tritschler, H.J.; Packer, L.; Rihn, B.H. α-Lipoic acid in liver metabolism and disease. *Free Radic. Biol. Med.* **1998**, *24*, 1023–1039. [CrossRef] [PubMed]

9. Cronan, J.E. Progress in the enzymology of the mitochondrial diseases of lipoic acid requiring enzymes. *Front. Genet.* **2020**, *11*, 510. [CrossRef]
10. Turkowicz, M.; Jastrzebska, I.; Hryniewicka, M.; Kotowska, U.; Gudalewska, D.; Karpińska, J. Investigation of lipoic acid—4-Methoxybenzyl alcohol reaction and evaluation of its analytical usefulness. *Food Chem.* **2020**, *309*, 125750. [CrossRef]
11. Dos Santos, S.M.; Romeiro, C.F.R.; Rodrigues, C.A.; Cerqueira, A.R.L.; Monteiro, M.C. Mitochondrial dysfunction and alpha-lipoic acid: Beneficial or harmful in Alzheimer's disease? *Oxid. Med. Cell. Longev.* **2019**, *2019*, 8409329. [CrossRef]
12. Viana, M.D.M.; Lauria, P.S.S.; Lima, A.A.; de Opretzka, L.C.F.; Marcelino, H.R.; Villarreal, C.F. Alpha-Lipoic Acid as an Antioxidant Strategy for Managing Neuropathic Pain. *Antioxidants* **2022**, *11*, 2420. [CrossRef]
13. Skibska, B.; Kochan, E.; Stanczak, A.; Lipert, A.; Skibska, A. Antioxidant and anti-inflammatory effects of α-lipoic acid on lipopolysaccharide-induced oxidative stress in rat kidney. *Arch. Immunol. Ther. Exp.* **2023**, *71*, 16. [CrossRef]
14. Karalis, D.T.; Karalis, T.; Karalis, S.; Kleisiari, A.S.; Malakoudi, F.; Maimari, K.E.V. The effect of alpha-lipoic acid on diabetic peripheral neuropathy and the upcoming depressive disorders of type II diabetics. *Cureus* **2021**, *13*, e12773. [CrossRef]
15. Teichert, J.; Hermann, R.; Ruus, P.; Preiss, R. Plasma kinetics, metabolism, and urinary excretion of alpha-lipoic acid following oral administration in healthy volunteers. *J. Clin. Pharmacol.* **2003**, *43*, 1257–1267. [CrossRef]
16. Gomes, M.B.; Negrato, C.A. Alpha-lipoic acid as a pleiotropic compound with potential therapeutic use in diabetes and other chronic diseases. *Diabetol. Metab. Syndr.* **2014**, *6*, 80. [CrossRef]
17. Capece, U.; Moffa, S.; Improta, I.; Di Giuseppe, G.; Nista, E.C.; Cefalo, C.M.A.; Cinti, F.; Pontecorvi, A.; Gasbarrini, A.; Giaccari, A.; et al. Alpha-Lipoic Acid and Glucose Metabolism: A Comprehensive Update on Biochemical and Therapeutic Features. *Nutrients* **2023**, *15*, 18. [CrossRef]
18. Seifar, F.; Khalili, M.; Khaledyan, H.; Amiri Moghadam, S.; Izadi, A.; Azimi, A.; Shakouri, S.K. α-Lipoic acid, functional fatty acid, as a novel therapeutic alternative for central nervous system diseases: A review. *Nutr. Neurosci.* **2019**, *22*, 306–316. [CrossRef]
19. Lalić-Popović, M.; Vuković, M.; Jovičić-Bata, J.; Čanji-Panić, J.; Todorović, N. Comparison of formulation characteristics of drugs and dietary supplements containing alpha-lipoic acid relevant to therapeutic efficacy. *Eur. Rev. Med. Pharmacol. Sci.* **2023**, *27*, 3159–3170. [CrossRef]
20. Pop, A.L.; Crișan, S.; Bârcă, M.; Ciobanu, A.M.; Varlas, V.N.; Pop, C.; Pali, M.-A.; Cauni, D.; Ozon, E.A.; Udeanu, D.; et al. Evaluation of dissolution profiles of a newly developed solid oral immediate-release formula containing alpha-lipoic acid. *Processes* **2021**, *9*, 176. [CrossRef]
21. Fogacci, F.; Rizzo, M.; Krogager, C.; Kennedy, C.; Georges, C.M.G.; Knežević, T.; Liberopoulos, E.; Vallée, A.; Pérez-Martínez, P.; Wenstedt, E.F.; et al. Safety Evaluation of α-Lipoic Acid Supplementation: A Systematic Review and Meta-Analysis of Randomized Placebo-Controlled Clinical Studies. *Antioxidants* **2020**, *9*, 1011. [CrossRef] [PubMed]
22. Teichert, J.; Tuemmers, T.; Achenbach, H.; Preiss, C.; Hermann, R.; Ruus, P.; Preiss, R. Pharmacokinetics of alpha-lipoic acid in subjects with severe kidney damage and end-stage renal disease. *J. Clin. Pharmacol.* **2005**, *45*, 313–328. [CrossRef] [PubMed]
23. Takeuchi, Y.; Miyamoto, T.; Kakizawa, T.; Shigematsu, S.; Hashizume, K. Insulin autoimmune syndrome Possibly Caused by Alpha Lipoic Acid. *Intern. Med.* **2007**, *46*, 237–239. [CrossRef] [PubMed]
24. Gullo, D.; Evans, J.L.; Sortino, G.; Goldfine, I.D.; Vigneri, R. Insulin autoimmune syndrome (Hirata Disease) in European Caucasians taking α-lipoic acid. *Clin. Endocrinol.* **2014**, *81*, 204–209. [CrossRef] [PubMed]
25. Lasoń, E.; Sikora, E.; Miastkowska, M.; Socha, P.; Ogonowski, J. NLC delivery systems for alpha lipoic acid: Physicochemical characteristics and release study. *Colloids Surf. A Physicochem. Eng. Asp* **2017**, *532*, 57–62. [CrossRef]
26. Bernkop-Schnürch, A.; Schuhbauer, H.; Clausen, A.E.; Hanel, R. Development of a sustained release dosage form for α-lipoic acid. I. Design and in vitro evaluation. *Drug Dev. Ind. Pharm.* **2004**, *30*, 27–34. [CrossRef] [PubMed]
27. Gleiter, C.H.; Schug, B.S.; Hermann, R.; Elze, M.; Blume, H.H.; Gundert-Remy, U. Influence of food intake on the bioavailability of thioctic acid enantiomers. *Eur. J. Clin. Pharmacol.* **1996**, *50*, 513–514. [CrossRef]
28. Amidon, G.; Lennernäs, H.; Shah, V.; Crison, J. A theoretical basis for a biopharmaceutic drug classification: The correlation of in vitro drug product dissolution and in vivo bioavailability. *Pharm. Res.* **1995**, *12*, 413–420. [CrossRef] [PubMed]
29. Brufani, M. Acido α-lipoico farmaco o integratore. Una panoramica sulla farmacocinetica, le formulazioni disponibili e le evidenze cliniche nelle complicanze del diabete. *Prog. Nutr.* **2014**, *16*, 62–74.
30. Maglione, E.; Marrese, C.; Migliaro, E.; Marcuccio, F.; Panico, C.; Salvati, C.; Citro, G.; Quercio, M.; Roncagliolo, F.; Torello, C.; et al. Increasing bioavailability of (R)-alpha-lipoic acid to boost antioxidant activity in the treatment of neuropathic pain. *Acta Biomed.* **2015**, *86*, 226–233. [PubMed]
31. DTU Food National Institute. Safety of Alpha-Lipoic Acid Use in Food Supplements. 2017. Available online: https://food.ec.europa.eu/system/files/2020-06/labelling-nutrition_vitamins-minerals_add_alpha-lipoic-acid_nfi-da.pdf (accessed on 29 June 2024).
32. Cremer, D.R.; Rabeler, R.; Roberts, A.; Lynch, B. Safety evaluation of α-lipoic acid (ALA). *Regul. Toxicol. Pharmacol.* **2006**, *46*, 29–41. [CrossRef]
33. Cremer, D.R.; Rabeler, R.; Roberts, A.; Lynch, B. Long-term safety of α-lipoic acid (ALA) consumption: A 2-year study. *Regul. Toxicol. Pharmacol.* **2006**, *46*, 193–201. [CrossRef] [PubMed]
34. EFSA Panel on Nutrition, Novel Foods and Food Allergens (NDA); Turck, D.; Castenmiller, J.; de Henauw, S.; Hirsch-Ernst, K.I.; Kearney, J.; Knutsen, H.K.; Mangelsdorf, I.; McArdle, H.J.; Naska, A.; et al. Scientific opinion on the relationship between intake of alpha-lipoic acid (thioctic acid) and the risk of insulin autoimmune syndrome. *EFSA J.* **2021**, *19*, e06577. [CrossRef] [PubMed]

35. Wagner, A.F.; Walton, E.; Boxer, G.E.; Pruss, M.P.; Holly, F.W.; Folkers, K. Properties and derivatives of α-lipoic acid. *J. Am. Chem. Soc.* **1956**, *78*, 5079–5081. [CrossRef]
36. FDA.gov. FDA Continues Taking Key Actions on Bulk Drug Substances Used for Compounding to Advance the Regulatory Framework Governing Compounded Drugs and to Protect Patients. Available online: https://www.fda.gov/news-events/press-announcements/fda-continues-taking-key-actions-bulk-drug-substances-used-compounding-advance-regulatory-framework (accessed on 23 May 2024).
37. Council of Europe. *European Pharmacopoeia*, 11th ed.; European Directorate for the Quality of Medicines & Healthcare; Council of Europe: Strasbourg, France, 2022.
38. GotI, P.P.; Savsani, J.J.; Patel, P.B. Spectrophotometric method development and validation for estimation of α-lipoic acid in tablet dosage form. *Int. J. Pharm. Pharm. Sci.* **2012**, *4*, 519–522.
39. Silverstein, R.M.; Bassler, G.C.; Morrill, T.C. *Spectrometric Identification of Organic Compounds*, 3rd ed.; John Willey and Sons, Inc.: New York, NY, USA, 1974.
40. Nikolic, R.S.; Krstic, N.S.; Nikolic, G.M.; Kocic, G.M.; Cakic, M.D.; Andelkovic, D.H. Molecular mechanisms of beneficial effects of lipoic acid in copper intoxicated rats assessment by FTIR and ESI-MS. *Polyhedron* **2014**, *80*, 223–227. [CrossRef]
41. Leane, M.; Pitt, K.; Reynolds, G.K.; Dawson, N.; Ziegler, I.; Szepes, A.; Crean, A.M.; Agnol, R.D.; Sy, T.M.C. Manufacturing classification system in the real world: Factors influencing manufacturing process choices for filed commercial oral solid dosage formulations, case studies from industry and considerations for continuous processing. *Pharm. Dev. Technol.* **2018**, *23*, 964–977. [CrossRef] [PubMed]
42. Todorović, N.; Čanji Panić, J.; Zavišić, M.; Krtolica, J.; Ratajac, R.; Petrović, J.; Bosiljčić, D.; Kladar, N.; Milošević, N.; Lalić-Popović, M. Compounding of Liquid and Solid Dose Adjustable Formulations with Pantoprazole: Comparison of Stability, Applicability and Suitability. *Pharmaceutics* **2023**, *15*, 717. [CrossRef] [PubMed]
43. Chiwele, I.; Jones, B.E.; Podczeck, F. The shell dissolution of various empty hard capsules. *Chem. Pharm. Bull.* **2000**, *48*, 951–956. [CrossRef] [PubMed]
44. Glube, N.; von Moos, L.; Duchateau, G. Capsule shell material impacts the in vitro disintegration and dissolution behaviour of a green tea extract. *Results Pharma Sci.* **2013**, *3*, 1–6. [CrossRef] [PubMed]
45. Brufani, M.; Figliola, R. (R)-α-lipoic acid oral liquid formulation: Pharmacokinetic parameters and therapeutic efficacy. *Acta Biomed.* **2014**, *85*, 108–115. [PubMed]
46. Jambhekar, S.S.; Breen, P.J. Drug dissolution: Significance of physicochemical properties and physiological conditions. *Drug Discov. Today* **2013**, *18*, 1173–1184. [CrossRef] [PubMed]
47. Braun, R.J.; Parrott, E.L. Influence of viscosity and solubilization on dissolution rate. *J. Pharm. Sci.* **1972**, *61*, 175–178. [CrossRef] [PubMed]
48. EMA. *Guideline on the Investigation of Bioequivalence*; (CPMP/EWP/QWP/1401/98 Rev. 1/Corr**); European Medicines Agency, Committee for Medicinal Products for Human Use (EMEA): Amsterdam, The Netherlands, 2010.
49. Sultana, M.; Butt, M.A.; Saeed, T.; Mahmood, R.; ul Hassan, S.; Hussain, K.; Raza, S.A.; Ahsan, M.; Bukhari, N.I. Effect of Rheology and Poloxamers Properties on Release of Drugs from Silicon Dioxide Gel-Filled Hard Gelatin Capsules—A Further Enhancement of Viability of Liquid Semisolid Matrix Technology. *AAPS PharmSciTech* **2017**, *18*, 1998–2010. [CrossRef] [PubMed]
50. Smith, A.; Lampard, J.F.; Carruthers, K.M.; Regan, P. The filling of molten ibuprofen into hard gelatin capsules. *Int. J. Pharm.* **1990**, *59*, 115–119. [CrossRef]
51. McTaggart, C.; Wood, R.; Bedford, K.; Walker, S.E. The evaluation of an automatic system for filling liquids into hard gelatin capsules. *J. Pharm. Pharmacol.* **1984**, *36*, 119–121. [CrossRef] [PubMed]
52. Hawley, A.R. Investigation of Thermosoftened Solid Dispersion Formulations of Ibuprofen for Hard Gelatin Capsules. Ph.D. Thesis, University of Sunderland, Sunderland, UK, 1993.
53. Fahr, A. *Voigt's Pharmaceutical Technology*; John Wiley & Sons: Hoboken, NY, USA, 2018; pp. 468–477.
54. Biglarian, N.; Rafe, A.; Shahidi, S.A.; Lorenzo, J.M. Rheological, textural and structural properties of dairy cream as affected by some natural stabilizers. *Chem. Biol. Technol. Agric.* **2022**, *9*, 96. [CrossRef]
55. Krstonošić, V.; Dokić, L.; Nikolić, I.; Milanović, M. Influence of xanthan gum on oil-in-water emulsion characteristics stabilized by OSA starch. *Food Hydrocoll.* **2015**, *45*, 9–17. [CrossRef]
56. Mandala, I.G.; Savvas, T.P.; Kostaropoulos, A.E. Xanthan and locust bean gum influence on the rheology and structure of a white model-sauce. *J. Food Eng.* **2004**, *64*, 335–342. [CrossRef]

MDPI AG
Grosspeteranlage 5
4052 Basel
Switzerland
Tel.: +41 61 683 77 34

Pharmaceutics Editorial Office
E-mail: pharmaceutics@mdpi.com
www.mdpi.com/journal/pharmaceutics

www.ingramcontent.com/pod-product-compliance
Lightning Source LLC
Chambersburg PA
CBHW040821250926
51850CB00007BA/1233
* 9 7 8 3 7 2 5 8 6 9 1 4 5 *